The Future of Long-Term Care

THE FUTURE OF LONG-TERM CARE

Social and Policy Issues

Edited by

ROBERT H. BINSTOCK, Ph.D.,

LEIGHTON E. CLUFF, M.D., and

OTTO VON MERING, Ph.D.

The Johns Hopkins University Press / *Baltimore and London*

© 1996 The Johns Hopkins University Press
All rights reserved. Published 1996
Printed in the United States of America on acid-free paper
05 04 03 02 01 00 99 98   5 4 3 2

The Johns Hopkins University Press
2715 North Charles Street
Baltimore, Maryland 21218
The Johns Hopkins Press Ltd., London

ISBN 0-8018-5320-6

Contents

Contributors

A. E. Benjamin, Ph.D., is professor of social welfare in the Department of Social Welfare, School of Public Policy and Social Research, University of California, Los Angeles. From 1977 to 1992 he was a member of the research faculty at the Institute for Health and Aging, University of California-San Francisco, where he was also associate director and professor in residence. His current research activities include a federally supported study of client and worker outcomes under alternative models of personal assistance services, evaluation of local initiatives to improve service systems for people with disabilities, funded under a national program supported by the Robert Wood Johnson Foundation, a review, funded by the same foundation, of state and local indicator systems for monitoring chronic care services, and an analysis of home care for persons with AIDS. He has published widely on home-based services and on issues in designing service systems for diverse client populations with chronic conditions.

Robert H. Binstock, Ph.D., is professor of aging, health, and society, at Case Western Reserve University. A former president of the Gerontological Society of America, he has served as director of a White House Task Force on Older Americans and as chairman or member of a number of advisory panels to the U.S. government, state and local governments, and foundations. He presently chairs the Gerontological Health Section of the American Public Health Association. Among his nineteen authored and edited books are four editions of the *Handbook of Aging and the Social Sciences*, the most recent (co-edited with Linda George) published in 1996. His awards and honors include the Kent and Brookdale awards from the Gerontological Society of America, the American Society on Aging Award, and the Key Award from the American Public Health Association.

James J. Callahan, Jr., Ph.D., is the director of the Policy Center on Aging, and research professor, Brandeis University, and director of the Robert Wood Johnson Foundation National Demonstrations on Linking Housing and Services, which are entitled "No Place Like Home" and

"Supportive Services in Senior Housing." He is also chair of the Steering Committee of the National Academy on Aging and principal investigator for the National Policy and Resource Center on Women and Aging. He has served in Massachusetts as the commissioner of the Department of Mental Health and the secretary of the Department of Elder Affairs. He has published widely in aging and social welfare journals on supportive services, delivery systems, and long-term care for the elderly. A frequently requested speaker and consultant who serves on numerous advisory committees, he was awarded the Gerontological Society of America's Maxwell Pollack Award for demonstrated excellence in bridging the worlds of research and practice.

Leighton E. Cluff, M.D., M.A.C.P., is professor of medicine and special advisor on health policy to the provost at the University of Florida. He was honored five years ago as a Veterans Administration Distinguished Physician. He is a former president and currently a trustee of the Robert Wood Johnson Foundation, where he is responsible for many programs dealing with long-term care for both older and younger individuals. He is the author or editor of nine books and has written articles and made presentations dealing with problems of chronically ill and disabled children, adults, and the elderly population. He is the founder of the University of Florida's National Health Forum, established in 1992. The subject of the first National Health Forum was long-term care.

Thomas R. Cole, Ph.D., is professor of history and medicine and graduate program director at the Institute for Medical Humanities, University of Texas Medical Branch in Galveston. He has published many articles and several books on the history of aging and humanistic gerontology. His book *The Journey of Life: A Cultural History of Aging in America* (1992) was nominated for a Pulitzer Prize. He was senior editor of *What Does It Mean to Grow Old?* (1986), the *Handbook of Humanities and Aging* (1992), *Voices and Visions: Toward a Critical Gerontology* (1993), and *The Oxford Book of Aging* (1994). He is currently completing two projects centering around mental illness, oral history, civil rights, and race relations in Texas.

Nancy Neveloff Dubler, LL.B., is professor of bioethics at the Albert Einstein College of Medicine and director of the Division of Bioethics in the Department of Epidemiology and Social Medicine at Montefiore Medical Center and the Albert Einstein College of Medicine. She has been a member of numerous federal panels and was co-chairperson of the Ethics Working Group on the National Health Care Reform Task Force for President Clinton. She is the author of *Ethics on Call: Taking Charge of Life-and-Death Choices in Today's Health Care System,* and numerous articles on such topics as geriatrics, termination of care, AIDS, and prisoners' rights to care.

Martha Holstein, M.A., has worked in the field of aging for over twenty years; for nearly fourteen of those years she was associate director of the American Society on Aging. Among her published work is the co-edited volume *A Good Old Age? The Paradox of Setting Limits* (with Paul Homer) and articles in journals such as *Gerontologist, Journal of Aging and Social Policy,* and *Research on Aging.* She is currently writing a historic account of Alzheimer disease and senile dementia and continues to teach and write in the area of ethics and aging. Ms. Holstein, currently finishing her doctorate, is Research Scholar at the Park Ridge Center for the Study of Health, Faith, and Ethics, in Chicago.

Robert L. Kane, M.D., holds the Minnesota Chair in Long-Term Care and Aging at the University of Minnesota School of Public Health, where he directs the university's Center on Aging and the Minnesota Area Geriatric Education Center. A health services researcher with a special interest in assessing the outcomes of care, he also directs the university's Clinical Outcomes Research Center. He has written widely about aspects of care for older persons, including co-authoring *Essentials of Clinical Geriatrics* and co-editing *Quality Care in Geriatric Settings.*

Dennis L. Kodner, Ph.D., is vice president of research and innovation at Metropolitan Jewish Health System, Brooklyn, New York, and executive director of its Institute for Applied Gerontology. Dr. Kodner's policy analysis and research interests are in the financing, organization, and delivery of care to the elderly and chronically ill, as well as in anticipatory gerontology, comparative long-term care, and integrated delivery systems. In addition to authoring numerous publications on these issues, he has served as a member of many advisory panels to governments, foundations, and national organizations. A pioneer in managed care of the elderly, Kodner was the first executive director of Eldercare, Inc., one of the four original social health maintenance organizations. Currently, he is working on a new home-centered model of care known as the Chronic Care Organization.

Mark R. Meiners, Ph.D., is associate professor and associate director for the Center on Aging at the University of Maryland. He is the director of the national program office of the Robert Wood Johnson Foundation (RWJF) Partnership for Long-Term Care and the new RWJF program, State Initiatives in Long-Term Care. In addition, he directs the RWJF Service Credit Program, an approach that encourages volunteers to provide informal care for the elderly in exchange for similar services if needed. Dr. Meiners is nationally recognized as one of the leading experts on financing and program development in long-term care. He has written numerous publications including articles on nursing home costs, long-term care insurance, and cost-of-illness analysis.

Mathy Mezey, Ed.D., R.N., F.A.A.N., is the Independence Foundation Professor of Nursing Education at New York University, Division of Nursing, in New York City. She is former director of the Robert Wood Johnson Foundation Teaching Nursing Home Program and current director of the Geriatric Nurse Practitioner Program at NYU. Dr. Mezey is editor of the Springer Series on Geriatric Nursing and co-editor of the *Encyclopedia of Aging* (1995) and *Advances in Long-Term Care* (1992). In recent years she has been engaged in research on decision making about life-sustaining treatment by older adults with questionable decision making capacity and their families.

Helena Temkin-Greener, Ph.D., is the director of research at the Community Coalition for Long-Term Care in Rochester, New York, a public-private partnership devoted to reforming service delivery and financing for persons with chronic conditions and disability. Currently, with funding from the Robert Wood Johnson Foundation, Dr. Temkin-Greener is directing the development of a demonstration program, for older impaired and unimpaired persons, aimed at integrating primary, acute, and long-term care services within a managed care, capitated environment. She also holds an appointment in the Department of Community and Preventive Medicine at the University of Rochester School of Medicine and Dentistry. Dr. Temkin-Greener is the author of a number of publications in the field of aging.

Otto von Mering, Ph.D., is professor of anthropology and professor of medicine at the University of Florida, as well as director emeritus of the university's Center for Gerontological Studies. A former president of the Association for Anthropology and Gerontology, he is a fellow of the Royal Society of Health, Royal Anthropological Society of England, and the Academy of Psychosomatic Medicine. Dr. von Mering is the author and editor of numerous publications, a *Who's Who in the World* biographee, and serves as a member of many different advisory boards in the field of aging. Recently he has been researching driving in the later years and its implications for the quality of life.

T. Franklin Williams, M.D., is professor of medicine emeritus at the University of Rochester and a Distinguished Physician with the Veterans Administration. He served as director of the National Institute on Aging, of the National Institutes of Health (1983–91), and presently serves as scientific director of the American Federation for Aging Research. His research and more than ninety publications have been concerned with metabolic diseases, including hereditary rickets and diabetes mellitus, and a variety of aspects of the care of chronically ill and aging persons. He is co-editor (with J. G. Evans) of *The Oxford Textbook of Geriatric Medicine* (1992) and co-editor (with T. L. Sprott and H. R. Warner) of *The Biology of Aging* (1993).

Preface

In February 1992, the University of Florida held its first National Health Forum. The topic under consideration was "Home Care: Legal, Ethical, and Policy Issues." Although this book covers a broader range of topics, and the chapters have been written especially for this volume, the forum provided the stimulus for ideas and planning that led to the fruition of this project. Several key participants in the forum contributed to this publication as well.

The first National Health Forum involved 110 invited participants: governmental officials from fifteen states with large elderly populations, representatives from twenty-six major national organizations concerned with the care of elderly people, and experts in home care. The forum was supported by the Robert Wood Johnson Foundation, the Kellogg Foundation, Gainesville Veterans Affairs Medical Center, Shands Hospital of the University of Florida, and others. The Robert Wood Johnson Foundation and the Kellogg Foundation also supported this volume, *The Future of Long-Term Care: Social and Policy Issues*. We acknowledge and appreciate their contributions. We also wish to express our appreciation to Marcia Bram, Karen Henderson, and Jenny Wilson, who provided the high-quality and loyal assistance that is essential in projects of this nature.

Overview of the Volume

The first part of this book comprises an introductory chapter and a historical analysis of long-term care in the United States as it has evolved to the present day. In Chapter 1, the editors explain why long-term care has emerged as an important issue in American society. They portray the growing population in need of long-term care, discuss the difficulties of paying for such care, and examine the problems involved in providing good-quality care.

In Chapter 2, Martha Holstein and Thomas R. Cole show how the characteristics of contemporary long-term care have been shaped by cultural forces, institutions, and policies dating from the colonial period through the present. Before 1820 — in the era of "outdoor relief" — the care (including medical care) of poor and ill persons was community based and flexible. From 1820 through the Civil War, a distinct shift took place toward the institutionalization of poor persons, although, except for the poorest, medical care was still provided at home. From 1865 until the New Deal, as institutional poor relief became harsher, older people were the dominant populations in almshouses, while hospitals became increasingly biased toward acute care. After World War II, federal policies shaped the modern long-term care system dominated by nursing homes, leaving the private sector relatively free to provide services even when substantial public funds are involved. In this analysis Holstein and Cole demonstrate how the features of today's long-term care system, and needs for reforming it, have been shaped by residual characteristics and cultural presuppositions of earlier eras as well as the modern policy of nourishing private-sector services with public dollars.

Part 2 deals with a range of factors that will shape the agenda for the future of long-term care. It focuses on contemporary populations of all ages who have need for care, the types of care they need and why they need it, projected future needs, and challenges that lie ahead in meeting those needs.

In Chapter 3, T. Franklin Williams and Helena Temkin-Greener focus on the older disabled population. They present demographic and "healthy life expectancy" projections and discuss current long-term care services and their shortcomings. They conclude with an analysis of the problems to be overcome in developing an improved system for providing chronic care services and they report on a series of experimental demonstration programs that are attempting to address those problems.

A. E. Benjamin adds to the picture of populations that need care. His analysis in Chapter 4 of nonelderly populations with disability includes persons with spinal cord injury and those with HIV infection/AIDS and illustrates the complexities of providing care to disparate populations. The similarities and differences between older and younger disabled populations become apparent with respect to long-term care requirements, and he draws out the implications that should be taken into account in future policies.

In Chapter 5, Leighton E. Cluff deals with the role of technology in long-term care. He discusses the emergence of a range of supportive and assistive technologies and their influence on the functional effectiveness of disabled young and old persons. Cluff presents three case vignettes of individuals with different types and degrees of disability, documenting their dependence on technologic support and emphasizing how this technology assists these individuals and how it affects those who care for them. He suggests that further improvements in the functional effectiveness of disabled persons will depend to a large extent on technologic developments, and he emphasizes the importance of electronic technology in this respect.

The part concludes with Mathy D. Mezey's discussion of the complexities of providing care for chronically ill persons. She begins by considering the goals of long-term care services and then identifies factors that make it difficult for services to meet those goals: the lack of primary care services and the difficulties in coordinating good-quality specialist care; arbitrary separation of primary care, acute care, and long-term care, as well as, more generally, health and social services; and the stresses experienced by caregivers. In addition, Mezey presents a series of promising models for delivering services more effectively. She rounds off her analysis with a discussion of the challenges involved in developing the capacities of the professionals and paraprofessionals who will be needed to provide adequate care.

Part 3 presents highly informed predictions regarding what the care in nursing homes and in home- and community-based settings will be like in the decades immediately ahead. Robert L. Kane analyzes the evolution of the American nursing home in Chapter 7. Carrying forward the historical themes delineated by Holstein and Cole earlier in the volume, he provides a comprehensive picture of how the nursing home is undergoing changes that are shaping its future. He starts with an analysis of the emergence of so-called managed care. Then he makes clear how nursing homes are taking on a variety of roles in dealing with diverse patient populations, are experiencing new modes for linking acute care and chronic care, and may increasingly "uncouple" or recombine traditional nursing home roles through programs such as "assisted living." Picking up on Cluff's discussion in Chapter 5, Kane predicts greater use of information technology. And he concludes with a consideration of broad issues that will affect the future of nursing homes: pressures for better accountability for the care they provide, changing health care ethics, and changes in what nursing homes get paid to do.

In Chapter 8, James J. Callahan, Jr., considers care in the home and other community settings. He takes us back some twenty-five years, recalling that few of the characteristics of today's long-term care system could have been forecast readily. To undergird his own prognostications, he reviews contemporary signs of the times that include portents of change over the next twenty-five years. Among these are different aspects of service use by persons of various disability characteristics and ages, changing living conditions of older persons, a shifting ethnic composition in the ranks of old persons, and, echoing Mezey, issues concerning the supply of formal service providers. On the basis of these signs and other data, he makes six predictions regarding the future of home and community-based care. Among them are that today's widely used measures of functional disability — activities of daily living (ADLs) and instrumental activities of daily living (IADLs) — will be supplemented by two additional measures, which he terms "professionally dictated activities of daily living" (PPDALs) and "appreciative activities of daily living" (AADLs).

Part 4 deals with a number of economic, political, ethical, and cultural factors that are bound up with the future of long-term care. In Chapter 9 Mark R. Meiners discusses the financing and organization of long-term care. At the outset he portrays the pivotal role that Medicaid presently plays in financing, and delineates three basic reform strategies that frame discussions about future financing: the social insurance model, means testing, and mixtures of public and private roles. With this background in place, he explicates the process through which the Clinton administration's proposal for long-term care was developed as part of the president's health care reform package in 1994, thereby unfolding what he terms the "latest 'new' thinking" about reform, the strategies devised to implement it, and the objections that various factions had to the proposal. Meiners then describes a demonstration program in which four states are engaging in partnerships with private insurance companies to jointly finance long-term care through a combination of Medicaid funds and insurance benefits, while protecting some of the assets of patients and their families. He also reviews demonstration projects that are attempting to integrate acute and long-term care, but, unlike the discussion of these experiments in Chapter 3, his detailed emphasis is on issues of financing. Finally, he discusses future initiatives that may be undertaken by state governments.

Starting in the late 1980s and continuing through President Clinton's 1994 proposal for health care reform, organized interest groups representing older and younger disabled populations were optimistic that some form of federal insurance for long-term care would be established. The failure of the Clinton plan, followed by a Republican takeover of Congress, substantially diminished that optimism. In Chapter 10, Robert H. Binstock assesses future prospects for such legislation. He depicts the present political context, in which the enactment of major policies to expand benefits to older people has become problematic. He draws particularly on lessons from the political saga of the Medicare Catastrophic Coverage Act, which was passed in 1988 and then largely repealed in 1989, to suggest that the enactment of a major program of public long-term care insurance will probably require broad grass-roots political support. Yet, Binstock argues, the older and younger constituencies of the disabled have difficulty finding common political ground. Moreover, he shows, older Americans themselves are far from a cohesive political force. He concludes with speculation about developments that could improve future prospects for public long-term care insurance.

Nancy Neveloff Dubler focuses on ethical issues in long-term care in Chapter 11. She begins by tracing the rise of the principle of "patient autonomy" in health care decisionmaking in recent decades and explores various interpretations of what the application of this principle means in different types of long-term care settings and situations. Then she relates the experience and thinking of the ethics working group that was assembled as part of the Clinton administration's National Health Care Reform Task Force in 1993, for whom the proposed legislation in long-term care raised a series of ethical issues. Drawing in part on the work of this ethics group, she discusses a range of ongoing ethical issues in long-term care, framing them as problems of conflict management and resolution.

In this part's last chapter, Otto von Mering portrays American culture and long-term care through the lens of an anthropologist. He starts with a discussion of age-grading in American society and how it shapes the culture of caregiving. He emphasizes the theme of self-reliance (as opposed to reliance on the public sector) in matters of personal economic and physical well-being. Von Mering goes on to discuss continuing care retirement communities, in which relatively affluent older persons receive formal and informal supports, and contrasts their situations with those of the "forgotten elderly," very poor and vulnerable older people who live in inner-city pockets or in rural areas who have little access to formal services. He then provides a picture of how even poor, inner-city elderly persons can band together in informal long-term care networks. He argues, optimistically, that such networks and other individualistic, non-bureaucratic manifestations of American culture can be "shape shifters" in framing the nature of long-term care in the future.

An epilogue by Dennis L. Kodner envisions what U.S. long-term care might look like in 2010. He presents a different approach to prediction from those undertaken by the authors of the preceding chapters. Through the Delphi methodology, he is able to aggregate expert opinion to derive a series of prognostications. First, Kodner presents six major factors that will affect the direction and shape of long-term care. Then he delineates important features of the future landscape, including financing, care coordination, settings for care, and measures to improve the quality of care. Finally, he draws out the implications of these forecasts in terms of the major challenges he believes will be involved in developing accessible, effective, and humane long-term care in the twenty-first century.

I

OVERVIEW AND HISTORY OF THE ISSUES

1

Issues Affecting the Future of Long-Term Care

Robert H. Binstock, Ph.D., Leighton E. Cluff, M.D., and Otto von Mering, Ph.D.

For most of this century, long-term care has been a comparatively drab backwater in the overall scene of U.S. health care. This has been the situation whether the persons needing such care have been older or younger, or afflicted by dementia, severe arthritis, cerebral palsy, spinal cord injury, severe mental illness, or any of a number of other chronic diseases and disabling conditions. Except for occasional nursing home scandals and fires — and subsequent ad hoc activities in response to such events — long-term care has received comparatively little attention from the medical profession and society at large. It has been eclipsed by the glamour and prestige of hospital-based medical care, which is inherently dramatic because it deals with acute episodes of illnesses and trauma, and their relatively "high-tech" and "quick-fix" dimensions of diagnosis and intervention.

In recent years, however, long-term care has begun to emerge as an important issue in American culture, in the health care arena, and among national, state, and local policymakers. A number of major societal dynamics — in demography, epidemiology, health care financing, family structure, politics, and medical advances — have contributed to this enhanced attention by increasing the needs and opportunities for long-term care and, at the same time, making its provision more problematic. As these dynamics continue to unfold, it is probable that dealing with the challenges of long-term care will become one of the more critical domestic problems American society faces.

This book examines the developments that have brought long-term care to the fore as an area of substantial concern, as well as the factors that will likely make it even more pressing in the future. It also explores and analyzes nascent organizational, policy, and professional developments and reforms that are being undertaken in the long-term care arena, and it delineates possibilities for further innovations. The goal of this volume is to acquaint its readers — policymakers, health care professionals, students, and the public in general — with the full range of issues involved in the future of long-term care in the United States and to stimulate thinking about the possibilities for coping with these issues in a timely and effective manner.

Overview of the Issues

The challenges of meeting long-term care needs in the twenty-first century will be substantial. The number of Americans requiring some form of long-term care is large now and will grow significantly over the next few decades. Financing such care is already very difficult for individuals, their families, and governments. Yet, indications are that the prices for services and their aggregate national costs will continue to escalate, while the role of governments in paying for care of an expanded disabled population may be curtailed. At the same time, the care that is provided is often inadequate, and social and economic factors suggest that family and service system capacities to provide quality care may be difficult to improve and, perhaps, will decline in the future.

The Growing Population Needing Care

The U.S. General Accounting Office (1994) reports that more than 12 million Americans need long-term care (we draw further on this report in the following discussion of care populations). Various other estimates yield somewhat different figures (as will become apparent in subsequent chapters of this volume), depending on their underlying definitions and assumptions regarding who needs care. Nonetheless, it is clear from all estimates that the population needing long-term care is large, diverse, and growing in size.

A person in need of long-term care is generally defined as someone who is functionally dependent on a long-term basis due to physical and/or mental limitations. Two broad categories of functional limitations are widely used by clinicians to assess need for care. One category is dependence in basic activities of daily living (ADLs) — getting in and out of bed, toileting, bathing, dressing, and eating. The other is limitations in instru-

Table 1.1

Services That May Be Needed by Disabled Individuals or Their Families

Diagnosis	Supervision
Acute medical care	Home health aide
Ongoing medical supervision	Homemaker
Treatment of coexisting medical conditions	Personal care
Medication, and elimination of drugs that cause excess disability	Paid companion/sitter
	Shopping
Multidimensional assessment	Home-delivered meals
Skilled nursing	Chore services
Physical therapy	Telephone reassurance
Occupational therapy	Personal emergency response system
Speech therapy	Recreation/exercise
Adult day care	Transportation
Respite care*	Escort service
Family/caregiver education and training	Special equipment (ramps, hospital beds, etc.)
Family/caregiver counseling	
Family support groups	Vision care
Patient counseling	Audiology
Legal services	Dental care
Financial/benefits counseling	Nutrition counseling
Mental health services	Hospice
Protective services	Autopsy

Source: Adapted from U.S. Congress, Office of Technology Assessment (1990), p. 16.

*Respite care includes any service intended to provide temporary relief for the primary caregiver. Other services in this list (e.g., homemaker, paid companion/sitter, adult day care), when used with such intention, constitute respite care.

mental activities of daily living (IADLs) — taking medications, preparing meals, financial management, doing light housework and other chores, being able to get in and out of the home, using the telephone, and so on. (Children and people with mental illness are often assessed by other criteria, such as the ability to attend school or problems in behavior.)

The range of services that may be needed by persons who have difficulties in carrying out their ADLs and IADLs, and by their primary caregivers, is extensive. A list of such services is presented in Table 1.1. In almost all cases, provision of the service is not limited by where the person resides — at home, in a nursing home, or in a residential setting such as a retirement community, board and care facility, adult foster home, assisted living facility, or other form of sheltered housing arrangement.

Popular perceptions are that most of the long-term care population is elderly and resides in nursing homes. However, this is not the case (see Table 1.2). People aged 65 or older make up only 55 percent of the long-term care population. Working-age adults account for 42 percent of the

Table 1.2
Number of Persons Needing Long-Term Care, by Age and Residence
(in thousands)

Age Group	In Institution	At Home or in Community Setting	Total Population
Children	90	330	420
Working-age adults	710	4,380	5,090
Elderly (ages 65+)	1,640	5,690	7,330
Total	2,440	10,440	12,840

Source: Adapted from U.S. General Accounting Office (1994).

total, and children the remaining 3 percent. Moreover, only 22 percent of the elderly population needing long-term care, and 19 percent of the total disabled population, resides in nursing homes and other institutions.

Although it seems apparent that the number of people needing long-term care will grow substantially in the future, reasonably precise predictions regarding the size of that population and its composition are difficult because of many factors that are involved. New and improved medical treatments and technological developments could help to prevent, delay, or compensate for various types of functional difficulties. Moreover, health-related lifestyle changes and environmental protection measures could markedly reduce rates of disabling diseases and injuries. On the other hand, medical advances could increase the need for long-term care. Lower death rates from heart disease and stroke, for example, could mean that more people will live longer with disabling conditions, and into the pathways of late-onset illnesses such as Alzheimer disease. Similarly, improvements in dealing with the complications of AIDS could engender longer periods of care for patients with this condition.

Future needs for providing and financing long-term care at older ages may also be affected by demographic factors. For instance, the cohorts that will reach old age in the next several decades will be better educated than their predecessors, and higher levels of education are associated with lower levels of disability and need for care (U.S. Bureau of the Census, 1992). Yet the ethnic composition of these same cohorts suggests that the need for care and the need for governmental subsidies to finance it may be even greater in the future than they are today. From 1990 to 2050 the proportion of Americans aged 65 or older that is nonwhite will more than double, from 9.8 percent to 21.3 percent. When they reach old age, these people may be highly dependent on public subsidies for their long-term care, if present patterns of economic resource distribution among racial and ethnic groups persist throughout the first half of the twenty-first century. Among persons aged 65 or older who have the lowest household incomes, nearly 40 percent are members of racial minorities, and their aggregate net worth is less than one-third that of older white persons (Crystal, 1996).

Even though precise projections are difficult, it does seems clear that there will be substantial increases in the number of disabled older people in the twenty-first century. When much of the baby boom — a large cohort of 74 million Americans born between 1946 and 1964 — reaches the ranks of old age in 2030, the absolute number of people aged 65 or older will have more than doubled, from about 31 million in 1990 to about 65 million. Moreover, the number of persons of advanced old-age will also more than double. The number of persons aged 75 or older will grow from 13 million to 30 million between 1990 and 2030, and those aged 85 or older will have increased from 3 million to 8 million (U.S. Bureau of the Census, 1992). As will be indicated in detail in this book, rates of disability increase markedly at these advanced old ages. One reflection of this can be found in the present rates of nursing home use in different old-age categories. About 1 percent of Americans aged 65 to 74 years are in a nursing home; this compares with 6.1 percent of persons ages 75 to 84, and 24 percent of persons aged 85 or older (U.S. Bureau of the Census, 1993). Similarly, disability rates increase in older old-age categories among older persons who are not in nursing homes: nearly 23 percent of those ages 65 to 74 experience difficulty with ADLs; 45 percent of those ages 85 and older do (Cassel, Rudberg, and Olshansky, 1992).

The tremendous growth expected in the older population in itself suggests that there will be millions more disabled elderly people in the decades ahead. Whether rates of disability in old age will increase or decline in the future, however, is a matter on which experts disagree, depending on their assumptions and measures (e.g., Fries, 1989; Manton, Corder, and Stallard, 1993; Schneider and Guralnik, 1990; Verbrugge, 1989). Assuming no changes in age-specific risks of disability, Cassel, Rudberg, and Olshansky (1992) calculated a 31 percent increase between 1990 and 2010 in the number of persons ages 65 and older experiencing difficulty with ADLs. Using the same assumption, the Congressional Budget Office (U.S. Congress, 1991) projected that the nursing home population would increase 50 percent between 1990 and 2010, double by 2030, and triple by 2050. But even those researchers who report a decline in recent years in the prevalence of disability at older ages emphasize that there will be large absolute increases in the number of older Americans needing long-term care in the decades ahead (see, e.g., Manton, Corder, and Stallard, 1993).

Predicting whether long-term care needs among people under age 65 will increase or decline is more difficult. One of the principal reasons is that reliable data bases for making projections are limited as compared with well-developed national and longitudinal sources available regarding the older population. Data collected on a state level vary widely with respect to rates for various types of disabilities (LaPlante, 1993). More-over, the numbers involved with respect to various disabling conditions — such as spinal cord injury, cerebral palsy, and mental retardation — are relatively small and much more susceptible to changing conditions.

Experts agree, however, that the number of younger disabled persons has grown in recent years, and this trend may well persist (Ross, 1994). New technologies and increased access to medical care continue to enable more people to survive injuries and other conditions that were heretofore fatal, and thus to live for many years with ADL limitations. For example, biomedical advances have enabled many more children with developmental disabilities and low birth-weight infants to survive much longer than in the past, and so to have extended years in which they need long-term care.

Paying the Costs of Care

The financial costs of long-term care are large and are likely to become much larger in the future. More than $100 billion was spent on long-term care in the United States in 1994 (U.S. General Accounting Office, 1994). The proportion spent on nursing home care is 72 percent and on home care 28 percent (Wiener, Illston, and Hanley, 1994). It is estimated that individuals and their families pay out of pocket for 44 percent of the total (Wiener and Illston, 1996). Private insurance pays only about 1 percent. The balance is paid by federal, state, and local governments. The Congressional Budget Office (U.S. Congress, 1991), using 1990 as a baseline year, projected that total national costs of long-term care will almost double by 2010 and more than triple by 2030.

An especially important factor in the growth of long-term care expenditures to date has been population aging, the increasing number and proportion of older people. Analyses that have focused on causes of *overall* increases in U.S. health care costs in recent decades have found that the impact of aging and other demographic changes has been dwarfed by the combined effects of such factors as increases in the intensity and utilization rate of health services, inflation in health-sector prices, and general

Table 1.3

Contribution of Aging to Real Increases in U.S. Health Care Spending, by Sector, 1987–1990

Sector	Annualized Rise in Costs due to Aging (%)	Annualized Rise in Total Real Costs (%)	Fraction of Total Rise in Real Costs due to Aging (%)
Hospital care	0.39	6.1	6.4
Physician care	0.33	7.0	4.7
Long-term care	1.42	6.5	21.8
Other care	0.23	7.5	3.1

Source: Data from Mendelson and Schwartz (1993).

inflation (Arnett et al., 1986; Mendelson and Schwartz, 1993; Sonnefeld et al., 1991). But, in the *long-term care sector*, aging has been a major contributor to annual cost increases. As can be seen in Table 1.3, between 1987 and 1990 population aging accounted for nearly 22 percent of the annualized rise in expenditures in long-term care, while it was a very small factor in increases in payments for hospital care, physician care, and other forms of care. A consensus among experts is that population aging will continue to contribute significantly to long-term care expenditure increases (see, e.g., U.S. Congress, 1991).

Dozens of federal programs and hundreds of state and local public and private agencies are sources of funding for long-term care services. Nonetheless, many patients needing long-term care services, and their family caregivers, find that they are ineligible for these programs and unable to pay out of pocket for services. In one study about 75 percent of unpaid informal caregivers for dementia patients reported that they did not use paid formal services because they could not afford them (Eckert and Smyth, 1988).

Paying the costs of long-term care out of pocket can be a catastrophic financial experience for patients and their families. The annual cost of a year's care in a nursing home averages $37,000 (Wiener and Illston, 1996) and ranges higher than $100,000. Although the use of a limited number of services in a home or other community-based setting is less expensive, noninstitutional care for patients who would otherwise be appropriately placed in a nursing home is not cheaper (Weissert, 1990), and it is sometimes more expensive. Out-of-pocket payments account for 51 percent of outlays for nursing home care and 26 percent of home care expenditures (Wiener, Illston, and Hanley, 1994).

Although Medicare pays for short-term, subacute nursing care, it does not cover the costs of long-term care, either in nursing homes or at home. Private long-term care insurance, a relatively new product, is very expensive for the majority of older persons, and its benefits are limited in scope and duration. The best-quality policies—providing substantial benefits over a long period of time—charged premiums in 1991 that averaged $2,525 for persons aged 65 and $7,675 for those aged 79 (Wiener and Illston, 1996). About 4 percent to 5 percent of older persons have any private long-term care insurance, and only about 1 percent of nursing home costs are paid for by private insurance (Wiener, Illston, and Hanley, 1994). A number of analyses have suggested that even when the product becomes more refined, no more than 20 percent of older Americans will be able to afford it (Crown, Capitman, and Leutz, 1992; Friedland, 1990; Rivlin and Wiener, 1988; Wiener, Illston, and Hanley, 1994). Although some studies suggest a potential for a higher percentage of customers, they assume quite limited packages of benefit coverage.

A variation on the private insurance policy approach to financing long-term care is continuing care retirement communities (CCRCs), which promise comprehensive health care services, including long-term care, to all members. CCRC customers tend to be middle- and upper-income persons who are relatively healthy when they become residents and pay a substantial entrance charge and monthly fee in return for a promise of "care for life." For older people who prefer to remain in their own homes rather than join age-segregated communities, an alternative product termed "life care at home" is also marketed to middle-income customers, with lower entry and monthly fees than those of CCRCs. Neither continuing care retirement communities nor life-care-at-home programs cover a significant number of people.

For those who cannot pay for long-term care out of pocket or through various insurance arrangements and who are not eligible for care through programs of the Department of Veterans Affairs, the available sources of payment are the federal and state Medicaid program, for which poor persons are eligible, and other means-tested programs funded by the Older Americans Act, Social Service Block Grants (Title XX of the Social Security Act), and by state and local governments. The bulk of such financing is through Medicaid, which paid an estimated 52 percent of total national nursing home expenditures in 1993, accounting for one-quarter of all Medicaid spending (Burner, Waldo, and McKusick, 1992).

Medicaid finances the care, at least in part, of about three-fifths of nursing home patients (Wiener and Illston, 1996). The program does not pay, however, for the full range of home care services that are needed by most clients who are functionally dependent. Most state Medicaid programs provide reimbursement for only the most "medicalized" services necessary to maintain a long-term care patient in a home environment; rarely reimbursed are essential supports such as chore services, assistance with food shopping and meal preparation, transportation, companionship, periodic monitoring, and respite programs for family and other unpaid caregivers.

Medicaid does include a special waiver program that allows states to offer a wider range of nonmedical home care services, if the total package provided to an individual is less costly than Medicaid-financed nursing home care. But the volume of services in these waiver programs — which in some states combine Medicaid with funds from the Older Americans Act, the Social Services Block Grant program, and other state and local government sources — is small in relation to the overall need (Miller, 1992).

Although many patients are poor enough to qualify for Medicaid when they enter a nursing home, a substantial number become poor after they are institutionalized (Adams, Meiners, and Burwell, 1993). Persons in this latter group deplete their assets in order to meet their bills and eventually "spend down" and become poor enough to qualify for Medicaid. Still others become eligible for Medicaid by sheltering their assets — illegally, or legally with the assistance of attorneys who specialize in so-called Medicaid Estate Planning. Because sheltered assets are not counted in Medicaid eligibility determinations, such persons are able to take advantage of a program for the poor without being poor. An analysis in Virginia estimated that the aggregate of assets sheltered through the use of legal loopholes in 1991 was equal to more than 10 percent of what the state spent on nursing home care through Medicaid in that year (Burwell, 1993). Asset sheltering has become a source of considerable concern to the federal and state governments, which are trying to contain their Medicaid outlays.

Many individuals needing long-term care, as well as their families, find this situation to be highly unsatisfactory. Out-of-pocket payments are steep. Private insurance policies are unaffordable for most people and generally provide inadequate coverage. People are anxious to avoid spending down their assets on long-term care, and many also seem concerned about the stigmatization of becoming dependent on welfare. Those who are eligible for Medicaid, or become so through spending down, fear that if they are Medicaid patients the quality of care they receive in nursing homes will be worse than the general standard of care. Moreover, if those eligible for Medicaid prefer to remain at home rather than enter a nursing home, they find that slots for receiving home- and community-based services provided through Medicaid waiver programs are limited in number, if available at all in their states.

Consequently, interest groups representing older people and younger disabled persons began in the 1980s to advocate for enactment of a new federal program of long-term care insurance. Although a number of bills to create long-term care insurance have been introduced in Congress since 1989, none has become law. The major reason is that any substantial version of such a program would cost tens of billions of dollars each year, just at the outset, and far more as the baby boom reaches old age.

Indeed, by the mid-1990s, legislative focus had shifted from creating a new program to curtailing the costs of long-term care. Medicaid expenditures, increasing rapidly, are projected to triple in the ten years from 1990 to 2000 (Burner, Waldo, and McKusick, 1992). A major policy agenda item in Washington and state capitals is how to curb the growth of Medicaid spending and, more specifically, the program's expenditures on long-term care.

The challenges of paying for long-term care, now and in the future, are becoming ever greater. Individuals and their families who pay out-of-pocket are likely to encounter rapidly increasing prices. Private insurance is not a panacea. Prospects for a new program of public insurance seem dim. And Medicaid, the largest payer of long-term care, is likely to be constrained by the federal and state governments from growing apace with future increases in the need for long-term care.

Providing Care

Even as the populations needing long-term care are likely to grow, and paying for care is becoming very difficult for most individuals, for their families, and for government, broad social and economic trends suggest that the provision of quality care may become increasingly problematic. Major concerns include both the informal, unpaid care provided by relatives and friends and the formal care provided by paid personnel in nursing homes and other residential settings, as well as what sort of formal service system we will have.

A number of research efforts have documented that about 80 percent of the long-term care provided to older persons outside of nursing homes is presently provided by family members — spouses, siblings, adult children, and broader kin networks. (No overall figure is available regarding informal care of younger disabled persons.) About 74 percent of dependent community-based older persons receive all their care from family members or other unpaid sources: about 21 percent receive both formal and informal services; and only about 5 percent use just formal services (Liu, Manton, and Liu, 1985). The vast majority of family caregivers are women (see Brody, 1990; Stone, Cafferata, and Sangl, 1987). The family also plays an important role in obtaining and managing services from paid service providers.

Unpaid caregiving is undertaken for a variety of reasons — principally emotional attachment, sense of obligation, and financial necessity. Regardless of the mixture of motivations, caregiving usually engenders substantial physical, mental, social, and financial strains for the caregivers, themselves, including conflicts with their other family responsibilities, with other relatives, and with their jobs.

A vast research literature has documented caregiver stress and explored factors that may mediate such stress (see Pearlin et al., 1996). Various programs, such as respite care and adult day care, have been developed for the purpose of reducing caregiver burdens. The federal Family and Medical Leave Act of 1993 established policies, applicable to large corporate employers, designed to reduce employees' short-term conflicts between job and caregiving. State governments and a number of businesses have established policies providing financial support and workplace benefits and programs designed to help caregivers with their burdens (Stern, 1995).

Despite the growing attention that has been given to moderating and alleviating caregiver stress, the capacities and willingness of family members to care for disabled older persons may decline when the baby boom cohort reaches old age, because of a broad social trend. The family, as a fundamental unit of social organization, has been undergoing profound transformations, which will become more fully manifest over the next few decades as baby boomers reach old age. The striking growth of single-parent households, the growing participation of women in the labor force, the high incidence of divorce and remarriage (differentially higher for men), all entail complicated changes in the structure of household and kinship roles and relationships. There will be an increasing number of "blended families," reflecting multiple lines of descent through multiple marriages and the birth of children outside of wedlock through other partners. This growth in the incidence of step- and half-relatives will make for a dramatic new turn in family structure in the coming decades. Already, such blended families constitute about half of all households with children (National Academy on Aging, 1994).

As such changes begin to coincide with the growth of three- and even four-generation families, what emerges will be a very complex picture, the ramifications of which have not yet been fully analyzed and understood. One clear implication, however, is that while kinship networks in the near future will become much more extensive than in the past, they will also become more complex, attenuated, and diffuse (Bengtson, Rosenthal, and Burton, 1990).

Early research evidence of a weakened sense of filial obligation in blended families does give cause for concern. If changes in the intensity of kinship relations significantly erode the capacity and sense of obligation to care for older family members when the baby boom cohort is in the ranks of old-age and disability, there is a distinct possibility that support for public long-term care insurance will become an issue on which most older Americans and their families will become united.

Even if more public funds are available to pay for services, issues concerning the work force that provides such services are likely to persist. Increasing efforts have been made to improve skilled care in nursing homes and to use technology in home care. But the quality of less skilled care — as Feldman (1994a) termed it, the "bed and body" care that provides personal assistance in toileting, bathing, and other ADLs — has received relatively little attention.

Recruiting, training, and retaining nursing home aides and home care aides to provide responsible, high-quality care is an ongoing problem for which no easy solutions are in sight; it is a problem shared by all industrialized countries. The functions performed by this work force are, on the whole, distasteful, boring, and physically and emotionally exhausting. Wages are low — worse than those of hospital aides (Crown, 1994) — and fringe benefits are generally unavailable for home care aides. These front line workers have little opportunity for advancement. Home care aides, especially, are isolated from their peers. Job burnout is frequent. The turnover rate has been estimated to be as high as 50 percent or more each year (Close et al., 1994).

Various strategies and trends have been identified that might deal with these problems (Feldman, 1994b). Improvements in training, managerial supervision, and other kinds of organizational supports could be of value in improving the quality of service provided by such workers. Broader changes in the health care arena, such as the spread of managed care, might lead to some reorganization of the functions performed by aides, with opportunities for upward mobility. In the last analysis, however, improvement in the work force of aides would probably require large infusions of financing into the service system for providing higher wages and benefits, as well as quality training and opportunities for advancement. The probability is small, however, that such changes will take place in the near future.

Even when high-quality and appropriate services are sufficiently available, many disabled persons and their families do not know about them and require help in defining their service needs and arranging for them to be met. The complexities of the health and social care arena are difficult to sort out. Delivery structures, public and private insurance mechanisms, and terms of benefits and eligibility are shifting every day. Most Americans are bewildered by the health care arena of independent practice associations (IPAs), preferred provider organizations (PPOs), health maintenance organizations (HMOs) and their social care variations (S/HMOs), geriatric assessment centers, ambulatory care units, skilled nursing facilities (SNFs), intermediate care facilities (ICFs), home health agencies, deductibles, co-insurance, "accepting assignment," Medicaid and Veterans Administration eligibility, private "Medigap" and long-term care insurance policies, and so on.

In this maze, when the need for long-term care arises, it is difficult for many individuals and their families even to begin the process of arranging for appropriate care. How and where will they be able to begin the process? From which of many agencies can they get help, and on what terms? What kinds of help will they get, and will it be appropriate and effective?

A pressing need now — and it will be far greater when the baby boom reaches old age — is a highly visible, distinctive agency in every community to which people can turn to begin arranging for appropriate services. Moreover, these agencies should be part of a nationwide network of similar agencies so that the efforts of adult children and other relatives who are trying to assist disabled elders in distant communities can be helped in an effective fashion.

A related problem, of course, is the fragmentation of the delivery system. Few units of organization integrate acute and long-term care in fashions that are optimal either for patient care or cost efficiency. Separate sources of financing for acute and long-term care, especially the separate streams of funding through Medicare and Medicaid and the incentives associated with them, tend to engender this fragmentation and, often, inappropriate care.

As will be delineated in subsequent chapters, experimental models for integrating financing and care for older patients have been developed and are being refined through field demonstrations. Each involves a mechanism of managed care, but their differences illustrate some of the issues and challenges generated by various sources of funding and different types of older patient populations. Such experiments have yet to involve younger disabled persons and their service needs.

In short, as is the case with most aspects of the U.S. health care delivery system, the characteristics of long-term care services and access to them are substantially shaped by the nature and extent of funding policies. Accordingly, success in reforming long-term care services to make them both adequate in supply and appropriate in quality and accessibility will largely lie in changing the nature of their funding.

References

Adams, E. K., Meiners, M. R., and Burwell, B. O. (1993). Asset spend-down in nursing homes: Methods and insights. *Medical Care* 31:1–23.

Arnett, R. H. III, McKusick, D. R., Sonnefeld, S. T., and Cowell, C. S. (1986). Projections of health care spending to 1990. *Health Care Financing Review* 7 (3): 1–36.

Bengtson, V., Rosenthal, C., and Burton, L. (1990). Families and aging: Diversity and heterogeneity. In R. H. Binstock and L. K. George, eds., *Handbook of Aging and the Social Sciences,* 3rd ed. (pp. 263–87). San Diego: Academic Press.

Brody, E. M. (1990). *Women in the Middle: Their Parent-Care Years.* New York: Springer Publishing.

Burner, S. T., Waldo, D. R., and McKusick, D. R. (1992). National health expenditures projections through 2030. *Health Care Financing Review* 14 (1): 1–29.

Burwell, B. (1993). *State Responses to Medicaid Estate Planning.* Cambridge, Mass.: SysteMetrics.

Cassel, C. K., Rudberg, M. A., and Olshansky, S. J. (1992). The price of success: Health care in an aging society. *Health Affairs* 11 (2): 87–99.

Close, L., Estes, C. L., Linkins, K. W., and Binney, E. A. (1994). *Generations* 18 (3): 23–27.

Crown, W. H. (1994). A national profile of homecare, nursing home, and hospital aides. *Generations* 18 (3): 29–33.

Crown, W. H., Capitman, J., and Leutz, W. N. (1992). Economic rationality, the affordability of private long-term care insurance, and the role for public policy. *Gerontologist* 32:478–85.

Crystal, S. (1996). Economic status of the elderly. In R. H. Binstock and L. K. George, eds., *Handbook of Aging and the Social Sciences,* 4th ed. (pp. 388–409). San Diego: Academic Press.

Eckert, S. K., and Smyth, K. (1988). *A Case Study of Methods of Locating and Arranging Health and Long-Term Care for Persons with Dementia.* Washington, D.C.: U.S. Congress, Office of Technology Assessment.

Feldman, P. H. (1994a). Introduction: "Dead end" work or motivating job? Prospects for frontline paraprofessional workers in long-term care. *Generations* 18 (3): 5–10.

Feldman, P. H., ed. (1994b). *Frontline Workers in Long-Term Care. Generations.* vol. 18, no. 3.

Friedland, R. (1990). *Facing the Costs of Long-Term Care: An EBRI-ERF Policy Study*. Washington, D.C.: Employee Benefits Research Institute.

Fries, J. F. (1989). The compression of morbidity: Near or far? *Milbank Quarterly* 67:208–32.

LaPlante, M. P. (1993). *Disability Statistics Report: State Estimates of Disability in America*. Washington, D.C.: National Institute on Disability and Rehabilitation Research, U.S. Department of Education, Office of Special Education and Rehabilitative Services.

Liu, K., Manton, K. M., and Liu, B. M. (1985). Home care expenses for the disabled elderly. *Health Care Financing Review* 7 (2): 52.

Manton, K. G., Corder, L. S., and Stallard, E. (1993). Estimates of change in chronic disability and institutional incidence and prevalence rates in the U.S. elderly population from the 1982, 1984, and 1989 National Long Term Care Survey. *Journal of Gerontology: Social Sciences* 48:S153–66.

Mendelson, D. N., and Schwartz, D. B. (1993). The effects of aging and population growth on health care costs. *Health Affairs* 12 (1): 119–25.

Miller, N. A. (1992). Medicaid 2176 home and community-based care waivers: The first ten years. *Health Affairs* 11 (4): 162–71.

National Academy on Aging (1994). *Old Age in the 21st Century*. Washington, D.C.: Syracuse University.

Pearlin, L. I., Aneshensel, C. S., Mullan, J. T., and Whitlatch, C. J. (1996). Caregiving and its social support. In R. H. Binstock and L. K. George, eds., *Handbook of Aging and the Social Sciences*, 4th ed. (pp. 283–302). San Diego: Academic Press.

Rivlin, A. M., and Wiener, J. M. (1988). *Caring For the Disabled Elderly: Who Will Pay?* Washington, D.C.: Brookings Institution.

Ross, J. L. (1994). *Long-Term Care: Demography, Dollars, and Dissatisfaction Drive Reform*. Testimony before the Special Committee on Aging, U.S. Senate, April 12. U.S. GAO/T-HEHS-94-140.

Schneider, E. L., and Guralnik, J. M. (1990). The aging of America: Impact on health care costs. *Journal of the American Medical Association* 263:2335–40.

Sonnefeld, S. T., Waldo, D. R., Lemieux, J. A., and McKusick, D. R. (1991). Projections of national health expenditures through the year 2000. *Health Care Financing Review* 13 (1): 1–27.

Stern, A. L. (1995). *A Multidimensional Assessment of Caregiving Outcomes*. Doctoral dissertation. Boston: University of Massachusetts, Boston.

Stone, R., Cafferata, G. L., and Sangl, J. (1987). Caregivers of the frail elderly: A national profile. *Gerontologist* 27:616–26.

U.S. Bureau of the Census (1992). *Sixty-five Plus in America*. Current Population Reports, Special Studies, P23-178. Washington, D.C.: U.S. Government Printing Office.

U.S. Bureau of the Census (1993). *Nursing Home Population, 1990*. CPH-L-137. Washington, D.C.: U.S. Government Printing Office.

U.S. Congress (1990). Office of Technology Assessment. *Confused Minds, Bur-*

dened Families: Finding Help for People with Alzheimer's Disease and Other Dementia. Washington, D.C.: U.S. Government Printing Office.

U.S. Congress (1991). Congressional Budget Office. Policy Choices for Long-Term Care. Washington, D.C.: U.S. Government Printing Office.

U.S. General Accounting Office (1994). Long-Term Care: Diverse, Growing Population Includes Millions of Americans of All Ages. GAO/HEHS-95-62. Washington, D.C.: U.S. Government Printing Office.

Verbrugge, L. M. (1989). Recent, present, and future health of American adults. In L. Breslow, J. E. Fielding, and L. B. Lave, eds., Annual Review of Public Health (vol. 10, pp. 333–61). Palo Alto, Calif.: Annual Reviews.

Weissert, W. G. (1990). Strategies for reducing home care expenditures. Generations 14 (2): 42–44.

Wiener, J. M., and Illston, L. H. (1996). Health care financing and organization for the elderly. In R. H. Binstock and L. K. George, eds., Handbook of Aging and the Social Sciences, 4th ed. (pp. 427–45). San Diego, Calif.: Academic Press.

Wiener, J. M., Illston, L. H., and Hanley, R. J. (1994). Sharing the Burden: Strategies for Public and Private Long-term Care Insurance. Washington, D.C.: Brookings Institution.

2

The Evolution of Long-Term Care in America

Martha Holstein, M.A., and Thomas R. Cole, Ph.D.

Long-term care, commonly understood today as a range of medical and social supports for older people and others with disabilities, is a relatively new phenomenon. For most of American history, families—primarily women—have taken care of their older relatives.

Until the last third of the nineteenth century, neither medicine nor hospitals had much to offer the ill or the disabled; and social services, as we understand them today, did not exist. Municipalities provided meager public support, not particularly for the sick or the frail, but for the indigent of all ages. In the middle third of the nineteenth century, poverty, not illness, triggered such support. Moralistic judgments and individualistic understandings about poverty and the poor gave rise to the poorhouse, a deliberately unpleasant institution initially intended to discipline and punish the poor, not to house the old.

In contrast to public facilities, private homes for the aged served "native-born women of good character" and some ethnic and racial minorities who could not be cared for at home. These private homes, sympathetic to their "worthy" clients but no less paternalistic toward them than were the almshouses, resembled supervised boarding houses more than modern nursing homes. In the twentieth century, the residues of these early Jacksonian and later Victorian attitudes and structures have continued to exert a subtle influence on long-term care policy development.

This chapter will divide the evolution of modern long-term care into four main periods. From the colonial period to 1820, care of the poor and the ill was community-based and flexible. The period from 1820 to 1865 marked a deliberate turn to institutional poor relief. Medical care, however, except for the poorest, still took place in the home. In the next period, from 1865 to 1935, institutional poor relief became harsher, hospitals increasingly biased toward acute care, and older people the dominant populations of the almshouse. This period also marked the dawning recognition that the aged might have special needs that almshouses could not meet. The period following the enactment of the Social Security Act in 1935 witnessed both the establishment of and the initial reaction to the modern long-term care system. This system is now the subject of reform agendas that range from efforts to improve conditions within facilities to experimentation with alternatives that move beyond both institutions and home care (see Retsinas, 1994).

The dominant story that we shall tell, recounted in public documents and private reports, focuses on the evolution of public policy and limited private not-for-profit initiatives. It is largely, though not entirely, told from the perspective of white, middle-class reformers, providers, and administrators, and concentrates primarily on long-term care in its institutional form. We have chosen this focus not because institutional long-term care is the only story but because it is the one that has, until recently, dominated public attention and activity.

What this story omits is in itself significant: how families, mostly women, have continued caring for their elderly relatives and friends, counting on one another and on occasional help from outsiders (Abel, 1991). Someday researchers will uncover many other stories of long-term care, refracted through the prisms of gender, race, class, age, ethnicity, and geographical region. We will address some of those other stories, though in an admittedly fragmentary way. Told in the voices of ethnic and racial minorities, who found ways to care for their own elders in the face of American nativism and systematic racial discrimination, their documentation is less extensive than the paper trail left by the white middle class.

Before turning to this history in detail, we want to alert the reader to some common themes — both ideological and practical — that have left indelible and often intractable marks on modern long-term care. Until the late twentieth century, policies that affected the chronically ill and the frail were "an afterthought, a side effect of decisions directed at other problems" (Vladeck, 1980, p. 31), such as indigence and acute illness. And even in the late twentieth century, concern about an older person's quality of life in institutional settings must compete with cost-containment efforts. We are now literally and figuratively paying the price for our earlier history, when policies were developed incrementally and in a piecemeal fashion, with little coordination and without adequate attention to their possible consequences.

In addition to these general themes in policy history, the development of long-term care also reflected and incorporated cultural norms about gender, indigence, and old age. These ideas, in turn, have intersected with the business cycle, the needs of the state, the shifting relationships among federal, state, and local governments, and the bias toward leaving the private sector relatively free to provide services, even when substantial federal funding is involved (Estes et al., 1984). Despite some recent shifts in thinking, the effect of these values and preferences on modern long-term care remains.

As we will illustrate in this chapter, modern long-term care cannot escape its history. While other more general features of American social welfare policy, such as the preference for creating private services with public dollars, have influenced the current shape of modern long-term care, the scars left by these earlier institutions, however residual and indirect, and the cultural presuppositions they incorporated have helped forge the conditions for and the boundaries of modern reform efforts.

The Colonial Period: The Dominance of "Outdoor" Relief

In early America, small, face-to-face, traditional communities offered poor relief in ways that generally did not stigmatize the poor nor rely upon rigid classification or eligibility criteria. Families provided virtually all care for poor and infirm elders. The problems communities sought to address were the residual, though serious, ones of poverty and destitution. The colonial system of "outdoor" (that is, noninstitutional) relief, modeled on the English Poor Law of 1601, held local government responsible for giving public relief to those who could not support themselves or obtain help from relatives, friends, or private philanthropy (Achenbaum, 1978; Quadagno, 1986).

Generally speaking, individuals of diverse economic and social backgrounds participated in caring for the indigent (Staples, 1991). In their turn, recipients of poor relief were expected to sew or knit or undertake other modest tasks in keeping with their level of physical infirmity. Communal values supported *both* rights and responsibilities of recipients. In addition, old bonds of personal loyalties, born in the medieval past, persisted into the public realm. A shared religious framework for understanding and manipulating the world reinforced a society structured through webs of personal relationships (Wood, 1992).

In the colonies and during the early years of the republic, the core moral values were communal and reciprocal. Fostered by homogeneity and the small size of communities, and as yet untouched by urban individualism or industrialization, early American communities saw poverty and ill-health as home-grown, familiar, and not morally blameworthy. Without romanticizing the early American attitude toward the poor, its personal qualities differentiated it sharply from what came later. Decisionmakers were local leaders; the poor had names and faces.

This attitude toward poverty, though supportive for most poor people in most communities, did not hold up universally. For example, strangers were "warned out," left to wander from town to town. The young and the able-bodied were often auctioned off to the highest bidder who would provide room and board in exchange for labor. Thus, although care of the poor and the old tended to be an accepted community function, communities were not beyond judging whom they would help and how generously.

When analyzing the growth first of nursing homes and then of other long-term care services, it is critical to remember that modern distinctions between poverty (welfare needs) and illness (medical care and social support needs) were generally absent through much of America's past. The most pressing social concern in colonial America, one that intensified in the nineteenth century, was poor relief. Poor relief might have included tending to the ill, but that was not its central goal. Thus, although those who were old *and* sick might require special forms of care, they were not singled out for categorical assistance. There was also little special that could be done for them, since medicine offered limited remedies. The few existing hospitals were hardly more than another form of poor relief (Rosenberg, 1987).

Relief Moves "Indoors": The Dominance of the Almshouse in an Era of Optimism, 1820–1865

These communal and religious values did not survive the rapid changes that overtook American society in the decades after the Revolution. Even in the mid-eighteenth century, a demographic explosion and economic changes unsettled old patterns and values, while commercial capitalism inserted the cash nexus into formerly hierarchical and personal relationships (see Wood, 1992). The Revolution itself sharply — and as it turned out irrevocably — challenged every form of authority and superiority (Wood, 1992), including religion. As the century advanced, growth in the number of immigrants from Southern and Central Europe created fears of disorder, which further ruptured the strong bonds that linked poor relief to religious, hierarchical, and communal values (Kutzik, 1979).

At the same time, Jacksonian Democrats, who saw unlimited possibilities in the vast American continent and in individual initiative, were less inclined than their Calvinist ancestors to accept poverty as an inevitable part of life. They thought poverty could be abolished, and they interpreted its presence as a sign of individual moral failure (Rothman, 1971). As a result, roughly between the Revolution and 1825, the apparently flexible and informal arrangements that had marked the earlier period began to break down (Staples, 1991).

Provoked by the young nation's first depression and the consequently escalated poor tax, both Massachusetts and New York commissioned major studies to analyze the causes of and remedies for poverty. The Quincy Report, published in 1821, and the Yates Report, issued in 1824, arrived at remarkably similar conclusions. Locating the causes of poverty squarely within the individual, particularly emphasizing intemperance and other forms of moral turpitude (Rothman, 1971; Staples, 1991), these reports had specific consequences for poor relief. In New York, the Yates Report led to the County Poorhouse Act of 1824; comparable legislation was rapidly adopted in other states (Butners, 1980; Kutzik, 1979; Rothman, 1971). The most dramatic result was the birth of an institutional solution to indigence. Alternatively labeled almshouses, poorhouses, or poor farms, such institutions developed rapidly, especially in the more industrialized cities on the Eastern Seaboard.

Designed by poor relief administrators to reform and punish the poor, these institutions housed the poor of all ages, as well as the sick, the retarded, the mentally ill, and the socially deviant. Although the reforming mission — to save people from themselves and therefore from poverty (Rosner, 1982) — required close supervision and instruction, the reformers also wanted the almshouses to serve as deterrents to, or punishment for, poverty. Therefore, these municipally supported facilities had minimal standards of comfort and cleanliness. The bad conditions and unsavory reputation of almshouses also met more subtle goals: to encourage people to accept any work at any wage and to strengthen a family's commitment to care for its needy members (Estes et al., 1984; Katz, 1984). But there was no parallel commitment to assist families in that task. The assumption that families would abandon their old if almshouse conditions were improved is, in its modern version, labeled the "woodwork effect."

Inevitably, the move toward almshouses affected older people if they were poor, infirm, and without adequate family support. By the mid-nineteenth century, those who could not be cared for at home had few options but the almshouse (Haber, 1993). As attitudes toward aging and old age became harsher in this period, the moral standards of "worthy" and "unworthy" theretofore reserved for younger, able-bodied inmates were also applied to the old. Until the middle third of the nineteenth century, many Americans still accepted sickness and dependency as inevitable dimensions of growing old. In contrast, Victorian moralists came to devalue those who experienced poverty, disease, and frailty in old age. Viewing these conditions as signs of personal moral failure, health reformers and ministers believed that one's economic and medical condition in old age was entirely within individual control (Cole, 1992).

Not unexpectedly, the dichotomy between those who aged "well" and those who did not often translated directly into "worthy" native-born American women versus unworthy "others." Thus, one's degree of worthiness had much to do with national origin, gender, and race. Blinded to the social and economic causes of poverty and ill health, many reformers accused poor men of profligacy and immigrants of slovenly work habits, lack of foresight, and other non-Protestant characteristics (Dieckmann, 1993). But even for the "worthy" poor, reformers were reluctant to expend resources. Why waste money on those who would be permanently disabled (Haber, 1993)? The aged poor were not immune from the rough edges of punitive "indoor" relief, whose advocates persisted in conceptualizing the causes of poverty in individual terms.

Alternative Responses to Indigence and Illness in Old Age

Also during the early nineteenth century, an alternative to the public almshouse emerged — the private home for the aged. White northern Protestant philanthropists developed these homes for "worthy" women of "appropriate caste and nativity," a trend that would accelerate after the Civil War (Butners, 1980). As early as 1814, the Association for the Relief of Respectable Aged Indigent Females was founded in New York City. It erected its first "asylum" in 1838 (Cole, 1975). With comparable motives, in 1817 Philadelphians founded the Indigent Widows' and Single Women's Society, which denied admission to anyone born and raised in poverty (Cole, 1987). In that same city, but 50 years later, Quakers and African Americans opened the doors to a home for "worthy and exemplary colored people," in a recognition that racism, not bad character, had made them poor (Haber, 1983).

During this period, as reformers tried to cope with poverty in terms of their particular ideological stance, large numbers of old and infirm African American men and women remained enslaved. We have few details about the care they received from their owners but it does seem clear that, as in traditional Africa, "slaves, including children, looked to the needs of their old people and treated them with respect and deference" (Genovese, 1974, p. 523). Enlarged social networks composed of real or fictive kin assumed responsibility for their elders. "The language of kinship expressed a broad range of mutual obligation": "brother," "sister," "aunt," "uncle" conferred the status of kin and the commensurate obligations on those unrelated by blood (Berlin, Miller, and Rowland, 1988). Such expectations, and the flexible and adaptable caregiving that followed, were built into community norms (Billingsley, 1992).

It is more difficult to generalize about how slave owners behaved toward their aging slaves. Treatment has been described as oppressive, barbaric, or at the best indifferent (Genovese, 1974; Martin and Martin, 1986), although in some instances old slaves were kindly and thoughtfully treated. Some old slaves were treated like "warn-out farm animals," and the practice of abandonment was widespread (Burnham, 1990, pp. 204–5).

The first benevolent society for blacks was founded by free African Americans in 1789. The Free African Society, born in the African Methodist Episcopal Church, dedicated itself to mutual support in sickness and in widowhood. The Prince Hall fraternal order, founded in 1787, offered social services, collected and distributed sick dues, and provided pensions to the elderly and companionship for the sick and disabled (Martin and Martin, 1986). By 1899, Philadelphia had approximately 106 benevolent societies enrolling one-half of the adult black population (Martin and Martin, 1986).

From Emancipation to 1935

The changes that occurred between 1865 and 1935 had momentous consequences for the development of modern long-term care. We will trace just a few of these changes. First, by the end of this period, older people had become the dominant population in almshouses. Second, the increasingly punitive nature of charity based on moral disapproval hampered significant changes in almshouse conditions, while growing pessimism about old age hindered the systematic development of alternative forms of care. Third, African Americans, facing solidifying racial barriers, could not obtain medical care or other services. In response, they turned to vigorous activism on behalf of their elders. Particularly through the churches and women's organizations, they founded numerous homes for the aged and strengthened their long history of mutual help. Fourth, other organizing efforts to found homes and strengthen mutual aid accelerated, especially among ethnic and racial minorities. And, fifth, health and welfare reformers became interested in more formalized postacute home care and the financing of care for chronic illness, yet both remained minor stories in this period.

The "Graying" of the Almshouses

By the mid-nineteenth century, the reformers' zeal for social improvement accelerated the growth of institutions specifically designed to reform, rehabilitate, and educate. More systematically than earlier in the century, reformers moved specific groups into separate institutions (Katz, 1986; Staples, 1991). The young went to orphanages, the insane to mental institutions, the physically handicapped to special schools, and the able-bodied to workhouses (Haber, 1983). By stripping away one group after another and leaving the elderly in place, these reformers unintentionally, but nonetheless effectively, transformed the almshouse into a residence for older, poor people (Katz, 1984), most of whom were foreign-born (Cole, 1992; Haber and Gratton, 1993). Because medicine held little hope for ameliorating the pathological conditions of old age, designing special institutions for the aged appeared futile (Haber and Gratton, 1993). Thus, the old became primary victims of a welfare strategy, and indirectly a health strategy, that accepted inadequate care as policy (Vladeck, 1980).

The emergence of curative medicine as the modern hospital's central activity reinforced the centrality of the almshouse as the institution most available for poor and chronically ill older people. Modern hospitals, dedicated to caring for the acutely ill, showed little tolerance for elderly people who were chronically impaired; they consumed beds and resources that could be put to "better" use (Haber, 1983; Rosenberg, 1987). As a result, the physically and mentally infirm were moved to the almshouse or to municipal hospitals. Like voluntary hospitals, private charities also declined to assist the old, whom they viewed as "nonredeemable" and therefore permanently dependent (Haber and Gratton, 1993; Quadagno, 1986). In these years, medical care came increasingly to mean acute care. Care of the chronically ill, who were either poor to start with or became poor as a result of their illness, was thus relegated to a welfare function.

As a result, and primarily by default, older people became the "natural" and principal inhabitants of the almshouse. Unlike the picture painted by Progressive era reformers, old people were not abandoned by their families, nor did poverty among the elderly increase significantly during this period. Close and instrumental kinship relationships persisted; families seem to have maintained a high degree of structural integrity despite the changes wrought by industrialization (Seward, 1978). They continued to honor two cultural norms: family responsibility and autonomous living (Haber and Gratton, 1993). Yet, caregiving was made more problematic. Geophysical mobility weakened bonds of kinship and community, and caregiving lost its earlier communal aspect; women became more isolated in this task (Abel, 1991).

Social Reform and Deteriorating Conditions in the Almshouse

In the last decades of the nineteenth century, conditions in the almshouses generally worsened. At the Home for Indigents in Philadelphia, prisoners composed the home's work force and substantially controlled the inmate's daily lives (Dieckmann, 1993). In New York State, conditions in the almshouses were so deplorable that a brief return to "outdoor" relief was attempted (W. Taylor, 1969).

Since all almshouses were municipally funded and operated, these worsening conditions were at least in part the result of the financial difficulties city governments were experiencing, but they were also a deliberate act of policy. If poverty was the result of an "inheritable" trait, as nativist and Social Darwinist thinking came to emphasize, it seemed foolhardy to invest large sums of scarce resources on remedial efforts (Rosner, 1982). As a result, the old conflict between compassion and deterrence in almshouse policy intensified. Some late-nineteenth-century "scientific" reformers went further. They often used their power to campaign against all public welfare, declaring it a promoter of pauperism, unless it had the singular aim of "curing" the individual (Butners, 1980; Rosner, 1982). In the thinking of late-nineteenth-century reformers, the subjective causes of poverty — bad character, immorality, and deviance — clearly trumped more objective causes such as illness, injury, unemployment, old age, and death of a spouse (Estes et al., 1984). These ideologically driven assumptions about poverty and ill health had a cascading effect on the aged and indirectly influenced American social welfare policy for generations.

While the charity reformers seemed to care little about the structural causes of poverty and ill health, some reformers, such as members of the State Charities Aid Association, founded in 1872, and the Charity Organization Society, founded in 1881, were concerned about the way almshouse policies affected the "worthy" aged. "Respectable" women, old and native born, differed from other inmates; therefore, they deserved the otherwise unheard of right to privacy (Clark, 1900).

In 1895, Mary Roberts Smith interviewed 228 women living in San

Francisco's almshouse. She deemed nine worthy; all but one were native-born Americans. "The clearly honest, deserving, and unfortunate, because they are so few, stand out in sharp distinction to the mass of the degenerate and unworthy" (Smith 1895, p. 258). The others — mostly foreign-born — deserved, in Smith's opinion, only minimal custodial care, penance for their earlier intemperate, immoral, and shiftless lives. Several years later, Smith recommended classifying inmates on the basis of their "habits, character, and degree of refinement" (Warner, 1908, p. 101).

Concern for the worthy poor rarely resulted in significant change; perhaps a library or religious services were added to the institution. But the reformers did expect all who could to work — to sew a rag rug, to wash the dishes — even if the work had to be done sitting down (Butners, 1980). Ironically, as nursing homes became more modern (and more medicalized), they also abandoned this earlier policy of responsibility and rough reciprocity.

The late nineteenth century, then, was a period of serious deterioration in almshouses: minimal physical care, no recreation, no attention to emotional needs, and the separation of husbands and wives (Kutzik, 1979). Cases of illness and insanity went untreated; filth and dilapidated conditions prevailed (Rothman, 1980). The early goals of the almshouse evaporated; instead custody replaced reform as the purpose of institutional life. The poorhouse became a symbol of brutality and corruption (Cole, 1992). As public sentiment became increasingly indifferent to the poor, the almshouses and their inhabitants were, in essence, abandoned.

Shifting Attitudes toward Aging and Old Age

The bad conditions in almshouses and the increasing presence of older residents did not escape all notice. In 1903, reformers like Homer Folks, New York's Commissioner of Charities, recommended, in an effort to lend dignity to older almshouse residents, that the city's almshouse be renamed the Home for the Aged and Infirm. This change did not radically alter care, but it did signify a changing perception of poverty and ill health in old age. Folks argued that it was time to recognize that the "inmates of almshouses were more nearly related to hospital patients than paupers" (Haber and Gratton, 1993, p. 277). Backed by studies such as Mabel Louise Nassau's 1913 study of almshouses, public welfare reformers sought to remove the stigma of old age poverty, blaming age itself as the source of problems. Though not returning full circle to the earlier Calvinist belief that dependency in old age was part of the human condition, these studies concluded that poverty often befell older men and women even when they had lived virtuously and worked hard all their lives (Cole, 1987).

Supported by late-nineteenth-century medical investigations that conflated pathology and old age, greater tolerance of, if not respect for, the elderly poor and ill emerged. To many physicians, aging itself became a disease, senile decline an inevitability. The Victorian concept of self-willed health and independence dissipated. The new myth of old age, conforming to the late-nineteenth-century medical model of senescence, suggested that no matter how one lived, most old people would eventually become patients (Haber, 1983). This new truism did not immediately result in specific efforts to determine how to best serve older people as patients, but it did begin to focus attention on the care given in almshouses and homes for the aging.

Earlier in the century, the "graying" of the almshouse had happened by chance, as reformers moved other population groups to specialized institutions. Now, many physicians and social reformers touted the almshouse as the best setting in which to care for impoverished and incapacitated elderly (Haber, 1983). Using a model of old age dependency, scientific reformers vigorously advocated for institutions as the appropriate location in which to care for the sick elderly. The almshouse gained a new status in the annals of scientific charity as the appropriate place to care for the sick elderly. "Care of the poverty-stricken elderly had come to be seen as the true function of the nation's poorhouses. . . . long-term care for the elderly, regardless of their mental condition, meant almshouse residency" (Haber and Gratton, 1993, p. 272, p. 7).

These widely held sentiments did not, however, remove the stigma associated with the almshouse. Older people and their families continued to fear the possibility of such incarceration. As a result, the almshouse became a powerful symbol in the struggle for old-age pensions. Hatred for the almshouse created a resistance to any public provision of nursing home care; thus, the almshouse and the heritage of nineteenth-century attitudes toward poverty that it enshrined indirectly but nonetheless forcefully led to the now-dominant proprietary nursing home industry.

African American Activism

There is another important story that marked these decades. The almshouses displayed the patterns of racial segregation that still persist in U.S. nursing homes. Either needy blacks were excluded from the almshouses or they moved into the older facilities. In 1866, the first African Americans entered the old Nashville poorhouse after extended negotiations between the municipality and the Freedmen's Bureau. As they arrived, white paupers relocated to new quarters (*Nashville Daily Press and Times,* 1867).

Hardening patterns of racial segregation, economic stagnation, and increasing impoverishment among blacks in the last third of the nineteenth century helped spawn concentrated social activism by African Americans, particularly on behalf of their elders and their youth (Carlton-LaNey, 1988; Hine, 1989). After Reconstruction, when blacks still resided primarily in the South, they were barred from most hospitals and dispensaries. The persistent fear of social reformers that the undeserving would benefit from public assistance was exacerbated by considerations of race. The Freedmen's Bureau did not intend to become a "pauperizing agency;" after 1862 it relied on enforced contributions from the able-bodied to support dependent blacks (Berkeley, 1990). The "interplay between white institutional racism and antagonisms within the Black community left former slaves with no alternatives but to rely on their own meager resources for survival" (Berkeley, 1990, p. 191). The postbellum atmosphere of discrimination and racism, the resentment of blacks to the white dominance of facilities that did admit blacks, and the strong traditions of survival and self-help embedded in the African American community together led to the voluntary creation of separate institutions for blacks (Salem, 1990).

African American women initiated these efforts, which, shaped by racism, had an insurgent edge. The women first organized into local clubs often associated with churches, and then into the National Association of Colored Women (NACW), founded in 1896 (Berkeley, 1990). Although affluent black women became the leaders of the clubs associated with the NACW, low-wage workers, such as domestics and laundresses, constituted two-thirds of the leadership of organizations affiliated with churches. Built in part on the historic tradition of self-help reflected in the older mutual aid and benevolent societies, these women's clubs founded homes for the aged, for working women, and for unwed mothers. They organized hospitals, programs of unemployment relief, and kindergartens (Firor-Scott, 1990).

In particular, these women turned to care for the aged. During the late nineteenth century, it became clear that aging ex-slaves had little means of support. Often their children could not care for them because of their own poverty or because of distance—the migrations north having separated many families (Carlton-LaNey, 1988). In 1905, black club women raised $2,000 to convert an antebellum mansion into an old age home; Harriet Tubman, an architect of the Underground Railroad, established a home for the elderly in her own home in Auburn, New York. Working-class blacks, organized by the "Tent Sisters," pledged one pound of food and at least 25 cents per year in cash and more when necessary, founded and maintained a nursing home in Raleigh, North Carolina (Pollard, 1978). Individuals also volunteered time and sometimes, well in advance of modern intergenerational programs, they combined the aged with orphans (Salem, 1990). Noting these accomplishments, W. E. B. DuBois described institutional care for the aged as the "first and best institutional work existing in black communities" (Salem, 1990, p. 68). The establishment of old people's homes, he noted, was the "most characteristic Negro charity" (DuBois, 1909, p. 65) in the postbellum period.

Such facilities, however, often encountered serious financial difficulties. White-operated institutions that accepted blacks presented blacks with the choice of accepting somewhat better endowed facilities that offered paternalistic, cold, and businesslike treatment and rejected black nurses and interns, or continuing to run their own, financially riskier, facilities. In most places, they continued to found their own homes. Although small, perhaps with sixteen beds, these homes for aged men and women were rooted in a community of women who had a vested interest in the fundraising and other activities that were necessary to keep them operating (Salem, 1990). The Cleveland Home for Aged Colored People, which opened in 1897, adopted as its motto: "Let us not be weary in well-doing" (Salem, 1990, p. 69). By the time of the great migration north of southern blacks, the home had moved to a new location and paid off its mortgage.

Homes founded for black elders, like those founded by other reformers, were quite concerned about the "worthiness" of their residents. Although no one expected these older people to work for their keep, their work history and record of thrift served as indicators of their worthiness. Membership in a benevolent or mutual aid society often served to demonstrate such "worthiness," such memberships may also have indicated that the person had some resources to contribute to their upkeep (Carlton-LaNey, 1988).

Other Organizing Efforts

In addition to homes founded and maintained by African Americans, throughout this period other philanthropic organizations, many ethnic in origin, also founded homes for the aged. For example, Jewish philanthropy began to be actively concerned with the welfare of older, poor Jews (Gold and Kaufman, 1970). Under varied auspices, private efforts — modest ones, by today's standards — supplemented public welfare. As the number of almshouses grew and public charity became more punitive, ethnic and racial minorities began systematic efforts to assist their own (Kutzik, 1979). Nursing staff were added to many facilities, and homes for the aged began their slow and fitful evolution into the now familiar nursing home or personal care homes with infirmaries (Dunlop, 1979). By the early twentieth century, there were over 1000 private homes for aged people in the United States (Pegels, 1988), many under the auspices of particular groups who sought to limit admission to older people who shared their faith or other background factors.

Mutual aid societies greatly expanded their membership and the diversity of their sponsorship. Like colonial poor relief, by helping families through rough times, they also facilitated family support of older members. Although immigrants from Scotland formed the first mutual aid societies, by the middle of the nineteenth century, Jews and blacks dominated the field. In Philadelphia, for example, deteriorating race relations, economic depression, and the resulting inaccessibility of "white" public assistance and organized charity "strengthened already strong motivations for blacks to care for themselves" (Kutzik, 1979, p. 41). In the South, a number of benevolent societies were founded. In Atlanta, one benevolent society's motto stated, "We assist the needy; we relieve our sick; we bury our dead" (*Atlanta Constitution*, 1871, quoted in Rabinowitz, 1974, p. 338). Among African Americans, this pattern of mutual aid and reliance on the community for the provision and subsidization of social services survived vigorously until the ravages of the Great Depression threatened their already fragile economic status and diminished their ability to assist families (McRoy, 1990).

Postacute and Chronic Illness Care

In the 1920s, several foundations, prominent physicians, and public health officials sought to examine more systematically the alternatives to acute-care hospitals and almshouses for the care of the chronically ill. Despite their resistance to admitting the chronically ill, acute-care hospitals still cared for a growing number on their wards. Although these experts considered home-based care, their preference was for specialized chronic-care hospitals (see Benjamin, 1993, for the first detailed look at the history of home care). In part, this decision reflected their reluctance to entrust care to the less well educated and the urban poor, although they also recognized that caregiving at home was difficult for both the patient and the family. During the 1930s and 1940s interest in home care continued, although no efforts were made to influence its direction.

Increased interest in care for the chronically ill also included discussions about financing such care. The first Blue Cross plans appeared during the Depression, in response to declining hospital revenues; but they did not respond to this new interest with any additional coverage, nor did the commercial insurance plans that followed them (Fox, 1989). As the Depression deepened, financing acute-care services in hospitals and assuring some measure of financial security in old age dominated reform agendas. Recounting the events that led to the passage of the Social Security Act is beyond the scope of this chapter, but two factors are specifically relevant. First, health security never achieved the wide public support won by economic security. Facing strong opposition from the American Medical Association and lacking pressure from a strong public constituency, Roosevelt dropped health security from the Social Security legislation, amidst rumblings that keeping a health program in the bill would scuttle the entire plan (Starr, 1984). Second, Social Security's contributory retirement and survivors' benefits did not prevent many older Americans from still needing help from the welfare system (Vladeck, 1980).

From 1935 to the Present

As a troubled icon, the almshouse became an important symbol in the struggle for old-age pensions (Haber and Gratton, 1993). If older people had a dependable source of income, so the reasoning went, they would no longer need the almshouse as a place of last resort. But as it turned out, the Social Security Act vanquished neither poverty nor the need for chronic-care services. In part to fill the two gaps in the programs and policies of the 1930s — the lack of health insurance benefits and the persistence of poverty despite contributory retirement and survivor's insurance — the modern nursing home industry evolved (Vladeck, 1980). Further, the need to free hospital beds, which chronically ill people continued to occupy, stimulated federal activism.

From the 1930s to the 1960s, six critical factors shaped the emergence of modern long-term care. First, direct Old Age Assistance welfare payments to poor old people or Old Age Insurance for its recipients allowed a portion of the elderly population to purchase some services. Second, federal payments made directly to facilities for older residents, which began in 1950, eased individual states' financial burdens and assured reliable sources of income for patient care (Dunlop, 1979). Third, the federal authorization of construction loans to private, nonprofit facilities through the Hill-Burton program (1954) and direct loan payments and loan guarantees to the proprietaries through the Small Business Administration

(SBA) in 1956 and the Federal Housing Authority (FHA) in 1959 led to new construction and the greater availability of more conventional construction loans. Indirectly, the FHA and SBA loan programs reinforced the businesslike attributes of nursing homes. While facilities received federal dollars, neither the SBA nor the FHA required that they be linked with other health care services. Fourth, the Kerr-Mills program extended federal financial participation for older people who were medically indigent. Fifth, the American Association of Nursing Homes emerged as a strong lobbying voice with vested interests in the new industry. And, sixth, in response to concerns by welfare advocates, the federal government began, in a very limited way, to develop federal standards for nursing homes. During this period, public homes languished, voluntary homes stabilized but did not expand greatly, and commercial homes proliferated (W. Taylor, 1969).

In 1940, 41 percent of institutionalized elders resided in a variety of nonmedical group quarters — boarding homes and board-and-care facilities, for example; in 1970 the percent had declined to 12 percent. In contrast, nursing home occupancy increased from 34 to 72 percent of all institutionalized persons in that same period. This accelerated development of nursing homes preceded the existence of Medicare and Medicaid, although those two programs, especially Medicaid, assured that nursing home growth would continue unimpeded.

The Social Security Act

The Social Security Act of 1935, arguably the most important U.S. social legislation of this century, did not contain provisions for health care. Nonetheless, the provision that no Old Age Assistance (OAA) funds, which were delivered in the form of matching grants to states, be extended to any person living in a public institution directly stimulated the already burgeoning commercial nursing home industry. The OAA program, set forth in Title I of the act, authorized federal matching grants for needy older people. This federal and state cash assistance permitted many elders, who were indigent but not infirm, to continue to live independently. Such payments also allowed individuals to purchase care in private domiciliary facilities.

The decision to deny OAA to residents of public institutions, and the unintended consequences of this policy, offers a particularly revealing example of how nursing home policy evolved through indirection and incomplete efforts to solve one problem — indigence — without addressing another problem — chronic illness. Pension advocates both within and outside government despised the almshouse. They reasoned that an assured income would enable individual older people to remain at home; the return of noninstitutional relief would thereby hasten the demise of the almshouse (Schell, 1993). Although financing care for chronic illness was a growing burden, one not willingly assumed by the Blue Cross plans or commercial carriers (see Fox, 1989 for a discussion of the struggles over the financing of chronic illness during this period), no governmental action was taken to address it specifically. As a result, Title I, by denying OAA payments to older people who lived in public facilities, inadvertently fostered the transfer of chronically ill older people who had no other means of care to proprietary and voluntary nursing homes.

Formal recognition of this problem occurred as early as 1938. The first issue of the *Social Security Bulletin* reported that "the advent of Social Security had little impact on the elderly residing in almshouses": pensions, as it turned out, were not a substitute for indoor relief (Vladeck, 1980, p. 37). Some of the elderly ill stayed in almshouses, and others went to local sanitariums (Haber, 1993), but most went to commercial nursing homes. Such homes, resembling board-and-care and other domiciliary facilities rather than current nursing homes, capitalized on need and people's ability to pay with OAA funds for at least some of the services they offered (Schell, 1993). Although state-supported mental institutions absorbed some of the almshouse residents who were reclassified as psychotic, commercial nursing homes, supported in part by public funds but without strong federal intervention or regulation, increasingly cared for mentally and physically frail older people (Haber, 1993). Thus, federal Social Security policy unwittingly encouraged the growth of a formal nursing home industry.

The Growth of the Proprietary Sector

After the passage of the Social Security Act, the number of private nursing homes grew rapidly (Haber and Gratton, 1993), while public facilities remained, as they have to this day, the "care setting of last resort . . . [serving] the poorest but also some of the sickest nursing home patients" (Dunlop, 1979, p. 100).

The first proprietary nursing homes, the prototypical "mom and pop" operation, seem to have begun when women, caring for their own ill or incapacitated husbands, took in other patients for a fee to help pay the bills (Vladeck, 1980). In the Depression's waning years, when money was scarce but large private homes were not, conditions permitted the proliferation of such small custodial facilities. Because local welfare officials desperately needed beds for impaired clients, they were forced to be rather lax in selecting facilities, a problem that persists for patients dependent upon Medicaid. Further, the level of cash assistance available through OAA determined where the person could be placed; choices were often restricted to the less desirable homes (Markus, 1972). Also, until the late 1940s and early 1950s, the distinction between facilities that provided only domiciliary care and those that offered nursing services was vague and variable (U.S. Senate, 1935). What became the modern nursing home industry thus started inconspicuously; it was difficult to distinguish from board-and-care facilities, and, as it turned out, frequently as class-based as the earlier poorhouse.

In the 1930s the number of older people in institutions declined by 10 percent, primarily because the almshouses emptied; by the 1940s, with the population of older people growing, the number in nursing homes and homes for the aged had risen by 38 percent (U.S. Senate, 1935). During the same period, welfare officials expressed deepening concern about the quality of care these homes were offering; they pointed to low federal payments as one cause of such inadequate care. Yet, while advocating for increased federal matching funds, they wanted assurance that improved standards of enforcement would accompany higher payments (Markus, 1972). In 1948, the Advisory Council on Social Security argued for a minimal standard of care and protection from fire hazards, unsanitary conditions, and overcrowding (Markus, 1972). To increase bed availability, it also requested that the ban on public assistance for patients in public nursing homes be lifted; that occurred in the 1950 amendments to the Social Security Act.

Post World War II to 1965

By the early 1950s, it was becoming quite clear that caring for the chronically ill was a serious national problem. Chronic disease hospitals added rehabilitation facilities and acute-care hospitals added beds to make lower-cost care available to the chronically ill (Hawes and Phillips, 1986). Although the developing private insurance industry gradually extended coverage for some chronic illnesses, it was reluctant to assume major responsibility for financing such care. Even then, insurance company leaders argued that the costs of care for the chronically ill should be spread widely, that is, supported by general taxation and only not by enrollees in insurance plans (Fox, 1989).

Until the 1950s, then, the federal government supported the costs of chronic illness (except for veterans) only through direct cash assistance to elderly recipients. In 1950, Congress authorized matching funds to states, through direct vendor payments, for services rendered to the aged poor and to the permanently and totally disabled in nursing homes. This vendor payment system and the funds it made available for nursing home care made the nursing home business attractive to entrepreneurs. Initiation of this payment system also gave the newly organized nursing home lobby a specific federal agency with whom to negotiate rates and regulations. "The vendor payment program thus shaped a system in which the cost, quality, and level of services are decided in a transaction between vendors (providers) and the state, creating the politics of long-term care" (Hawes and Phillips, 1986, p. 495).

In 1953–54, the U.S. Public Health Service and the Commission on Chronic Illness surveyed the long-term care facility situation in ten states and found it seriously inadequate (Markus, 1972). In response, a 1954 amendment to the Hill-Burton program — the Medical Facilities Survey and Construction Act — provided construction grants to nonprofit nursing homes and other nonproprietary long-term care facilities. This amendment also set in motion the further medicalization of such facilities by redefining "skilled nursing" and requiring that any facilities constructed with Hill-Burton funds be affiliated with a hospital. The Public Health Service, which administered Hill-Burton, also "formulated the first standards on physical plant design and construction, as well as staffing in nursing homes, further transforming these institutions into more medically oriented settings" (Hawes and Phillips, 1986, p. 495). Thus, Hill-Burton not only influenced bed supply but also shaped licensure standards, notions of bed need, and health planning (Dunlop, 1979). In the end, however, many of the long-term care beds added to general hospitals by means of Hill-Burton funds "appear to have been used for patients requiring acute care" (Fox, 1989, p. 274).

Because Hill-Burton excluded proprietary facilities, Congress responded to vigorous lobbying from the American Association of Nursing Homes by authorizing two additional loan programs. In 1956, they authorized the Small Business Administration to make direct or participatory loans to proprietary nursing homes. In 1959, the Federal Housing Administration offered loan guarantees for up to 90 percent of construction costs to developers of nursing homes. Such loans helped open the way for such institutions to receive more conventional mortgages and fostered the development of an industry relatively isolated from other medical care institutions: unlike Hill-Burton, which required nursing homes to operate in conjunction with hospitals, neither the SBA nor the FHA imposed any such requirements. Nursing homes constructed with SBA or FHA loans operated as freestanding business operations. Their numbers expanded rapidly (Vladeck, 1980).

In the late 1950s, as a result of Hill-Burton requirements, not-for-profit nursing homes began their gradual transition from "homes for the aged" to more hospital-like medical care facilities. This transition made it easier for physicians to trust them as sources of care for their patients. The comparable medicalization of commercial homes took another decade. But SBA and FHA loans made nursing homes an increasingly attractive business venture. Even before the passage of Medicare and Medicaid, new entrepreneurs appeared.

The only alternative to nursing home care considered during this period was formally organized home care, but efforts made on its behalf remained meager. At this time, home care lacked a constituency, as well as a clear notion of how benefits should be covered or what they should be (Benjamin, 1993). The only consensus appeared to be the link with hospitalization, that home care should be viewed as a substitute for hospitalization for the severely incapacitated patient. In this way, it conformed to the thinking that later structured the Medicare long-term care benefit program. Although its advantages to the patient and family could not be denied, the real motivation was to reduce the costs of hospital care (Benjamin, 1993).

Federal assistance for home care, first made available indirectly through OAA after 1935, was increased after the passage of the Kerr-Mills Act in 1960. Intended to expand vendor payments under OAA to meet the needs of older people who were not categorically eligible for OAA assistance, Kerr-Mills fell far short of its goals. It was not a mandated program, and few states chose to participate. It did, however, facilitate home care by covering a wide range of services and by making federal payments contingent upon state coverage of noninstitutional as well as institutional services (Benjamin, 1993).

The U.S. General Accounting Office estimated that during the 1960s, despite the three construction loan programs, the shortage of long-term care beds would be between 250,000 and 500,000 (Hawes and Phillips, 1986). While Medicare and Medicaid incubated, the problem of beds for chronic illness loomed large, particularly as the costs of hospital care increased substantially. The response by Medicare would be limited; it would address only the problem of postacute convalescent care. Nursing homes, therefore, received little attention except as a means to reduce the costs of hospitalization and to limit the liability of public and private insurers (Fox, 1989). Medicare would pay for the last stage of convalescence from a protracted illness in an "extended care facility" (Vladeck, 1980).

The Era of Medicare and Medicaid

In the years immediately preceding the adoption of Medicare and Medicaid in 1965, Congress turned again to the issue of quality of care (Markus, 1972). Yet, even after the implementation of Medicare, program officials did little to uphold the standards they had written into the extended-care statutory requirements. Regulators overlooked noncompliance for three primary reasons: the vague belief that some nursing homes would "do better," the fear of escalating costs if higher standards were strictly enforced, and the perceived need for beds. Instead, they licensed facilities as long as they were in "substantial compliance," a new category that implied facilities were "somewhat close" to meeting the requirements and expressed the intention to improve (Vladeck, 1980). Nonetheless, nursing homes that did not meet these higher requirements rarely lost their certification.

Since Medicare nursing home costs soon far exceeded the original actuarial assumptions, in 1969 the Bureau of Health Insurance tightened eligibility criteria for extended care. In addition to requiring that the patient have the potential for rehabilitation, which effectively eliminated payments for terminal illness, Intermediary Letter 371 instructed Medicare's fiscal intermediaries to "err on the side of denying rather than approving benefits" (cited in Vladeck, 1980, p. 57). It reaffirmed the intention that Medicare not support custodial care; it was to be only a medical benefit. Extended care did not mean care for an extended period but rather an extension of inpatient care (Vladeck, 1980). Not surprisingly, the American Association of Nursing Homes opposed this instruction; in this case their interests overlapped those of patients. Retroactive denials often took months and left families with huge bills, often long after the patient had died; some patients were evicted from nursing homes; and many homes simply dropped out of the Medicare program.

Despite these limits, Medicare had the effect of accelerating the growth of proprietary nursing homes. By limiting the time between hospitalization and nursing home placement to fourteen days (in 1972, this requirement was eased under special circumstances), this regulation again inadvertently supported the larger, for-profit facilities, which tended to have shorter waiting lists than the voluntary homes (Dunlop, 1977).

Medicaid, which provided medical coverage to all people who received cash welfare benefits or met the established criteria for medical indigence, became the most important source of federal support for care in skilled nursing homes (later Medicaid was also used to support care in intermediate care facilities [ICFs]). Again, it appears that little forethought went

into the program design. Vendor payments continued with little definition, without a budget ceiling, and without strict enforcement of standards (Hawes and Phillips, 1986; Stevens and Stevens, 1974; Vladeck,
1980). While fearing the potential costs associated with strict enforcement
of standards, Medicaid planners ignored what would become a major
contribution to high costs: there was no cap on federal matching payments to states (Vladeck, 1980). Costs continued to escalate for care that
was often marginal at best. Even when Congress added the ICF program,
as a means to meet the needs of those who did not require skilled nursing
care and to reduce costs, states and facility owners were able to work
around the regulatory requirements. Patients were reclassified as needing
skilled nursing care. Homes that could not meet the standards for a skilled
nursing facility (SNF) were admitted as ICFs, and states included public
facilities and mental institutions under the ICF program (Markus, 1972).

The number of older people occupying nursing home beds continued to
climb. This increase occurred not only because more older people sought
services but also because states began to transfer patients from state-
supported institutions, such as mental hospitals, to nursing homes in
order to take advantage of the federal funding stream (Caplow, 1975;
Dunlop, 1979; Hawes and Phillips, 1986; Vladeck, 1980). While the number of older people in nursing homes rose 58 percent between 1950 and
1960, during the next decade it climbed 107 percent.

Notwithstanding many efforts to enforce standards during the past
twenty years, the quality of care in nursing homes has remained a center of
contention, and nursing homes have not changed substantially. Earlier, in
the years immediately following the enactment of Medicare and Medicaid, nursing homes rarely achieved the visibility to become a center of
contention and to inspire systematic reform. Such activism finally came in
the 1970s, but even then reform operated within the pre-existing structural constraints.

Neither Medicare nor Medicaid responded adequately to the growing
burden of chronic illness care. For their architects, such as Wilbur Cohen,
the custodial type of care that many older people required belonged to the
welfare and not the medical care system. Yet, the welfare system offered
little to older people for whom the line between "custodial" needs and
medically related needs was often indistinct and shifting. With limited
public benefits, few had sufficient resources to purchase services. Their
only recourse was the Medicaid program; that generally meant nursing
home placement. That many had to take such a path in order to obtain
financial assistance helps to explain the overuse of skilled nursing facili-

ties. This overuse has been costly in psychological as well as financial terms for people who do not require that level of care.

The federal law's unintended bias toward private, for-profit facilities had particularly important repercussions for African Americans. Patterns of segregation led blacks into overcrowded county facilities, state-run mental institutions, and unregulated personal care homes. Even Medicare and Medicaid did not substantially alter the historic patterns of segregation. Neither pressure from President Lyndon Johnson's administration nor the actions of regulators pushed nursing homes to integrate (D. S. Smith, 1979). In a much-quoted study published in 1981, the Institute of Medicine reported that ethnic or racial factors continued to influence health care "in ways that are not in the interests of the groups affected. . . . a pattern of discrimination *seems* to be the cause" (Institute of Medicine, 1981, p. 28). Although admitting that the evidence was scanty, the Institute of Medicine concluded that user rates varied primarily because of differential access and not because of ethnic social preferences. Recent scholarship (Headen, 1992; R. J. Taylor, 1988, among others) calls into question the easy assumption that African American families do not use institutions *solely* because family support norms are so powerful.

In sum, roughly from 1935 to 1975, the development of nursing homes occurred almost by chance. When pension reform did not alleviate the need for almshouselike facilities, legislators, welfare professionals, and advocates had few options — or so it seemed — besides support for private nursing homes. Because demand was exceeding bed supply and almshouses (or public facilities) had been roundly rejected as appropriate caregiving venues, the state, inadvertently and with little forethought of consequences, increased its financial participation for patients in private nursing homes. Federal funds, offered with few strings, transformed the nascent home for the aged into a burgeoning business enterprise. Rather than demand for nursing home care being reduced, as reformers had anticipated, it increased almost immediately. Demographic shifts, changing patterns of morbidity and mortality, and the transfer of patients from other institutions to nursing homes fueled such demand. The federal response in the form of increased funds to pay for such care, favorable reimbursement rates, and lax enforcement of standards all encouraged the growth of an ill-controlled nursing home industry (Hawes and Phillips, 1986).

For the past twenty years, nursing homes have been the subject of sustained debate and study. It took scandals, increased advocacy for and by the elderly, escalating costs, and more vigorous interest in chronic illness and frailty to achieve this focused attention. Regulatory reform was the first task undertaken, but regulations that address one or more problems may also create new ones. For example, as fire and safety standards improved, many smaller nursing homes could not afford the added costs, so they left the field and larger homes came to dominate the industry. Whether this outcome is good for the residents' quality of life is at best debatable.

In the past decade, nursing homes have come under continued scrutiny. The public response has included tougher enforcement of standards, new regulatory measures, in particular those emerging from the Omnibus Budget Reconciliation Act of 1987, and new forms of advocacy, such as the Ombudsman program. The reformist agenda has also led to more refined definitions of quality and further efforts at enforcement, to new measures aimed at guaranteeing patient's rights, and to an emphasis on patient autonomy. Yet, as with the earlier fire and safety codes, these responses have had more than one effect. While intended to protect vulnerable people from the dangers of unscrupulous care, they also can directly and indirectly limit personal choices. Relative protection has generally trumped relative freedom; older residents, living their lives according to a care plan, have few opportunities to exercise choices that are meaningful in the context of their own lives and their frameworks of meaning (see Agich, 1993; Diamond, 1992; Lidz, Fischer, and Arnold, 1992). Once again, if history teaches us anything it is that unintended consequences deserve close attention.

Summary

Long-term care, as we understand it today, developed almost haphazardly. Despite the growing interest in chronic illness since the 1920s and the recognition that such illnesses often require ongoing medical and social care, no coherent planning or overall policy review has been devoted to long-term care. It is not entirely clear why so little happened. The struggle for old-age pensions may contain one explanation. For pension advocates, the almshouse symbolized the inevitable and dreaded alternative to pensions (Haber and Gratton, 1993). The almshouse's other function, as a "home for the aged," as Homer Folks had observed three decades earlier, was ignored. Thus, the advocates' efforts to empty the almshouses and to "solve" the problem of income security by providing direct financial assistance inadvertently left the field of long-term care open to entrepreneurial interests.

Choices made in the past inevitably structure and limit later policy options (Vladeck, 1980). Vested interests develop, which reduces the space within which reform can take place. Remedies are targeted at specific problems while the conditions that give rise to those problems remain untouched. Case management, for example, emerged as an acceptable response to a fragmented system of care (Maddox, 1992). Earlier choices become starting points for debates about their replacements. "Policy debates are regularly informed by ideas about how best to correct the perceived imperfections of past policy, rather than simply how best to respond to social conditions as such" (Orloff, 1988, p. 42). Modern nursing home reform is predicated on historically conditioned structural arrangements and normative values that reformers may not share but within whose borders they must negotiate.

Our final comments concern the often subtle relationship between ideology and policy development in America's past. The residues of this interaction are, in part, why reform of long-term care is so central to the current agenda on aging and why long-term care is so intractable to change. As we have illustrated, ideological presuppositions about poverty, worthiness, gender, and old age led to the development of specific approaches to indigence and indirectly to chronic impairment. For example, the role of women in the nineteenth century largely excluded them from the public sphere, leaving them available for caregiving. Those earlier assumptions regarding gender still provide the tacit substructure for long-term care policy (Walker, 1983). In addition, the burden of caregiving affects families differentially, since low-income individuals cannot purchase assistance (Walker, 1983). These dimensions of care have only recently entered the public conversation. What families — mostly women — provided was simply assumed, and therefore largely unexamined; state responsibility was residual, directed at the very poor and isolated.

Reformers in the 1920s and 1930s believed that solving the problems of indigence would allow older people to buy the care they needed. For many people this actually happened. Old Age Assistance, however meager the benefit levels, did help to replace the domiciliary role that almshouses had played. It could not, however, adequately respond to medical and social needs that families could not meet. As a result, many older people turned to existing "rest homes." There they could receive some care and use their OAA money as payment. In the period immediately following the passage of the Social Security Act, however, the need for beds outpaced the supply. As a result, these largely unregulated homes proliferated without a clear link to other health or social services. During the 1950s, as federal financial participation increased, the distinction between public and private blurred; federal dollars supported private construction and private services with minimal interference. Regulations, even when they existed, were rarely enforced and, when they were, they unintentionally drove the smaller "mom and pop" homes out of business. Homes grew larger, more bureaucratized, more medicalized, and soon more corporatized. Bad conditions led to even more regulation, and regulation inspired further bureaucracy.

In this manner, a particularly American solution to long-term care needs emerged. It rested on the traditional distrust of a large and activist government, interest group politics, and the continued need for care otherwise unavailable. By the 1970s, institutionally based structures would become the standard around which alternatives would be created. These alternatives were assessed principally in terms of their cost-saving potential. Only recently have many questioned if large, proprietary, and bureaucratically organized nursing homes best respond to the needs of the chronically ill aged; but for all the reasons noted above, that system is particularly resistant to change. Modern long-term care, to this day, uneasily and incompletely responds to the needs of chronically ill elders and their families.

References

Abel, E. (1991). *Who Cares for the Elderly? Public Policy and the Experiences of Daughters.* Philadelphia: Temple University Press.

Achenbaum, A. (1978). *Old Age in the New Land.* Baltimore: Johns Hopkins University Press.

Agich, G. (1993). *Autonomy and Long-Term Care.* New York: Oxford University Press.

Atlanta Constitution (1871). Quoted in H. N. Rabinowitz (1974). From exclusion to segregation: Health and welfare services for southern blacks. *Social Services Review* 48:327–54.

Benjamin, A. E. (1993). An historical perspective on home care policy. *Milbank Quarterly* 71:129–66.

Berkeley, K. (1990). Colored ladies also contributed: Black women's activities from benevolence to social welfare, 1866–1896. Reprinted in D. Hine, ed. *Black Women in U.S. History* (vol. 1, pp. 61–84). Brooklyn: Carlson.

Berlin, I., Miller, S., and Rowland, L. (1988). Afro-American families in transition from slavery to freedom. *Radical History Review* 42:89–121.

Billingsley, A. (1992). *Climbing Jacob's Ladder: The Enduring Legacy of African-American Families.* New York: Simon and Schuster.

Burnham, D. (1990). The life of the Afro-American woman in slavery. In D. Hine, ed. *Black Women in U.S. History.* Brooklyn: Carlson.

Butners, A. (1980). *Institutionalized Altruism and the Aged: Charitable Provision for the Aged in New York City, 1865–1930,* Ph.D. dissertation, Columbia University.

Caplow, T. (1975). Foreword. In Manard, B., Kart, C., and van Gils, D., eds. *Old-age Institutions.* Lexington, Mass.: D. C. Heath.

Carlton-LaNey, I. (1988). Old folks' homes for blacks during the Progressive period. *Journal of Sociology and Social Work* 15:43–60.

Clark, M. (1900). The Almshouse. *Proceedings of the National Conference of Charities and Corrections.* National Conference of Charities and Corrections.

Cole, T. (1975). *An Essay on Aging in Modern America.* Master's thesis, Wesleyan University.

Cole, T. (1987). Class, culture, and coercion: A historical perspective on longterm care. *Generations* 11 (4): 9–15.

Cole, T. (1992). *The Journey of Life.* New York: Cambridge University Press.

Diamond, T. (1992). *Making Gray Gold.* Chicago: University of Chicago Press.

Dieckmann, J. (1993). From almshouse to city nursing home. *Nursing History Review* 1:217–28

DuBois, W. E. B. (1909). *The Social Betterment among Negro Americans.* Atlanta: Atlanta University Press.

Dunlop, B. D. (1979). *The Growth of Nursing Home Care.* Lexington, Mass.: Lexington Books.

Estes, C., Gerard, L., Zones, J., and Swan, J. (1984). *Political Economy, Health, and Aging.* Boston: Little, Brown.

Firor-Scott, A. (1990). Most invisible of all: Black women's voluntary associations. *Journal of Southern History* 56:3–22.

Fox, D. (1989). Policy and epidemiology: Financing health services for the chronically ill and disabled, 1930–1990. *Milbank Quarterly* 67 (suppl. 2, pt. 2): 257–87.

Genovese, E. (1974). *Roll Jordan Roll.* New York: Random House.

Gold, J., and Kaufman, S. (1970). Development of care of the elderly: Tracing the history of institutional facilities. *Gerontologist* 10:262–74.

Haber, C. (1983). *Beyond Sixty-five.* New York: Cambridge University Press.

Haber, C. (1993). Over the hill to the poorhouse: Rhetoric and reality in the institutional history of the aged. In K. W. Schaie and W. A. Achenbaum, eds. *Societal Impact on Aging: Historical Perspectives* (pp. 90–113). New York: Springer.

Haber, C., and Gratton, B. (1993). *Old Age and the Search for Security: An American Social History.* Bloomington: Indiana University Press.

Hawes, C., and Phillips, C. (1986). The changing structure of the nursing home industry and the impact of ownership on quality, cost, and access. In B. Gray, ed. *For-Profit Enterprise in Health Care.* Washington, D.C.: National Academy Press.

Headen, A. E. (1992). Time costs and informal social supports as determinants of differences between black and white families in the provision of long-term care. *Inquiry* 29:440–50.

Hine, D. (1989). *The State of African-American History: Past, Present*. Baton Rouge: Louisiana State University Press.

Institute of Medicine (1981). *Health Care in the Context of Civil Rights*. Washington, D.C.: National Academy Press.

Katz, M. (1984). Poorhouses and the origins of public old age homes. *Milbank Memorial Fund Quarterly/Health and Society* 62 (1): 110–40.

Katz, M. (1986). *In the Shadow of the Poorhouse*. New York: Basic Books.

Kutzik, A. (1979). American social provision for the aged: An historical perspective. In D. Gelfand and A. Kutzik, eds. *Ethnicity and Aging: Theory, Research, and Policy*. New York: Springer Publishing.

Lidz, C., Fischer, L., and Arnold, R. (1992). *The Erosion of Autonomy in Long-term Care*. New York: Oxford University Press.

Maddox, G. L. (1992). Long-term care policies in comparative perspective. *Aging and Society* 12:355–68.

Markus, R. (1972). *The Nursing Home and the Congress*. Washington, D.C.: Congressional Research Service.

Martin, E., and Martin, J. (1986). *The Black Extended Family*. Chicago: University of Chicago Press.

McRoy, R. G. (1990). A historical overview of black families. In S. Logan, E. Freeman, and R. McRoy, eds. *Social Work Practice with Black Families*. New York: Longman.

Nashville Daily Press and Times (1867). Quoted in H. N. Rabinowitz (1974). From exclusion to segregation: Health and welfare services for southern blacks. *Social Services Review* 48:327–54.

Orloff, A. (1988). The political origins of America's belated welfare state. In M. Weir, A. S. Orloff, and T. Skocpol, eds. *The Politics of Social Policy in the United States* (pp. 37–80). Princeton: Princeton University Press.

Pegels, C. (1988). *Health Care and the Older Citizen: Economic, Demographic, and Financial Aspects*. Rockville, Md.: Aspen.

Pollard, W. (1978). *A Study in Black Self-help*. San Francisco: R and E Assoc.

Quadagno, J. (1986). The transformation of old age security. In D. Van Tassel and P. Stearns, eds. *Old Age in a Bureaucratic Society* (pp. 129–55). New York: Greenwood.

Retsinas, J. (1994). Can Vladeck's HCFA deliver loving care? *Aging Today* (Jan.–Feb.): 1–2.

Rosenberg, C. (1987). *The Care of Strangers: The Rise of America's Hospital System*. New York: Basic Books.

Rosner, D. (1982). Health care for the truly needy. *Milbank Memorial Fund Quarterly/Health and Society* 60:355–85.

Rothman, D. (1971). *The Discovery of the Asylum*. Boston: Little, Brown.

Rothman, D. (1980). *Conscience and Convenience: The Asylum and Its Alternatives in Progressive America*. Boston: Little, Brown.

Salem, D. (1990). *To Better Our World: Black Women in Organized Reform, 1890–1920*. Brooklyn: Carlson.

Schell, E. (1993). The origins of geriatric nursing: The chronically ill elderly in almshouses and nursing homes, 1900–1950, *Nursing History Review* 1:203–16.

Seward, R. (1978). *The American Family: A Demographic History*. Beverly Hills: Sage.

Smith, D. S. (1979). Life course, norms, and the family system of older Americans in 1900. *Journal of Family History* 4:285–98.

Smith, M. R. (1895). Almshouse women: A study of two hundred and twenty-eight women in the city and county almshouse of San Francisco. *American Statistical Association* 8:258. Cited in Butners, 1980.

Staples, W. (1991). *Castles of Our Conscience: Social Control and the American State, 1800–1985*. New Brunswick, N.J.: Rutgers University Press.

Starr, P. (1984). *The Social Transformation of American Medicine*. New York: Basic Books.

Stevens, Robert, and Stevens, Rosemary (1974). *Welfare Medicine in America: A Case Study*. New York: Free Press.

Taylor, R. J. (1988). Aging and supportive relationships among black Americans. In J. Jackson, ed. *The Black American Elderly: Research on Physical and Psychosocial Health*. New York: Springer.

Taylor, W. (1969). *Nursing Homes and Public Policy: Drift and Decision in New York State*. Ithaca: Cornell University Press.

U.S. Senate (1935). Committee on Labor and Public Welfare. *The Aged and Aging in the United States: A National Problem: Summary and Recommendations*. Washington, D.C.: 86th Congress, 2nd session.

Vladeck, B. (1980). *Unloving Care*. New York: Basic Books.

Walker, A. (1983). Care for elderly people: A conflict between women and the state. In J. Finch and D. Groves, eds. *A Labor of Love: Women, Work, and Caring* (pp. 106–28). London: Routledge and Kegan Paul.

Warner, A. (1908). *American Charities*. (Rev. by Mary Roberts Coolidge). New York: Thomas Crowell. Cited in Butners, 1980.

Wood, G. (1992). *The Radicalism of the American Revolution*. New York: Alfred Knopf.

II

POPULATIONS NEEDING CARE AND ISSUES OF PROVIDING CARE

3

Older People, Dependency, and Trends in Supportive Care

T. Franklin Williams, M.D., and
Helena Temkin-Greener, Ph.D.

This chapter focuses on projected changes in dependency among older persons and on expected future needs for supportive care. After summarizing the major demographic projections, we turn to examining the availability of and the problems with current services. This is followed by a discussion of the possible ways to meet future care needs, emphasizing the importance of system building and integration of care delivery. Innovative approaches already underway are discussed.

Tomorrow's Older Population

Demographic Trends

The trends in dependency and needs for supportive care among older persons must be considered against the background of the overall demographic trends in the older population. In the United States, the 1990 census documented 31.1 million persons ages 65 and older, accounting for 12.6 percent of the total population. The Bureau of the Census projects approximately 52 million persons over the age of 65 by the year 2020, which will be approximately 20 percent of the total population. However, projections from other sources vary considerably. For example, the demographer Kenneth Manton (1991), based on his estimates of further reductions in mortality through control of the major risk factors, projected over 84 million persons ages 65 and older by the year 2020.

Of more immediate interest in relation to the incidence and prevalence of dependency, and needs for support, are data on very old persons, defined in different analyses as those 80 years and older or 85 years and older. As of 1990, approximately 7 million persons in the United States were aged 80 or over; by the year 2025, Census Bureau projections indicate that this will increase to more than 14 million persons. This absolute increase of more than 100 percent is impressive, but, due to the aging of the baby boom population in these next 35 years, the actual proportion of those over 65 who are age 80 or over will change very little, from 22.4 percent now to 23 percent in the year 2025. The impact of baby boomers becoming very old (i.e., ages 80 and above) will not be felt until after 2025 and before 2050. Projections based on further potential reductions in morbidity and in risk factors that contribute to earlier mortality indicate substantial increases in the numbers of those surviving to age 80 and beyond.

An important consideration in these general data on older population changes, as well as in comments that follow about dependency and needs for services, is the extensive variation and diversity in the older population. Geographic, ethnic, and cultural differences have major impacts on the characteristics of dependency and care needs and on the suitability of services. In the United States, of those presently aged 80 or older, 87 percent are Caucasian, 8 percent African American, 4 percent Hispanic, and 1 percent Asian. Approximately 1 million of U.S. residents aged 65 or older do not speak English. By the year 2050, major changes in ethnic distribution will have occurred, with the Hispanic population increasing to 16 percent of all Americans, African-Americans to 10 percent, Asian Americans to 8 percent, and the proportion of Caucasians aged 80+ decreasing to 67 percent (U.S. Bureau of the Census and National Institute on Aging, 1993, chap. 2). Currently, with each year above the age of 65, an increasingly larger proportion of the population is female, such that among those aged 85 or older the female to male ratio exceeds 3:1.

In 1990, 30.5 percent of persons in the United States ages 65 and older were living alone (U.S. Bureau of the Census, 1993, chap. 6). In all countries the preponderance of those living alone are women, and poverty rates are higher among this subpopulation than any other.

Another important characteristic of the profile of the elderly population is the availability of adult family members to provide support for their older relatives. In 1990, approximately two-thirds of all persons ages 50–60 in the United States had living parents. Another way to look at this relationship is the "parent support ratio," which has been reported in terms of the numbers of persons ages 80 and older per 100 persons ages

50-64. In 1990, this ratio was 23 for Caucasians (i.e., 23 Caucasian persons aged 80 or older per 100 Caucasians ages 50–64). Ratios for other American ethnic groups ranged from 9 to 16. By the year 2050, the large increase in the 80+ population will be reflected in much higher ratios: 58 Caucasians aged 80 or older per 100 Caucasians ages 50–64, and ratios of 27–38 for other ethnic groups (U.S. Bureau of the Census and National Institute on Aging, 1993, chap. 6). These increasing numbers of very old persons in relation to middle-aged persons are important to the consideration of family and other sources of informal support for those who need services.

Healthy or Active Life Expectancy

A major phenomenon of the past 10 to 20 years has been the increasing number of older persons who are living into late years with reasonably good health and function. A number of studies (e.g., Williams, 1992) have shown that humans are capable of maintaining most organ functions and meeting most requirements of personal and social living into very late years, including, at least for some, into the second century of life.

Such capabilities depend on healthful life styles and on being fortunate enough not to inherit or acquire one or more of the chronic disabling conditions that are indeed still common. Even in terms of these disabling conditions, however, there are certainly grounds for hope and for the expectation that, through further scientific advances and more effective therapies to control diseases and restore function, we will see even more decreases in the burdens from chronic illness. We have already seen striking decreases in mortality from stroke; we know much about how to minimize or even reverse the course of osteoporosis; we can decrease considerably the risks of coronary artery disease; there are exciting advances in our understanding of the causes and risk factors for cancers and conditions like Alzheimer disease. Although in our projection for the future we must consider conservative assumptions about the benefits of further advances, we should also, as Manton (1991) and others suggest, consider what the future for old and very old populations may be like if we do indeed make further advances in dealing with these and other chronic conditions.

The terms *healthy life expectancy* and *active life expectancy* have been developed to describe and project the number of years of life that can be anticipated to be healthy and essentially fully functional. The difference between the total life expectancy and the healthy or active life expectancy is the years during which one or more dependency needs are likely to exist.

At present in the United States, the Bureau of the Census (1993, chap. 2) calculates total life expectancy for persons at age 65 as 14.4 years for males and 18.6 years for females. Working from the National Long-Term Care Survey, Manton and Stallard (1991) calculated active life expectancy at age 65 as 11.9 years for males and 13.6 years for females. At age 85, males have a total life expectancy of 5.15 years and an active life expectancy of 2.55 years; females have a total life expectancy of 6.44 years and an active life expectancy of 2.25 years. Of note is the fact that, whereas among "young old" persons (ages 65–74) females have a measurably higher active life expectancy (as well as total life expectancy) than males, by age 85 the active life expectancy for males begins to exceed slightly that of females.

Branch and colleagues (1991), in a communitywide analysis of populations in East Boston, New Haven, and rural Iowa, examined information that included both improvements in function and loss of function over time. They found that approximately 25 percent of older persons who had acquired some disability subsequently had improvement in function. From their analyses of the Caucasian populations in these three settings,[1] Branch and colleagues estimated total life expectancy at age 65 to be 13.2–16.7 years for males, and 18.5–21.4 years for females, the higher figures reflecting the rural Iowa population.* Of these years, the range of active life expectancy for males was estimated at 11.3–12.9 years and for females at 15.4–17.1 years. Overall, the percent of remaining years of projected independence in activities of daily living (i.e., active years) was estimated as 80–85 percent at age 65 and was essentially identical for men and women in all three sites. Interestingly, while the researchers found a slow decline in the percentage of active years for later ages, there was also an apparent rise in active life expectancy in the New Haven male population beyond age 75 and in males in East Boston and Iowa beyond age 85.

Very recent studies (e.g., Perls et al., 1993) of persons living beyond age 100 suggest that for persons reaching this age there are lesser degrees of both mental and physical incapacitation (except for limitations in vision and hearing) and thus, again, a higher proportion of the few remaining years as active years. Figure 3.1 illustrates this relative improvement in very late years.

---

*There were too few non-Caucasians in these studies to permit estimates on ethnic groups other than Caucasians. An ongoing National Institute on Aging study based in the Durham area of North Carolina will be providing specific data on African Americans. A similar study is being undertaken in Texas which will provide data on Hispanic Americans.

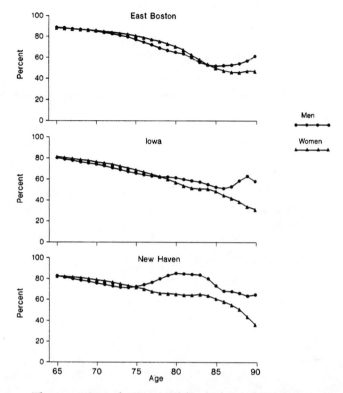

Figure 3.1. The percentage of remaining life which is independent in activities of daily living. Reprinted, by permission of the Gerontological Society of America, from Branch et al. (1991), p. M148.

Based on data from national surveys, detailed calculations and projections have been made of the extent of dependency (i.e., need for help from others or for assistive devices). In 1991 Manton and Stallard, for example, estimated that for those age 85 there would be 0.7–0.9 years of moderately impaired life expectancy. The number of years of heavily impaired life expectancy would be approximately the same for males and females still residing at home. For those in long-term care institutions, impaired life expectancy would be about 0.8 years for males and 1.7 years for females.

Kunkel and Applebaum (1992) projected the numbers of persons ages 65 and older likely to have various degrees of disability, depending upon (1) a scenario based on current rates of mortality and disability, (2) a scenario of longer life and lower disability, (3) a scenario of longer life and higher disability, and (4) a scenario of longer life and moderate disability (their best guess). Moderate disability they define as impairment in at least

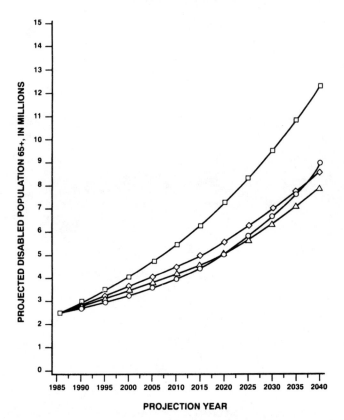

Figure 3.2. Total projected population 65 and older with severe disability (in millions), 1986 to 2040. Key to different mortality and disability assumptions: △ Constant; ○ Longer life, less disability; □ Longer life, higher disability; ◇ Moderately longer life, moderately higher disability. Figure and caption reprinted, by permission of the Gerontological Society of America, from Kunkel and Applebaum (1992), p. S258.

one but no more than two activities of daily living. Figure 3.2 illustrates their projected disabled populations depending on the different scenarios. In their best guess, by the year 2020, of 52 million persons in the United States over the age of 65, there would be 5.4 million with severe disabilities and another 5.3 million with moderate disabilities, or a combined total of 22 percent of the older population. As the graph indicates, the range of possibilities is considerable. This may be compared with the current estimates of 5–6 million, about 20 percent, of persons ages 65 and older in the United States with any degree of disability.

Thus, we see variations in estimates of life expectancy and in active life expectancy, depending on the populations studied and on how *active* and *healthy life expectancy* are defined. By the year 2025, older Americans (ages 80 and older) may have a life expectancy of 5–8 years, of which approximately 4 will be essentially independent years and approximately 2 will be years requiring some help because of disabilities. Based on such gross overall estimates, and again keeping in mind considerable individual and community variations, one might state that, by the year 2025, at any one time approximately one-third of persons aged 80 or older, or 4.7 million persons, will be needing assistance of some degree. Projections for all persons aged 65 or older appear to approximately double the expected number of those with some degree of dependency within the next 20 to 25 years.

Chronic illness can affect people throughout the life span, although the likelihood of suffering from a chronic illness or a disabling condition increases substantially with age. More than four out of five persons age 65 or older have at least one chronic condition (Altcare, 1990). In the course of their chronic illness, affected persons may experience acute episodes of illness requiring hospitalization and rehabilitation as well as periods of stability or of deterioration that may require primary health care and community-based or institutional long-term care.

Today, over 50 percent of acute hospital beds are occupied by persons age 65 or older being treated, for the most part, for chronic conditions. This is a significant change from the 30 percent of beds being so used just a decade ago, and this rate of increase is expected to continue well into the twenty-first century (Altcare, 1990). Three chronic illnesses — stroke, cancer, and heart disease — are responsible for 20 percent of doctor visits and 40 percent of hospital days (Altcare, 1990).

Current and Projected Use of and Need for Supportive Services

Types of Supportive Care

A wide range of types of supportive services have evolved to meet the needs of persons with varying types and degrees of disability and handicaps, and they are still evolving and changing. These supportive services include: informal care at home by family members and friends; help purchased directly; services provided by formal home care agencies; congregate living and assisted living settings; day programs with varying degrees of social and health-related supportive services; residential health care facilities, including those providing limited health care services and those providing a range of skilled nursing services; rehabilitation settings; and hospice care.

Throughout the United States and, indeed, in other developed countries, the definitions and mixes of services available in different living settings vary and are changing. Perhaps the epitome of blurring of the distinction between living settings and supportive services is the move underway in Denmark to incorporate nursing homes into an overall home support service system (Wagner, 1989). Each nursing home is being redefined such that each room is the private residence of its occupant, and all services are negotiated with that person, or family, just as would be done in any other community living setting.

A number of studies have documented that 80–90 percent of supportive care needed by chronically disabled older people is provided on an unpaid basis, informally, by relatives and friends in the person's own home or the home of a relative or friend (Hanley, Wiener, and Harris, 1992). The sources of payment for formal home health care provided by an agency are reported as 12.2 percent out-of-pocket, 14.3 percent by private insurance, and 73.5 percent by Medicare or Medicaid (Helbing, Sangl, and Silverman, 1992).

A relatively new development in this country — although well established in a number of other countries — is a cash allowance to chronically disabled persons or to their family members, from government or other insurance sources, for the purchase of such services, rather than direct payment to a formal agency (Cameron, 1994).

Congregate living is a term applied to residential settings of various sizes in which frail or otherwise disabled persons live together with housekeeping and meals provided but with the expectation that each person will be generally independent. These settings may range from private dwellings accepting a few such residents to much larger hotel or apartment-house-type dwellings. Expenses are met through private payment or through such sources as Supplemental Security Income and housing subsidization.

A relatively new development is the so-called "assisted living" setting. These residences serve frail and modestly disabled persons who, in addition to housekeeping and meal services, require some degree of supervision in such aspects as medication use and daily living schedules, and may need limited help in personal care (Kane and Wilson, 1993; Regnier, 1994). Assisted living is seen as a service for persons who need a residential setting other than their own home, and it fills in the gap between congregate living and skilled nursing settings. A few states, such as Oregon, are actively encouraging the development of such living arrangements.

The Program of All-inclusive Care for the Elderly (PACE) is an innovative approach to care, modeled after the original On Lok service in San Francisco (discussed below), in which persons with substantial functional losses, physical and/or mental, of the extent that would qualify them for care in a skilled nursing facility, are helped to continue living in their own home settings. This is accomplished through a highly developed day program that includes health, rehabilitative, and social supports and is integrated with supervised home care services. PACE will be discussed in more detail below.

Perhaps the best documentation of the current extent of use of supportive services applies to licensed nursing facilities, now professionally termed residential health care facilities but still popularly called nursing homes. In 1990, approximately 1.6 million elderly persons in the United States were living in nursing homes. Forty-two percent of residents were aged 85 or older, and 75 percent were women (U.S. Bureau of the Census, 1993, chap. 6).

Murtaugh, Kemper, and Spillman (1990) showed that approximately 50 percent of all men aged 85 or older, and almost 70 percent of older women, will reside for some period in a nursing home. Studies of the Established Populations for Epidemiologic Studies of the Elderly, of the National Institute on Aging, indicate considerable variability in nursing home residence rates depending on whether the subject population was urban or rural and on other community differences. The use of nursing homes is much higher, for example, among persons living in rural Iowa counties, where organized home care services would be difficult to provide, than in East Boston, where family and other supportive services are strong and use of nursing homes is much lower. Projections for the future indicate that by 2005 there will be 3.3 million nursing home residents in the United States; by the year 2020, 4 million.

An example of the consolidation and integration of services as needed over the course of later years is the continuing care retirement community (CCRC), now reasonably well developed in this country in a number of settings. Persons who choose to and can afford to move into such communities while they are still reasonably healthy may expect to receive, as later needed, any type of supportive service. Services range from personal care in their own residential apartments on through more supportive personal care units and into skilled nursing units.

Problems with Current Services

Even though a wide range of supportive services has evolved, a major problem is a fragmentation of services that includes lack of integration of primary, preventive, and acute health care services with a full range of choices for chronic supportive care. A major unfortunate result of this general fragmentation is the likelihood of inappropriate choice of service and, in particular, the overuse of highly expensive hospital services. Perhaps the best example of the difference a more integrated approach can make, even for persons with high degrees of disability, can be seen in some of the PACE sites: there has been as high as an 80 percent reduction in rehospitalizations of very frail persons being cared for in the PACE program. A lighter utilization of services also occurs in continuing care retirement communities, although the self-selection of relatively healthy and well educated persons who live in these settings makes broader comparisons difficult.

An obvious type of organized care into which long-term care services could be integrated is the health maintenance organization (HMO). Stimulated by the Tax Equity and Fiscal Responsibility Act (TEFRA) of 1989, a limited number of HMOs have enrolled older, Medicare-eligible persons for the usual types of care provided by HMOs, with reimbursement from Medicare on a capitation basis. However, only a few Medicare HMOs have undertaken to extend their services to include long-term care. One of the best examples is the Fallon Clinic in Worcester, Massachusetts, which has developed networks of organized home care services for the Medicare-insured persons enrolled in that HMO. Proposals by a variety of provider organizations have been made to incorporate a full panoply of long-term care services, including the PACE or On Lok model, into HMOs, with negotiated capitation reimbursement by Medicare and Medicaid. To date, however, no comprehensive trials of such arrangements have been initiated.

Given the very high frequency of multiple health and social problems affecting chronically ill older individuals, it is clear that comprehensive, multidisciplinary geriatric assessment and ongoing care management is a necessity for such persons, and they have been shown, within the institutions of the Veterans Administration as well as in other settings, to be beneficial in both medical and functional outcomes and in lowering the use and cost of services (Stuck et al., 1993). Multidisciplinary geriatric assessment and ongoing care management need to be built into any integrated approach.

Future Care Needs: System Building for Chronic Care

It can be argued, we think persuasively, that long-term care is best addressed in the framework of comprehensive and effective chronic care.

Long-term care exists to meet the needs of persons who have chronic problems. Their needs may extend into all aspects of health and social services, and they must be addressed as interrelated.

The prevalence of chronic diseases and disabilities has been rising steadily and consistently since at least the middle of this century. Today, chronic diseases account for 80 percent of all deaths and 90 percent of all morbidity (Goldsmith, 1989). To date, great strides have been made in pharmaceutical therapies, and significant technological advances have occurred in imaging, permitting earlier diagnosis. Other technologically elegant tools are likely to emerge. However, for the most part, our health care system has not kept pace with the changes in people's illness experiences.

Health care delivery and financing are heavily dependent on the highly skilled medical practitioners who seek to cure or stabilize presenting problems through high technology and short-term interventions. Chronic care, on the other hand, requires providers to integrate their various disciplines and to work collaboratively and over a longer period of time. It requires the integration of services into the home and community by health care providers, extensive involvement of patients and their families, and new and innovative ways of financing of services.

Integration of Care Delivery

Caring for the chronically ill requires a blurring of the boundaries between acute and long-term care. From the perspective of a chronically ill client, the distinctions between the two are artificial and disruptive, since most chronically ill persons usually and often simultaneously need both types of care. The average nursing home patient spends 11.3 days annually in an acute-care hospital, and 60 percent of hospital discharges to nursing homes are patients who originally were admitted to the hospital from a nursing home (Eggert, 1984). On the other hand, the average hospital patient requires transitional and long-term care. A RAND Corporation study reported that 20 percent of Medicare discharges from short-stay hospitals used either skilled nursing or home health care after discharge (Neu and Harrison, 1986). A more recent study, from Rochester, New York (an area where hospital and nursing home bed ratios are low, and occupancy rates are very high), shows that 27 percent of the Medicare-only elderly and 64 percent of those who are dually eligible for Medicare and Medicaid used some form of long-term care within 100 days after a hospital discharge (Temkin-Greener et al., 1994). The findings of this study further emphasize the frequency of transitions between acute and long-term care. As Table 3.1 shows, up to 32 percent of those whose

Table 3.1
Hospital Readmissions, depending on Use or
Nonuse of Long-Term Care Services after Initial
Discharge, Monroe County, New York, 1990–91

Long-Term Care	Medicare Only (%)	Medicare and Medicaid (%)
Not used	15	13
Used	32	26

initial hospital discharge was followed by the use of long-term care were subsequently readmitted to the hospital, as contrasted with only 13 to 15 percent of readmissions among those who did not use long-term care services following a hospital discharge.

A chronically ill older patient typically suffers from multiple, interrelated problems, from medical conditions that need treatment, from functional impairments that prevent functional independence, and often from some degree of cognitive impairment. Many chronically ill older persons have limited income and less-than-adequate support services and housing. For example, according to the Clinton administration (1993), 60 percent of persons who need assistance with three or more activities of daily living, or have severe cognitive impairments, are poor or near poor (income of under $15,000 per year for single persons, and under $20,000 for couples).

A chronically ill older patient typically requires many interrelated services: medical care, assistance in the home, adaptive housing, transportation, nutrition, and social support. Each individual service provider has some capacity for coordination of care, for example, through discharge planners. But such coordinators work primarily within their own agency's set of services, and arrangements for care transitions are often minimal at best. For instance, while nursing home or home care services are planned and provided for on discharge from a hospital, this often happens without full knowledge of a patient's prior treatment or of other ongoing medical interventions. Rehabilitation services, which are often begun in a hospital setting, are rarely linked to services outside of the hospital. Patients move between providers, such as hospital, nursing home, home care, and others, with each provider having little knowledge as to the extent of care, or the cost of care, being provided elsewhere. Without a mechanism for integrating all needed services, a chronically ill patient makes do with what is accessible, not necessarily with what is appropriate or cost-effective.

Chronic care requires an expanded view of care episodes. Acute-care professionals need to move beyond viewing patients in terms of their medical conditions, while long-term care professionals need to move beyond viewing patients strictly in terms of functional status. Chronic care requires that a multidisciplinary team of professionals be involved in the patient's care, following the entire course of chronic illness and working together to optimize personal well-being and functional independence. Chronic care also requires extensive involvement of patients, their families or caregivers, and paraprofessionals. Care must take into account what patients and families want and how they make care decisions.

The last decade has brought the new recognition that management of chronic illness can be addressed effectively only when preventive, primary, acute, long-term, and supportive aspects of care are encompassed (National Chronic Care Consortium, 1991; Zawadski, 1984). A number of local and national demonstrations have been implemented to learn how to coordinate and integrate care for the chronically ill. Most of the demonstrations have relied, at least to a degree, on case management as means of coordinating and controlling services. Not all of the approaches have managed to achieve care integration or to be wholly successful.

Demonstrations of community-based long-term care (CBLTC) that relied on a case manager to assess needs and arrange or broker services include: Triage, Project OPEN, the Multipurpose Senior Services Project, South Carolina Community Long Term Care, ACCESS, and the National Channeling demonstration. Reviews of these and other CBLTC studies suggest that few of these attempts were found to be cost-effective (Weissert and Hedrick, 1994). To some extent, failure to achieve cost savings has been attributed to poor "targeting" of patients (i.e., inability to correctly identify high-risk patients for whom additional benefits and intervention would be most cost-effective). In most of these demonstrations, structural integration, that is, the merging of different services into a single system, did not, for the most part, include integration of funding sources. This, undoubtedly, has contributed to the failure to achieve cost-effectiveness.

Another approach to integration of services has been through a direct service model, or consolidated model. Unlike the brokerage model, most consolidated models establish a single pool of funds and integrate diverse funding sources from which payment for all services is made. In these models, it is the providers of care rather than the funding sources who control individual services. Examples of consolidated approaches to service integration include social health maintenance organizations (S/HMOs), On Lok/PACE programs, some models of continuing care retirement communities, life care at home models (LCAH), EverCare, and capitated Medicaid experiments. Of these consolidated models, S/HMOs, On Lok/PACE programs, CCRCs, and LCAH arrangements are community-based; they are discussed in the next section of this chapter.

EverCare, on the other hand, is a nursing home — based approach to care integration. It currently runs programs in Minneapolis — St. Paul and Chicago and seeks to replicate the model in multiple sites nationwide. Using HMO Medicare risk contracts, EverCare manages the acute care financing and care delivery for nursing home patients. EverCare is financially at risk for primary and hospital services, as well as Medicare reimbursable skilled nursing home care. Like Medicare, it does not cover the costs of custodial long-term care (Malone, Chase, and Bayard, 1993). EverCare enrollees exhibit much lower use of acute hospital care (1,582 days per 1,000 residents) than the average for all nursing home residents (3,462 days per 1,000).

Another approach to care integration has been undertaken by the Arizona Health Care Cost Containment System, a Medicaid demonstration operating since 1982 and providing acute care. In January 1989 the long-term care component, called the Arizona Long-Term Care System, for the older and physically disabled population was also implemented. Benefits covered under this long-term care system include acute care as well as care in skilled nursing facilities, intermediate-care facilities, intermediate care mental retardation facilities, and home- and community-based services (within a spending cap). Varied degrees of service integration have been achieved by program contractors, some of whom provide and manage a continuum of all services, while others are still developing their provider networks (Laguna Research Associates, 1992).

The National Chronic Care Consortium (NCCC), consisting of leading providers of acute and long-term care, was established in 1990, as an effort to build momentum and support for chronic-care reform. The NCCC has identified several areas that represent major barriers to integrating the policies, administrative systems, and delivery of chronic care services (National Chronic Care Consortium, 1993). The barriers include:

1. *Lack of vision.* For the most part, policymakers, payers, providers, and consumers view health care reform from their own narrow perspectives. Yet, chronic conditions require a multidisciplinary, flexible, and ongoing approach to care that results in a seamless continuum of preventive, primary, acute, and long-term care that is responsive to patients' needs. The NCCC recommends the establishment of such chronic care networks within a prospective capitated reimbursement.

2. *Public and private policy barriers.* The existing multiple layers of policies that govern acute and long-term care (for example, with respect to eligibility, benefits, and financing) are often contradictory and incompatible with care needs that cross various federal mandates and private program approaches.

3. *Financing barriers.* Payers tend to micromanage provider behavior rather than encourage global budget targets that allow for provider flexibility and innovation. In the absence of global budgets, providers have no incentive to integrate care for patients with multiple and complex chronic care needs.

The NCCC advocates programs where care is managed across time, place, and profession, with an emphasis on primary care and disability prevention and with patient involvement in the care process. Provider networks that deliver all aspects of a person's care should be encouraged to do so within a predefined, capitated rate.

Community-Based Integrated Care

There is clearly a critical need for programs designed to meet a variety of levels of care within a community and at home. These programs need to address the heterogeneity of the older population and its care needs, which are often complex and ongoing. Although there already exists a wide array of community-based services, ranging from skilled medically related services to housing and social support, in their current configuration these programs cannot effectively meet the needs of the chronically ill older population.

What is still not sufficiently addressed and developed are community-based comprehensive and coordinated systems of care. By this we mean programs that: (a) bring together a continuum of services that best meet the needs of the individual; (b) focus on delivery of care that will reduce or delay institutional care and maintain an optimal level of physical and mental functioning; and (c) strive to coordinate both the diverse services and the reimbursement into a more rational integrated system. In this section, we provide brief descriptions of existing systems and of some currently under development.

The social health maintenance organizations were funded by the federal government in 1982 as a demonstration designed to bring service providers and funding streams (Medicare and to some degree Medicaid) together under one umbrella. The S/HMOs were expected to provide a significant measure of cost control to long-term care. The concept of the demonstration was to combine the ideas of case management and social support with capitated payment and to enroll a cross-section of the older population, including both well persons and functionally impaired persons. Within the consolidated care management system of the S/HMOs, nurses or social workers serve as case managers or resource coordinators, assessing the individual's need for services and providing service coordination. Each S/HMO has contractual arrangements with long-term care providers. While some plans have built delivery systems with reasonable levels of care coordination, others exhibit little evidence of service integration (Yordi, 1988).

The four S/HMO sites are in Brooklyn, New York; Portland, Oregon; Long Beach, California; and Minneapolis, Minnesota. All four have faced some developmental and operational problems, including ones related to management and control of utilization and costs of basic Medicare services and expanded care. The sites have experienced high hospital expenditures, and only two of the four S/HMOs have been able to keep hospitalization levels as low as the U.S. average for the Medicare population, while the other two sites have exceeded that figure (Harrington and Newcomer, 1990). In addition, the S/HMOs appear to have had problems controlling the use of ambulatory visits, specialty services, and emergency room visits. Although community-based long-term care utilization and costs within S/HMOs do not appear to have been a problem, by 1992 the coverage of nursing home care had been cut (at three of the four sites) to between 14 and 21 days per spell of illness. Today, the S/HMOs nursing home benefit is not "a significant solution to long-term nursing home costs" (Leutz et al., 1993).

The On Lok model originated in San Francisco in the early 1970s, and by 1979 it had developed into a Medicare capitated system of community-based care for older persons eligible for nursing home care (Ansak and Zawadski, 1984). At the heart of this model is a multidisciplinary team of professionals and paraprofessionals who manage and provide care. Their functions include assessment and periodic reassessment of participants' needs, development of care plans, management of care, and delivery of all services (Zawadski and Eng, 1988).

By 1983, On Lok had obtained Medicaid waivers, in addition to Medicare waivers, and had become the first fully capitated program to integrate acute and long-term care for the nursing home eligible older patients. In 1990 On Lok was granted its first set of waivers to replicate the program elsewhere. Today, there are eleven PACE programs across the country, and many more are in various stages of the replication process.

Unlike the S/HMOs, PACE provides a very broad long-term care benefit package, in addition to preventive, rehabilitative, primary, and acute care and transportation and nutrition services for nursing home eligible enrollees. Similarly to the S/HMOs, On Lok/PACE receives special federal waivers that permit combining capitated funds from Medicare and Medicaid into a single reimbursement pool. This integration of financing gives programs the flexibility to provide services that are appropriate and needed, as opposed to reimbursable, and to control the volume of those services and the overall cost of care.

While the formal evaluation of the PACE programs has not yet been completed, preliminary findings indicate that this approach to integration of delivery and financing has produced both cost-savings and reductions in hospital and nursing home care. Overall public savings resulting from the PACE programs are conservatively estimated at between 5 percent and 15 percent of current public expenditures for a comparable population not enrolled in the PACE program (Shen and Iversen, 1992). For privately paying PACE members, the cost of care in the program is estimated at 60 percent of the cost of a private pay nursing home bed, with no additional cost for drugs, copayments, and deductibles (Program of All-inclusive Care for the Elderly, 1994). An examination of hospital use shows that, in 1992, hospital days per 1,000 PACE enrollees (age 65+), all of whom were frail and nursing home eligible, was 2,777. By comparison, the national average for Medicare enrollees (age 65+), including those who were well and nonusers of health services, was 2,845 days per year per 1,000 (Program of All-inclusive Care for the Elderly, 1993). An independent evaluation, funded by the John A. Hartford Foundation of New York City, of the Rochester, New York, PACE site, Independent Living for Seniors, shows consistently high levels of satisfaction with the program and with the perceived quality of life among the program's participants and their caregivers (Center for Governmental Research, 1994).

Although today the PACE programs are limited both by the availability of waivers and because they generally serve only older patients, the PACE of the future may have a broader application. Massachusetts is in the process of replicating PACE statewide, and New York State is also moving in this direction. In 1993, the Robert Wood Johnson Foundation funded three PACE sites, to extend their integrative approach to care to other populations, such as patients who are HIV positive (the site in East Boston), children with chronic illnesses and disabilities (Columbia, South Carolina), and chronically ill patients under age 55 (Bronx, New York).

Continuing care retirement communities combine financing and delivery of long-term care and may include — in addition to housing and social and recreational services — hospitalization coverage, skilled and custodial care, emergency response systems, therapies, and prescriptions. However, faced with the rapidly growing population of "older old" (i.e., those ages 85 and above), and with rapid increases in the cost of health care, these communities' original promise of "care for life" has become more and more difficult to fulfill. Today, there are approximately 1,100 retirement communities nationwide that meet the criteria of CCRCs, and they serve a total of 250,000 persons, with the heaviest concentration in Pennsylvania, California, Florida, Ohio, and North Carolina (Emerson and Gillespie, 1993). However, only 40 percent of CCRCs offer their residents contracts that provide for a full and coordinated continuum of care, including long-term care, in exchange for their entrance fee and monthly fee. Another 30 percent of CCRCs offer modified contracts which, in exchange for a lower entrance fee and a monthly fee, provide shelter, services, and a specified amount of nursing home care. The remaining CCRCs offer nursing home care at a fee-for-service daily rate.

Hospital utilization by residents of CCRCs appears to be lower than for a comparable general population of the same age. While this may not be surprising, since CCRC members represent a self-selected, healthier population, CCRC's care management does probably keep the utilization in check. The use of skilled nursing and personal care beds by CCRC residents was estimated at 20.2 percent, with a considerably lower figure for communities offering full-care contracts (15.6% for skilled care, and 13.1% for personal care) (Cohen and Sloan, 1993). This suggests that CCRCs that offer full contracts within an integrated continuum of care and financing have incentives to provide residents with cost-effective and appropriate care alternatives to those offered in institutional settings.

Traditionally, CCRCs have been most popular with middle- and upper-middle-class individuals who can afford both the admission and the monthly fee. A sluggish real estate market and decreasing property values have made affordability an issue. Only about 10 percent of older persons, it was estimated in 1988, could afford to join a continuing care retirement community (Cohen, 1988). Most older persons, however, prefer to stay in their own homes and do not like the idea of age-segregated living.

Life care at home, an off-campus alternative to the CCRC, was developed in 1987 (Tell, Cohen, and Wallack, 1987) and was originally targeted at the healthy, middle-income older population. This approach is designed to allow older persons to maintain their own living arrangements while receiving a life-long care contract similar to that offered in full-guarantee CCRCs. Lower entry fees and monthly fees make LCAH a lower-cost alternative to the CCRC life-care model. Today, there are only three LCAH programs operating in the country, covering almost 500 people (Callahan and Somers, 1994).

The Long-Term Care Options Project (LTCOP) is a demonstration program of the Minnesota Department of Human Services. LTCOP was funded by the Robert Wood Johnson Foundation in 1992 to design and provide a continuum of health and social services to seniors who are eligible for both Medicare and Medicaid. Program participants may reside either in the community or in a nursing home. The project seeks to combine all services and funding sources under a single umbrella, providing a single point of access for the participants. For the community residents, the project seeks to maintain maximal independence and prevent or delay the need for institutional care. For nursing home residents, the project aims to reduce hospital admissions and to facilitate return to the community, if feasible. Just approved by the Health Care Financing Administration, this demonstration will constitute the first time a state will have offered a combined Medicare/Medicaid insurance package.

Continuing care networks (CCNs) are also in the developmental phase. They attempt to bridge primary, acute, and long-term care, and they focus on older persons, including those who are chronically ill and/or disabled, living either in the community or in a nursing home. This project, undertaken by the Community Coalition for Long Term Care, in Rochester, New York, was funded by the Robert Wood Johnson Foundation for a three-year period beginning in 1994. The demonstration's objectives are to implement continuing care networks designed to improve access to services, create an integrated continuum of preventive, primary, acute, and long-term care, and to reduce both the overall cost of care and the use of services, with incentives of prospective capitated reimbursement.

System Building and Health Care Financing

The integration of acute and chronic care systems has been extremely hard to achieve under the existing reimbursement arrangements. These arrangements give the participants in the systems — the professional caregivers, the institutions, and the patients — a grab bag of incentives, few of which promote efficiency and cost-effectiveness. Consolidation of the existing multiple funding streams is one approach to developing a more appropriate and cost-effective way of delivering and managing care. This can be achieved by pooling funds from different reimbursement streams in a single fund for delivery of all services. Because so often "form follows finance," the integration of funding is critical to the elimination of service fragmentation, maximization of provider incentives for cost-effectiveness, and reduction of administrative costs. This new model of health care reimbursement has begun to emerge in demonstrations that use prospective, capitated payments and in which providers assume financial control and risk. Although some critics argue that capitated reimbursement systems can lead providers to skimp on care so as to stay within budgets, there is virtually no evidence to support that assertion. On the other hand, there is ample evidence of inappropriate use and overuse of services in fee-for-service systems.

To date the biggest impediments to risk-based reimbursement have been the providers' unwillingness to assume financial risk and the government's reluctance to grant waivers, which make capitation possible. As mentioned, there are only four S/HMO sites currently operating under federal waivers. Through the 1990 Omnibus Budget Reconciliation Act, Congress permitted an addition of four new S/HMO sites. On Lok/PACE currently holds a limited number of waiver slots for PACE replications. Further expansion of this demonstration will depend on future availability of waivers.

Although community-based integrated delivery and financing systems have not been fully or formally evaluated, and each program has its weaknesses, for the most part the existing models do demonstrate better success in providing coordinated and cost-effective care than the more traditional stand-alone programs. Integrated care systems, with a single payer and a broad control over a spectrum of settings, have organizational incentives that encourage appropriate, timely, and cost-effective use of service. The projected growth of older populations experiencing a high prevalence of chronic illness and disability and needing appropriate care requires innovative and cost-effective strategies. According to Manton and colleagues (n.d.), a 33 percent reduction in the incidence of dementia, a 75 percent reduction in arthritis, and a 50 percent reduction in chronic heart disease (excluding heart attacks) could reduce Medicare costs by \$8.1 billion (in 1991 expenses), or 7.5 percent of total cost. On the other hand, according to Gruenberg, Rumshishkaya, and Kaganova (1993), PACE programs are already producing Medicare savings ranging from 13 to 39 percent. While the latter is clearly a more immediately achievable strategy, future approaches must focus both on the prevention and treatment of chronic illness and on building a coherent, integrated system of care.

Acknowledgment

The editorial assistance of Jeanne Soderberg is appreciated.

References

Adams, K., Meiners, M. R., and Burwell, B. (1993). Asset spend-down in nursing homes: Methods and insights. *Medical Care* 31:1.

Altcare (1990). *Chronic Care . . . Independence through Innovation*. Bloomington, Minn.: Altcare Corporation.

Ansak, M. L., and Zawadski, R. T. (1984). On Lok CCODA: A consolidated model. In R. T. Zawadski, ed., *Community-Based Systems of Long Term Care*. New York: Haworth.

Branch, L. G., Guralnik, J. M., Foley, D. J., Kohout, F. J., Wetle, T. T., Ostfeld, A., and Katz, S. (1991). Active life expectancy for 10,000 Caucasian men and women in three communities. *Journal of Gerontology: Medical Sciences* 46: M145–50.

Callahan, D. (1987). *Setting Limits: Medical Goals for an Aging Society*. New York: Simon and Schuster.

Callahan, J. J., and Somers, S. A. (1994). Life care at home: The experience and the issues. *Compensation and Benefits Management* 10 (2): 49–60.

Cameron, K. (1994). *International and Domestic Programs Using "Cash and Counseling" Strategies to Pay for Long-Term Care*. Washington, D.C.: United Seniors Health Cooperative.

Center for Governmental Research (1994). *Independent Living for Seniors: A Three-Year Assessment of Perceptions and Impact of Program*. Rochester, N.Y.: Center for Governmental Research.

Chellis, R. D., and Grayson, P. J. (1990). *Life Care: A Long-Term Solution?* Lexington, Mass.: Lexington Books.

Clinton Administration (1993). Presentation of the Health Security Act by Mary Harahan. Rochester, N.Y. November 11.

Cohen, G. D., and Sloan, F. (1993). Responses to Emerson and Gillespie. In *Care in the Long Term: In Search of Community and Security*. Washington, D.C.: Institute of Medicine.

Cohen, M. (1988). Life care: New options for financing and delivering long-term care. *Health Care Financing Review*, ann. suppl.

Coward, R. T. al. (1993). *Old and Alone in Rural America*. Washington, D.C.: American Association of Retired Persons.

Eggert, G. M. (1984). Reforming long term care: A proposal for a catastrophic, managed care plan. Rochester, New York.

Emerson, J. F., and Gillespie, A. E. (1993). Expanding the boundaries of the continuing care retirement community. In *Care in the Long Term: In Search of Community and Security*. Washington, D.C.: Institute of Medicine.

Goldsmith, J. (1989). The paradigm shift: Transforming from an acute to chronic care model. In *Decisions in Imaging Economics*.

Gruenberg, L., Rumshishkaya, A., and Kaganova, J. (1993). *An Analysis of Expected Medicare Costs for Participation in the PACE Demonstration*. Cambridge, Mass.: Long Term Care Data Institute.

Hanley, R. J., Wiener, J. M., and Harris, K. M. (1992). Will paid home care erode informal support? *Journal of Health Politics, Policy and Law* 16 (3): 507–21.

Harrington, C., and Newcomer, R. J. (1990). Social Health Maintenance Organizations as Innovative Models to Control Costs. *Generations* 14:49.

Helbing, C., Sangl, J. A., and Silverman, H. A. (1992). Home health agency benefits. *Health Care Financing Review, Medical and Medicaid Statistical Supplement.*

Japan Aging Research Center (1991). *Aging in Japan.* Tokyo: Jarc's Sasakawa Memorial Information Center/International Publication Series, no. 2.

Kane, R. A., and Wilson, K. B. (1993). *Assisted Living in the United States: A New Paradigm for Residential Care for Frail Older Persons?* Washington, D.C.: American Association of Retired Persons.

Kunkel, S. R., and Applebaum, R. A. (1992). Estimating the Prevalence of Long-Term Disability for an Aging Society. *Journal of Gerontology: Social Sciences* 47:S258.

Laguna Research Associates (1992). Evaluation of the Arizona health care cost containment system demonstration. Report prepared for the Health Care Financing Administration.

Leutz, W., Abrahams, R., Altman, S., Capitman, J., Gruenberg, L., Hallfors, D., and Ritter, G. (1993). Design of second generation social health maintenance organization sites. Final report prepared for the Health Care Financing Administration.

Malone, J. K., Chase, D., and Bayard, J. L. (1993). Caring for nursing home residents. *Journal of Health Care Benefits* Jan–Feb:51.

Manton, K. G. (1991). The dynamics of population aging: Demography and policy analysis. *Milbank Quarterly* 69:309–38.

Manton, K. G., and Stallard, E. (1991). Cross-sectional estimates of active life expectancy for the U.S. elderly and oldest-old populations. *Journal of Gerontology, Social Sciences* 46:S170–82.

Manton, K. G., Stallard, E., and Vertrees, J. C. (n.d.). Estimates of costs of medical conditions in elderly populations. Durham, N.C.: Duke University, Center for Demographic Studies (unpublished ms).

Murtaugh, C. M., Kemper, P. G., and Spillman, B. C. (1990). The risk of nursing home use in later life. *Medical Care* 28:952–62.

National Chronic Care Consortium (1991). Capacity building in geriatric chronic care. Application to the John A. Hartford Foundation of New York City. Bloomington, Minnesota.

National Chronic Care Consortium (1993). Health Care Reform: Barriers to Integration. Working document. Bloomington, Minnesota.

Neu, C. R., and Harrison, S. (1986). *Prospective Payment for Medical Post-Hospital Services: Some Empirical Considerations.* RAND/UCLA Center for Health Care Financing Policy Research.

Perls, T. T., Carey, J. R., Vaupel, J. W., Manton, K. G., and Allard, M. (1993).

Selective survival of the oldest old: A cohort of successfully aging individuals. *Gerontologist* 33, special issue 1, October, p. 1.

Program of All-inclusive Care for the Elderly (1993). Progress report on the replication of the On Lok model.

Program of All-inclusive Care for the Elderly (1994). Sixth Annual PACE Forum. Washington, D.C.

Preston, S. H. (1993). Demographic changes in the United States, 1970–2050. In K. G. Manton, B. H. Singer, and R. M. Suzman, eds. *Forecasting the Health of Elderly Populations.* New York: Springer Verlag.

Regnier, V. A. (1994). *Assisted Living Housing for the Elderly: Design Innovations from the U.S. and Europe.* New York: Van Nostrand Reinhold.

Scitovsky, A. A. (1988). Medical care in the last twelve months of life: The relation between age, functional status, and medical care expenditures. *Milbank Quarterly* 66:640.

Shen, J., and Iversen, A. (1992). PACE: A capitated model towards long-term care. *Henry Ford Hospital Medical Journal* 40:41.

Somers, A. R., and Spears, N. L. (1992). *Continuing Care Retirement Community.* New York: Springer Publishing.

Spence, D. A., and Wiener, J. M. (1990). Estimating the extent of Medicaid spend-down in nursing homes. *Journal of Health Politics, Policy and Law* 15:607.

Stuck, A. E., Siu, A. L., Wieland, G. D., Adams, J., and Rubenstein, L. Z. (1993). Comprehensive geriatric assessment: A meta-analysis of controlled trials. *Lancet* 342:1032–36.

Tell, E. J., Cohen, M. A., and Wallack, S. S. (1987). New directions in LifeCare: An industry in transition. *Milbank Quarterly* 65:71.

Temkin-Greener, H., Meiners, R. M., Petty, E. A., Szydlowski, J. S. (1992). The use and cost of health services prior to death: A comparison of the Medicare-only and the Medicare-Medicaid elderly populations. *Milbank Quarterly* 70:679.

Temkin-Greener, H., Meiners, R. M., Petty, E. A., Szydlowski, J. S. (1993). Spending-down to Medicaid in the nursing home and in the community: A longitudinal study from Monroe County, New York. *Medical Care* 8:663.

Temkin-Greener, H., Meiners, M. R., and Naples, K. J. (1994). Analysis of chronic illness episodes: Medicare-only and Medicare/Medicaid older persons: Preliminary results. Unpublished.

U.S. Bureau of the Census (1993). *An Aging World II.* International population report P95/92–3. Washington, D.C.: U.S. Government Printing Office.

U.S. Bureau of the Census and National Institute on Aging (1993a). *Profiles of America's Elderly: Racial and Ethnic Diversity of America's Elderly Population.* No. 3. Washington, D.C.: U.S. Government Printing Office.

U.S. Bureau of the Census and National Institute on Aging (1993b). *Profiles of America's Elderly: Living Arrangements of the Elderly.* No. 4. Washington, D.C.: U.S. Government Printing Office.

Wagner, L. (1989). A proposed model for care of the elderly. *International Nursing Review* 36 (2): 50–60.

Weissert, W. G., and Hedrick, S. (1994). Lessons learned from research on effects of community-based long-term care. *Journal of the American Geriatrics Association* 42 (3): 348–53.

Williams, T. F. (1992). Aging versus disease. In R. L. Sprott, H. R. Warner, and T. F. Williams, eds. *The Biology of Aging,* special issue of *Generations* 16 (4): 21–25.

Yordi, C. L. (1988). A consolidated model of long-term care: Service utilization and cost impacts. *Gerontological Society of America* 25:389.

Zawadski, R. T. (1984). *Community-Based Systems of Long Term Care.* New York: Haworth.

Zawadski, R. T., and Eng, C. (1988). Case management in capitated long-term care. *Health Care Financing Review,* ann. suppl.

4

Trends among Younger Persons with Disability or Chronic Disease

A. E. Benjamin, Ph.D.

As a society, we have been struggling for much of this century with how to address the care needs of people with chronic conditions (see Benjamin, 1993). Soon after the passage of Medicare and Medicaid in 1965, policymakers found themselves confronting a host of new challenges related to the organization and financing of what came to be called long-term care. For much of the 1970s and 1980s, long-term care was considered synonymous with services for older persons, and specifically with nursing home care for older adults. As is made clear throughout this volume, much has changed in recent years with respect to data, perspectives, and proposed reforms related to long-term care, even while the seemingly intractable problems of financing such care persist.

Among the most important changes in chronic (or long-term) care perspectives in recent years is the growing recognition of the diversity of those who are limited in functioning by chronic illnesses and conditions. Although older persons constitute the majority of the population with serious chronic care needs, and the risk of disability increases with age and reaches its apex among the very old, chronic conditions are not the exclusive province of older persons. Significant numbers of people requiring chronic care services are under age 65. For policymakers, this younger population is characterized by daunting diversity and complexity. Moreover, these groups bring growing numbers and increasingly sophisticated political organizations to a debate about the future direction of chronic care policy—a debate once dominated by those representing the interests of elderly people.

The increased attention now being paid to the chronic care issues of nonelderly persons with disabilities is the result of several developments. First, the demographics of chronicity are changing as developments in medical science have dramatically increased the prospects for survival of persons disabled by disease or injury. As a result, the number of younger persons living with disabilities has grown and will continue to do so.

Second, the "deinstitutionalization" movement has had an impact well beyond old-age relevant concerns for developing home and community-based alternatives to nursing homes. Many nonelderly persons with disabilities have been shifted (often "dumped") into the community, making much more visible the care needs of various people once confined to institutional settings.

Third, in the past decade new disability lobbies and coalitions have emerged to work for passage of the Americans with Disabilities Act. With that success to celebrate, they have turned eagerly to other issues. Services to people with disabilities in the home and community have become the new policy focus of these organizations, and this new focus has helped to redefine the cast and content of the larger chronic care debate.

Fourth, an active minority within the aging lobby, led by the Gray Panthers, has long been calling for a view of long-term care that embraces more than the needs of older persons. Hence, the broader scope and the small body of literature that purveyed it (Mahoney, Estes, and Heumann, 1986; Minkler, 1990) were familiar to the field as other pressures grew for a collaborative perspective on aging and disability.

Finally, more than a decade of budget crises at the federal and state levels has sobered many policy actors about the political risks created when competing groups with similar needs struggle for a share of a shrinking budget pie. While the impact on advocacy organizations of deficit politics can be exaggerated, there is growing anecdotal evidence that policymakers who are the targets of chronic care advocacy are now insisting that diverse interests collaborate in formulating their policy demands.

This chapter describes in broad strokes nonelderly persons with disabilities, with attention to the primary subgroups that compose this diverse population. I consider two groups in some more detail, persons with spinal cord injuries and persons with HIV disease/AIDS, highlighting the service needs of each and the ways these are specified and addressed. Next, an attempt is made to synthesize themes that cut across service planning and advocacy for elderly and nonelderly persons (the common ground) and those that suggest important differences and sources of conflict. I close with some thoughts on the policy implications of diversity and the challenges it represents.

Overview of Younger Disabled Populations

In the world of health statistics, various measures are used to describe the size and character of the American population with chronic care needs. The broadest estimates suggest that in 1989 approximately 14 percent (34 million) of all Americans living in the community had an activity limitation due to a chronic condition, and that a little more than two-thirds of those were under the age of 65 (LaPlante, Rice, and Kraus, 1991).

This broad estimate, however, tells us very little about the subset of persons with significant care needs, the group of primary relevance for public policy. For this, we turn to data on people with difficulty in performing basic life activities, including both activities of daily living (ADLs), such as bathing and dressing, and instrumental activities of daily living (IADLs), such as meal preparation and laundry. As the data in Table 4.1 suggest, an estimated 9.5 million Americans living in the community have difficulty performing basic life activities. Of these, about 3.9 million (41%) are under the age of 65 (see column 2). In other words, about four in ten of those persons most in need of assistance for chronic disability are not elderly. Although the likelihood of having difficulties doubles with each succeeding age group, chronic disability is a problem for persons of all ages (Feder and Scanlon, 1992; LaPlante and Miller, 1992). The sheer magnitude of the nonelderly population (about 87% of the citizenry) means that, even with the comparatively low prevalence of disability among children and younger adults, the absolute numbers are significant.

Relatively little work has been done to project the future of chronic disability among younger populations, because there are so many and such diverse subsets to consider and because the sources of disability are so complex. Predicting, for example, the number of victims of firearms injuries that will survive with spinal cord and head injuries that are disabling is very speculative, not to mention sobering (Max and Rice, 1993). Unlike aging, which itself plays some measurable role in explaining the prevalence of chronic needs, there are no common causal threads on which to build solid projections for the younger disabled population. As the population ages, the relative share of those with chronic care needs who are under age 65 will probably decline, even as the actual number is likely to grow. While the percentages shift, the policy (and human) challenges will not soon go away.

Because we have only very recently begun to consider the broad range of nonelderly persons living with disabilities, no single framework for describing these diverse groups has been developed (Feder and Scanlon,

Table 4.1
Persons Having Difficulty Performing Basic Life Activities, by Age

Age	Total Population by Age Group (in thousands)	Number with Any Difficulty (in thousands)	Percentage of Age Group	Percentage of Total with Any Difficulty (N = 9,511)
0–17	63,900	195	0.3	2.1
18–44	101,609	1,524	1.5	16.0
45–54	22,427	848	3.8	8.9
55–64	22,046	1,324	6.0	13.8
65–74	16,886	1,993	11.8	21.0
75–84	8,750	2,315	26.5	24.3
85+	2,274	1,310	57.6	13.8
Subtotals				
0–64	209,981	3,893	1.9	40.9
65+	27,909	5,619	20.1	59.1
Total	237,890	9,511	4.0	100

Source: Adapted from LaPlante and Miller (1992), 1987 National Medical Expenditure Survey, Round 1.

1993). Viewed broadly, there are at least six subsets of the nonelderly population with disabilities. Most, if not all of them, are as diverse internally as the population over age 65 with disabilities (see Newcomer and Benjamin, 1995, and individual chapters therein on these populations).

First, about 2 percent of children have severe functional limitations that require sustained, supportive care. Known as "children with special health needs," this population has grown as medical technology has made it possible to save children who only a decade or two ago would have died at or soon after birth (Stein, 1989).

Second, medical science has greatly improved the likelihood that adults with physical disabilities caused by disease and injury will survive and, with required support, lead long and productive lives (Trieschmann, 1988). Visual impairment and impaired mobility are among the chronic conditions included under the rubric "adults with physical disabilities."

Third, the "chronically medically ill" includes persons with chronic illnesses, such as cancer, heart disease, rheumatoid arthritis, and HIV infection, that require ongoing medical monitoring. It is the illness component, and the prominent need for medical care, that distinguish persons with rheumatoid arthritis and persons with the human immunodeficiency virus from other adults with chronic care needs.

Fourth, from 2 to 3 percent of Americans are identified as mentally retarded or developmentally disabled during their preadult years. A much smaller number (perhaps one-half of one percent) are considered moderately to profoundly retarded into adulthood and in need of supportive care (Lakin et al., 1989; Thornton, 1990).

Fifth, the chronically mentally ill include an estimated 1 percent of the adult population of all ages with recurrent episodes of mental illness, most notably schizophrenia (Mandersheid and Sonnenschein, 1992). This population requires a blend of clinical, rehabilitative, and supportive services to address what can be severe limitations in functioning.

Sixth, we are now aware of a (still inadequately defined) number of long-term users of alcohol and drugs whose needs for supportive services have much in common with those of more traditional recipients of chronic care services. While relatively little is known about these "chronic alcohol and drug abusers," it is apparent that some small percentage of users are not amenable to current treatment interventions and require tailored versions of chronic care (Institute of Medicine, 1990).

Such cryptic descriptions of complex populations barely hint at the diversity of care needs involved or the commonalities among those needs. To provide some needed texture to a broad overview, let us next consider in more detail those service needs and issues associated with two subsets of younger adults with disabilities: persons with spinal cord injuries and persons with HIV disease. While it is difficult to argue that these two groups are truly representative of all younger adults with disabilities, a more thorough examination of them does reveal issues that should inform any discussion of the service needs of the nonelderly and the potential for collaborative approaches to service system reform.

Persons with Spinal Cord Injuries

Using persons living with spinal cord injuries (SCI) as an example makes sense for several reasons: their assistance needs tend to be profound and complex; these needs have been the subject of a great deal of research in the rehabilitation and postrehabilitation fields; and persons with SCI are very visible within the leadership of the disability rights movement, so that their assistance needs have been well articulated and debated.

Informed estimates of the number of Americans currently living with SCI who have significant neurological deficit range between 177,000 and 220,000 (DeJong and Batavia, 1991; Harvey et al., 1990). Annually, an estimated 7,000 to 8,000 persons incur a traumatic spinal cord injury, about half resulting from motor vehicle accidents and most of the rest from falls, violence (primarily gunshots), and sports (primarily diving)

(National Spinal Cord Injury Association, 1992). In the light of the sources of injury, it is not surprising that most of the newly injured are young and male. Relatively little data are available on the incidence or prevalence of disease-induced SCI.

Over the past half century, advances in medicine have significantly improved the survival and longevity of persons who have sustained SCI. Modern trauma and rehabilitation centers ensure that most persons who survive the initial trauma will complete the acute and rehabilitation phases of care and reenter the community to live with a disability, most for many years (Trieschmann, 1988). Dramatic advances in the prospects for survival and longevity, however, have not been matched by attention to the service needs and quality of life of these persons in the community following discharge from rehabilitation (Eisenberg and Saltz, 1991; Sims, Manley, and Richardson, 1993).

The service needs and locales for care of persons with SCI are similar to those of persons with severe mobility limitations attributable to polio, cerebral palsy, and other conditions. First, most persons with SCI are discharged to home following rehabilitation; only a small percentage go to a nursing home. Second, persons with SCI are very vulnerable to a variety of acute conditions, such as pressure sores and infections of the urinary and respiratory tracts, any of which can become life threatening. Third, recovery and recuperation from such acute conditions are likely to take longer for persons with SCI than for others. Fourth, as people with SCI age, they are increasingly vulnerable to new chronic conditions, such as cardiovascular diseases. Fifth, most persons with SCI rely on assistive equipment and other technologies, and their equipment needs are likely to change over time. Finally, from half to two-thirds of this population requires continuing assistance with some or all basic life activities (ADLs and IADLs), both to enhance their independence and to monitor and maintain their health status (DeJong, Brannon, and Batavia, 1993; Yarkony et al., 1990).

As a result of disability and the features described above, persons with SCI are heavy users of medical care, in terms of unscheduled hospitalizations, length of hospital stay, and number of visits to medical practitioners. They are also regular users of prescription medications as a part of their daily regimen and frequent users of nonprescription drugs. People with SCI rely on a range of adaptive equipment, including leg braces, wheelchairs, and canes. Not surprisingly, they also depend heavily on other persons, mostly family members and friends, for assistance in personal care, homemaking, and other in-home activities (DeJong and Batavia, 1991; DeJong, Brannon, and Batavia, 1993).

Four broad clusters of resources and services often are needed by those with SCI: acute rehabilitative care, long-term medical management, long-term services for daily living, and other "essential living resources" (De-Jong, Brannon, and Batavia, 1993; Feder and Scanlon, 1992; Sims, Manley, and Richardson, 1993). The acute and postacute phases of SCI can be managed only to the extent that specialized personnel and facilities are available and timely. To the extent that these resources are available, the costs of care are heavy in meeting the acute and rehabilitation needs of persons with SCI.

Primary care is essential to successful long-term medical management. The supply of primary care physicians and other health professionals trained to work with people with physical disabilities is growing. However, inadequate numbers and uneven distribution continue to represent barriers to appropriate management and treatment of persons with disabilities and to monitoring the medical complications that attend impaired mobility (DeJong and Batavia, 1991).

At the core of services designed to support daily living for people with SCI are personal assistance services (known as personal care services in other contexts) (Batavia, DeJong, and McKnew, 1991; Litvak and Kennedy, 1991). They include assistance in personal or bodily functions (ADLs) and household maintenance activities (IADLs). For persons with SCI, personal assistance has become the *sine qua non* for remaining in the community and achieving some degree of long-term independence. Access to personal assistance is not readily available, and its availability depends on financial resources, place of residence, and eligibility for Medicaid and state and federal social services programs.

Because persons with disabilities are more likely to have lower incomes than those who are able-bodied, persons with SCI are often lacking "essential living resources," that is, the income, shelter, and insurance resources necessary to live securely and safely. This means they are comparatively likely to be excluded from the work force, be limited in affordable housing options, and be dependent on public programs for income support and health insurance. Income support programs that tie eligibility to inability to work may present barriers to independence and an adequate standard of living for those who would prefer to be employed (Feder and Scanlon, 1992). Traditional vocational rehabilitation programs are only partially responsive to the needs of persons with SCI who want to work.

An important response to these issues has been the development of an independent living movement among persons with disabilities. It assumes that the primary barriers to living independently in the community are social and environmental and that persons with disabilities can be self-directed consumers of services, fully capable of managing their own lives (Batavia, DeJong, and McKnew, 1991). The movement has developed a national network of centers for independent living. The local organizations are run by persons with disabilities and provide services to a range of clients, including many with SCI. They are funded under the federal Rehabilitation Act of 1973 (Nosek, Roth, and Zhu, 1990). In many communities, these centers have become the primary source of social services and advocacy for persons with disabilities. At the same time, the independent living movement has raised some issues that challenge prevailing ways of thinking about long-term care for the elderly and others with chronic care needs; these issues will be discussed below.

Persons with HIV Infection/AIDS

Persons with AIDS constitute one subset of those who are chronically medically ill. "HIV infected" is a term that describes persons carrying the human immunodeficiency virus. Because an HIV-weakened immune system is vulnerable to numerous opportunistic infections, virtually everyone with HIV eventually develops AIDS. AIDS is most commonly characterized as a disease with acute episodes and progressive deterioration, and most policy debate focuses on preventing the spread of the virus and finding effective treatment and vaccines. Considerably less attention has been paid to the chronic character of the disease and its service requirements (Fee and Fox, 1992).

As of June of 1995, just under 480,000 Americans had been diagnosed with AIDS since the epidemic was first identified a decade earlier. Of this number, about 60 percent had died, and about 180,000 persons were living with AIDS (U.S. Centers for Disease Control and Prevention, 1993). Estimates indicate that 1.5 to 2.0 million others are currently infected with the HIV virus and that the median latency period from infection to clinical AIDS is about 10 years (Mann, 1991). The challenge of responding to the service needs of persons living with AIDS is long term.

Median life expectancy estimates for persons diagnosed with AIDS in the late 1980s have been between 12 and 15 months. The continuing development of new treatment modalities, especially drug therapies, is likely to extend life expectancy for persons diagnosed in the 1990s, with estimates from some local data suggesting median survival times of 22 months (Hellinger, 1992; Lemp, Hirozawa, et al., 1992, Lemp, Payne, et al., 1990). While there is debate about the impact of early medical intervention and of specific medications, such as AZT, designed to delay the onset of certain opportunistic infections, there is little doubt that life ex-

pectancy has improved. But variations in survival time among those diagnosed are substantial, ranging from one month to eight years or more. In
all likelihood, continuing development of more effective treatments will
moderate the prevalence and severity of acute conditions, extend the average duration of chronic illness associated with AIDS, and increase the
need for community-based care (Feder and Scanlon, 1992).

Several features of living with AIDS are important in shaping and defining the chronic care needs of those affected. First, while AIDS can be
considered chronic, debilitating, and terminal, it is also acute, medically
complex, and episodic. The onset of one or several opportunistic infections may be followed by complications or remission, so the course of the
disease is frequently nonlinear and unpredictable. Persons with AIDS may
experience periods in which they are near death and then move into periods in which they are relatively well and self-reliant. This contrasts with
the typical person with SCI who, while vulnerable to acute episodes, is
able to limit their occurrence with appropriate prevention and care.

Second, most persons with AIDS (like most persons with chronic illness) live at home and spend a majority of their time outside the hospital
and the physician's office. This reflects both the course of the disease and
increasing efforts by health care providers to shift from inpatient to outpatient treatment.

Third, the course of illness is characterized by wide variations in functional dependency among people at similar stages of the disease and for a
given person over time (O'Dell et al., 1991). Such fluctuations are far less
common among persons with SCI, because that chronic condition typically limits the range of possible functional variation.

Fourth, one reservoir of the AIDS virus in the human body is the central
nervous system, and this can be manifested as dementia (Ho et al., 1987).
As it does in elderly patients, dementia in people with AIDS greatly com-
plicates the provision of long-term care.

There are wide variations in the demographics of persons with HIV
infection. While the largest subset of those with AIDS continues to be
among homosexual men, the most dramatic growth in prevalence is
among injecting drug users, minorities, women, and children. This shift
poses policy implications that flow from the socioeconomic status and
available resources of those affected. An AIDS diagnosis and subsequent
illness often disrupts the material fabric of life in significant ways. Many
with the disease are unemployed. Others face the risk of losing their jobs
and, thus, their primary source of income and health insurance as well as
the disruption of established living arrangements and informal care networks. One consequence has been a growing dependency by persons with

AIDS on welfare, especially Supplemental Security Income (SSI) and Medicaid (Fleishman and Mor, 1993; Green and Arno, 1990).

Current service utilization patterns within this population generally reflect the features of illness associated with AIDS (and to a lesser and still uncertain extent, those associated with the period of HIV disease before an AIDS diagnosis). Persons with AIDS are relatively heavy users of medical care, including hospitalization, despite continuing efforts to expand outpatient care alternatives (Hellinger, 1992). Not surprisingly, those diagnosed with AIDS are relatively heavy users of prescription and nonprescription medications. Many who are living in the community frequently need assistance with routine activities of daily living and are therefore dependent on either family members, volunteers, or publicly subsidized supportive services. Reliance on volunteers and formal service providers is especially heavy for the quarter to a third of persons with AIDS who live alone (Mor, Piette, and Fleishman, 1989). These patterns parallel those noted earlier for persons with SCI, but the period of disability with AIDS is much shorter and the incidence of life-threatening episodes on average is much higher.

The essential elements of a service model for persons with AIDS resembles that for people with SCI, although there are some important differences. The model includes specialized acute and long-term medical care and management, long-term supportive living services, coordination of care, and appropriate living resources. Specialized medical care is important for early intervention, acute medical treatment following diagnosis, and ongoing medical monitoring. Frequent diagnostic monitoring, drug therapy, and ongoing primary care, including prevention and home health (primarily nursing) services, are among the important elements of this care. Specialized AIDS medical care, while very unevenly distributed within and across communities, is relatively well developed in many "high impact" cities. Less is known about ongoing medical care for persons with SCI, but advocates for people with physical disabilities suggest that for these groups appropriate primary care, outside of rehabilitation medicine, is less well articulated and far less available than that for AIDS.

Supportive living services are essential to maintaining persons with AIDS at home or in other community settings, thereby providing alternatives to lengthy hospital stays. Central among them are in-home care, including personal assistance and homemaking services, meals and transportation, hospice services, nursing home care, respite care, and psychosocial services (Benjamin, 1989; Merzel et al., 1992; Benjamin, 1989; Mor, Piette, and Fleishman, 1989). In comparing services for those with SCI and AIDS, there is little difference in the categories of services required, but there are some important differences in how they are conceptualized and used. For example, home care services to persons with SCI are designed to restore or maintain the independence of those expected to live long lives with relatively stable physical disabilities. The services are designed to be continuous and to eliminate or minimize the impact of those disabilities. In contrast, home care for persons with AIDS tends to be more intermittent and episodic, reflecting the course of illness, and to be more concerned with medical interventions.

Coordination of services is an important issue in any form of chronic care. Because AIDS involves a complex and erratic clinical picture, it has drawn particular attention to issues of case management (Benjamin, Lee, and Solkowitz, 1988; Fleishman, Mor, and Piette, 1991; Mor, Piette, and Fleishman, 1989). For the AIDS population, the case manager plays a medical monitoring function that requires expertise and experience with the various opportunistic infections and symptoms associated with the disease, as well as with the range of community, residential and institutional services that may be needed. While this kind of medically sophisticated case management is not unknown in other areas of chronic care, it is essential to managing the care of persons affected by HIV-related illnesses.

Another feature of AIDS, commonly, is the deterioration or absence of essential resources for daily living. AIDS can diminish the ability to generate income through work and to maintain employer-based health insurance coverage. For those with already low incomes, living with an AIDS diagnosis means a shortage of jobs, medical and social services, housing, transportation, and available drug abuse treatment. These resource issues are complicated by the stigma associated with the disease.

The extension of "presumptive disability" to persons with AIDS under the Supplemental Security Income program and the access to Medicaid eligibility that this classification makes possible, has put a partial floor under the declines in income and health insurance coverage that are common for those with this illness. The value of this floor, of course, varies in accordance with differences among state governments in welfare benefit policies.

Housing is an especially pressing need for persons with AIDS, because most have low or declining incomes (Andrews et al., 1989; Benjamin and Bennett, 1991; Mor, Piette, and Fleishman, 1989). Living with the illness often means finding new housing that is affordable and amenable to supportive services. Such housing is generally in short supply; but in most communities, suitable housing for persons known to have HIV disease is especially limited. For many chronically ill populations, a traditional public sector response to this problem has been to expand the supply of nursing home beds. For a host of reasons, however–including nursing home industry reluctance to alienate its primary constituency (i.e., elderly persons and their families)–the supply of beds for those with AIDS has grown very slowly, despite widespread public sector efforts to encourage its expansion (Andrews et al., 1989; Benjamin and Swan, 1989; Swan and Benjamin, 1993).

Common Ground for Long-Term Care

Brief profiles of these two younger populations with chronic conditions or disease suggest a number of similarities and a broad common ground on which to construct collaborative approaches to services for all persons with chronic long-term care needs (Binstock, 1992; Zola, 1988). For those familiar with policy and services for elderly persons, the service needs of persons with spinal cord injuries and HIV disease evoke many familiar themes (Ansello and Eustis, 1992).

Across groups and with increasing conviction among diverse chronic care interests, there is recognition that most persons with chronic long-term care needs live in the community. Moreover, most if not all of those who do not would be able to if only provided the necessary supportive services (Eustis and Fischer, 1992; Zola, 1988). For many, nursing homes are considered restrictive and unloving (Vladeck, 1980), if not the enemy in the struggle for independence and self-reliance. At the same time, there is broad recognition that deinstitutionalization is not enough, as experiences in the community of the chronically mentally ill and other groups have demonstrated.

Advocates for various long-term care groups seem to agree that primary medical care is a critical resource for prevention, managing acute symptom episodes, and monitoring self-care in the community. For the most part, however, they have little conviction that medical professionals need to play a central role in planning for community services. They are also aware, of course, that whatever the population and its insurance status, medical care nearly always is better insured and more available than assistance with community living.

The various long-term care populations, also have a common dependence on, and thus a shared interest in, SSI and Medicaid, the primary sources of income and of health insurance, respectively, for many persons with disabilities. (They also share an interest in Social Security Disability Insurance and Medicare, programs that have been more restrictive with respect to eligibility). Any efforts to restrict, expand, or otherwise reform the SSI and Medicaid programs are certain to attract common attention across these groups. Medicaid waivers for home- and community-based services are one case in point; they have become an important mechanism for service innovation not only for elderly persons but also for persons with AIDS (Merzel et al., 1992), mental retardation (Miller, 1992), and increasingly, for children and adults with physical disabilities.

The concept of a continuum of care has found its way into the discourse of these long-term care populations. The labels used to describe component services have many similarities, and some categories are virtually universal, including home-based services, personal assistance, supportive housing, service coordination and integration, and respite services. Underlying the labels is a shared conviction about the importance of nonmedical care, and the need to move beyond curative medicine to a broader conception of community living and services that make independence feasible and productive.

One other development is important in considering the extent of common ground among populations with chronic care needs. Because of steady increases in life expectancy, growing numbers of persons now counted among the younger disabled are approaching old age. Consequently, cohorts of persons disabled by SCI, polio, mental retardation and developmental disabilities, chronic mental illness, and other chronic conditions, are now developing conditions and needs associated with aging that complicate self-management of their primary disability. New subfields in the study of these populations have emerged that address issues of aging with a disability, as well as aging among the parents of younger persons with disabilities and a concomitant erosion of their capacities to provide supportive care (Kemp, Brummel-Smith, and Ramsdell, 1990; Trieschmann, 1987). Over time, as persons with diverse disabilities and experiences enter the elderly population, they may alter future expectations about living with disability in old age.

Diversity and Conflict

While there are significant commonalities in service needs and perspectives among younger and older persons with chronic conditions and diseases, there are also some notable differences in needs and the ways these are interpreted by different affected groups. These differences are important both because they have implications for services policy and because they shape the way each group views the others.

At the most general level, groups like persons with SCI and persons with AIDS have specialized care needs that differ from those of the elderly (and from each other). For example, younger populations with disabilities historically have been very concerned about employment-related issues (Berkowitz, 1987). These may include the retention of employment after the onset of illness (as in HIV infection), the adaptation by the employer of working conditions to accommodate the changing needs of the employee with a chronic condition (SCI, HIV), or the preservation of employment-related benefits after impairment makes continued work difficult or impossible (HIV, and persons with degenerative conditions like multiple sclerosis). The salience of employment issues for many younger adults with disabilities also means that service needs usually associated with the home must also be addressed in the workplace and that pressures will grow to extend home care services to diverse community settings beyond the primary residence (Eustis and Fischer, 1992).

In an era of medical complexity and specialization, the medical needs of diverse populations vary considerably, and one consequence is requirements for specialized personnel, treatments, and procedures. In the case of AIDS, this involves, among other things, an array of prescription drugs and protocols for their application that must be integrated with the delivery of community-based care. As suggested earlier, this sort of complexity is hardly unknown among elderly persons or persons with SCI, but with AIDS the monitoring of rapidly changing medical conditions becomes part of the everyday business of case management and home-based and nursing home care, among other services. The medical needs of persons with AIDS drive the delivery of chronic-care services to them to a far greater degree than is true for most other chronically ill populations. This highlights the need in future reform to address more thoroughly the integration of acute and chronic care, not only for the medically chronically ill, like persons with AIDS, but also for a range of populations with disabilities, including elderly people.

The role of nursing home care is more prominent in the continuum and more "mainstream" for the elderly, on balance, than for younger groups with disabilities. An exception to this is found in what may seem like surprising parallels between the care options available to the frail elderly and to intravenous drug users (IDUs) diagnosed with AIDS. In many cities where the number of AIDS cases has grown rapidly among IDUs, nursing homes have become the most feasible and affordable form of long-term care for them, since many are living in marginal neighborhoods and have few resources and little workable informal support. To the extent that nursing home care continues to be a viable care option for the frail elderly, institutional services will play an important role among available, publicly supported care options for both groups. (This is not to say that facility administrators believe that the elderly and their families would agree to fully integrated services within the nursing home, although in a few public facilities the two groups reside in separate units within the same building [Benjamin and Swan, 1989].)

A major conflict among the long-term care groups with respect to nursing home policy emerges because nursing homes are anathema to many persons with SCI and to many younger, middle-class persons with AIDS. Leaders of these groups perceive that advocates for older people encourage the steady expansion of nursing home coverage under public and private insurance, are concerned foremost with asset protection for the middle-class (Binstock, 1992), and tolerate the enormous fiscal bite that nursing homes take out of the public long-term care budget. The most outspoken of disability advocates, led by persons with SCI, call for the evacuation of all younger disabled persons from nursing homes and the reallocation of at least 25 percent of all federal funds for these institutions to expanded personal assistance services at home for persons with disabilities living independently in the community (DeJong, Brannon, and Batavia, 1993). The perception is that older people, by contrast, have accommodated to nursing home placement and are "soft" on service alternatives that support and maintain independence.

This emphasis on independence suggests another important difference in outlook between younger and older disabled populations that is likely to affect future reform debate. Certainly *independence* is a familiar part of the language of services to the aging, most notably those related to community care. However, the term is the core of a philosophy, independent living, that unites many persons with SCI and other physical disabilities. Whether disabled at birth or later in life, these persons have traditionally challenged societal expectations that they are incapable of a productive or enjoyable life and that they should therefore be confined and protected from a world designed for and run by the able-bodied. In response, advocates for persons with disabilities argue that the issue is not their disabilities but the ways in which society responds, or fails to respond, to them. Persons with disabilities are able to lead productive, economically and socially rewarding lives using what are now well-understood models of personal assistance in daily activity, appropriate adaptations of the physical environment of the home and community to make them accessible to everyone, and equal opportunities for education, employment, and recreation (Batavia, DeJong, and McKnew, 1991; Berkowitz, 1987).

These younger groups interpret services for the elderly as intended to achieve something considerably less, because community-based care of frail older persons is primarily designed to maintain them in their homes. But independent living advocates view the home as a potential prison, not unlike the nursing home. From their perspective, the measure of independence is the ability of the person with a disability to pursue life goals in and out of the home with minimal barriers and without restrictive expectations on the part of others. They feel that age differences and philosophy matter a great deal in shaping what services are provided and what they are designed to achieve. At the least, current and future debate about home care policy will need to integrate flexible models of home care that acknowledge differences in the definition and goals of care.

Conclusions

Increasingly, scholars and advocates traditionally concerned with frail elderly persons will need to come to terms with the range of younger groups with disabilities now making competing demands for long-term care resources. As they do so, they will be confronted with both new and familiar themes that challenge conventional thinking about services for those with severe disabilities (Simon-Rusinowitz and Hofland, 1993). Among these are consumer choice and the importance of consumer preferences versus the customary family and professional ones; social and economic perspectives on services versus medically related ones; and a view of independent living that focuses on removing physical barriers and strengthening consumer direction over personal assistance as crucial elements of service planning.

As chronic services come to be understood in terms of a range of population groups, the importance of flexible financing, planning, and delivery will become more apparent. The structuring of such flexibility may be the greatest challenge of all confronting public policy, and a failure to incorporate flexibility will make it difficult to respond to the diversity of needs within and across populations.

In the Pepper Bill of 1987 (H.R. 2762), the Pepper Commission Report in 1990 (U.S. Congress, 1990), and the Health Security Plan of the Clinton administration in 1993 (White House Domestic Policy Council, 1993), policymakers have attempted to forge home- and community-based service programs aimed at both elderly and nonelderly persons with disabilities. These proposals have included a range of benefits for all persons who meet a generic standard of functional need—in the Clinton proposal, need for assistance in three or more ADL areas—regardless of age or type of disability. In the process of working on national health care reform, the

American Association of Retired Persons offered its proposal to the Consortium for Citizens with Disabilities, which includes about 45 organizations representing children and adults with disabilities, for review. The result was some significant changes in language and emphasis to accommodate nonelderly disability groups, as well as an apparent willingness on both sides to collaborate on future proposals.

While these developments are significant, they erase neither the tendency of American social and health policy to deal with groups on a categorical basis nor the territoriality of categorical interests that, in turn, have labored long and hard for their share of the budgetary pie (Torres-Gil and Pynoos, 1986). This is not such a bad thing. The service needs of various groups seem to differ in substance, emphasis, and style.

What seems especially promising is new and comparative research and analysis that considers service issues across disability groups. Such an approach brings into play both the commonality and the diversity across populations, and it can highlight new and creative ways of thinking about how to provide services to the frail elderly and to younger persons with disabilities.

References

Andrews, R., Preston, B., Howell, E., and Keyes, M. (1989). A comparative analysis of AIDS service demonstration projects in Los Angeles, Miami, New York, and San Francisco. Report submitted to the Health Resources and Services Administration. Washington, D.C.: SysteMetrics/McGraw Hill.

Ansello, E. F., and Eustis, N. N. (1992). A common stake? Investigating the emerging "intersection" of aging and disabilities. In E. F. Ansello and N. N. Eustis, eds. *Aging and Disabilities: Seeking Common Ground* (pp. 1–8). Amityville, N.Y.: Baywood Publishing.

Batavia, A. I., DeJong, G., and McKnew, L. B. (1991). Toward a national personal assistance program: The independent living model of long-term care for persons with disabilities. *Journal of Health Politics, Policy and Law* 16 (3): 523–45.

Benjamin, A. E. (1988). Long-term care and AIDS: Perspectives from experience with the elderly. *Milbank Quarterly* 66 (3): 415–43.

Benjamin, A. E. (1989). Perspectives on a continuum of care for persons with HIV illness. *Medical Care Review* 46 (4): 411–37.

Benjamin, A. E. (1993). An historical perspective on home care policy. *Milbank Quarterly* 71:129–66.

Benjamin, A. E., and Bennett, T. (1991). Chronic care for persons with HIV disease. Unpublished report to the American Foundation for AIDS Research.

Benjamin, A. E., Lee, P. R., and Solkowitz, S. N. (1988). Case management of persons with acquired immunodeficiency syndrome in San Francisco. *Health Care Financing Review,* ann. suppl.:69–74.

Benjamin, A. E., and Swan, J. H. (1989). Nursing home care for persons with HIV illness. *Generations* 13 (4): 63–64.

Berkowitz, E. D. (1987). *Disabled Policy, America's Programs for the Handicapped: A Twentieth Century Fund Report.* New York: Cambridge University Press.

Binstock, R. H. (1992). Aging, disability, and long-term care: The politics of common ground. In E. F. Ansello and N. N. Eustis, eds., *Aging and Disabilities: Seeking Common Ground* (pp. 165–75). Amityville, N.Y.: Baywood Publishing.

DeJong, G., and Batavia, A. I. (1991). Toward a health services research capacity in spinal cord injury. *Paraplegia* 29 (6): 373–89.

DeJong, G., Brannon, R., and Batavia, A. I. (1993). Financing health and personal care. In G. G. Whiteneck et al., eds., *Aging with Spinal Cord Injury* (pp. 275–94). New York: Demos Publications.

Eisenberg, M. G., and Saltz, C. C. (1991). Quality of life among aging spinal cord injured persons: Long-term rehabilitation outcomes. *Paraplegia* 29 (8): 514–20.

Eustis, N. N., and Fischer, L. R. (1992). Common needs, different solutions? Younger and older homecare clients. In E. F. Ansello and N. N. Eustis, eds., *Aging and Disabilities: Seeking Common Ground* (pp. 25–37). Amityville, N.Y.: Baywood Publishing.

Feder, J., and Scanlon, W. (1992). People with disabilities: A review of current knowledge. Unpublished report. Washington, D.C.: Georgetown University, Center for Health Policy Studies.

Fee, E., and Fox, D. M., eds. (1992). *AIDS: The Making of a Chronic Disease.* Berkeley: University of California Press.

Fleishman, J. A., Hsia, D. C., and Hellinger, F. J. (1993). Correlates of medical service utilization among people with HIV infection. Unpublished paper.

Fleishman, J. A., and Mor, V. (1993). Insurance status among people with AIDS: Relationships with sociodemographic characteristics and service use. *Inquiry* 30 (2): 180–88.

Fleishman, J. A., Mor, V., and Piette, J. (1991). AIDS case management: The client's perspective. *HSR: Health Services Research* 26 (4): 447–70.

Green, J., and Arno, P. S. (1990). The 'medicaidization' of AIDS: Trends in the financing of HIV-related medical care. *Journal of the American Medical Association* 264 (10): 1261–66.

Harvey, C., Rothschild, B. B., Asmann, A. J., and Stripling, T. (1990). New estimates of traumatic SCI prevalence: A survey-based approach. *Paraplegia* 28: 537–44.

Hellinger, F. (1992). Forecasts of the costs for medical care for persons with HIV, 1992–1995. *Inquiry* 29 (3): 356–63.

Ho, D., Pomerantz, R. J., and Kaplan, J. C. (1987). Pathogenesis of infection with human immunodeficiency virus. *New England Journal of Medicine* 317 (5): 287–86.

Infeld, D. L., and Southby, R. M. F. (1989). *AIDS and Long-Term Care: A New Dimension*. Owings Mills, Md.: National Health Publishing.

Institute of Medicine (1990). *Broadening the Base of Treatment for Alcohol Problems*. Washington, D.C.: National Academy Press.

Kemp, B. J., Brummel-Smith, K., and Ramsdell, J., eds. (1990). *Geriatric Rehabilitation*. San Diego: Pro-Ed Publishers.

Krause, L. E., and Stoddard, S. (1989). *Chartbook on Disability in the United States*. Washington, D.C.: U.S. National Institute on Disability and Rehabilitation Research.

Lakin, K. C., Hill, B. K., Chen, T.-H., and Stephens, S. A. (1989). Persons with mental retardation and related conditions in mental retardation facilities: Selected findings from the 1987 National Medical Expenditure Survey. Minneapolis: Center for Residential and Community Services, University of Minnesota.

LaPlante, M., and Miller, K. (1992). Disability statistics abstract. Disability Statistics Program, Institute for Health and Aging, School of Nursing, University of California, San Francisco.

LaPlante, M., Rice, D. P., and Kraus, L. E. (1991). Disability statistics abstract. Disability Statistics Program, Institute for Health and Aging, School of Nursing, University of California, San Francisco.

Lemp, G. F., Hirozawa, A. M., Cohen, J. B., Derish, P. A., McKinney, K. C., and Hernandez, S. R. (1992). Survival for women and men with AIDS. *Journal of Infectious Diseases* 166 (1): 74–79.

Lemp, G. F., Payne, S. F., Neal, D., Temelso, T., and Rutherford, G. W. (1990). Survival trends for patients with AIDS. *Journal of the American Medical Association* 263 (3): 402–6.

Litvak, S., and Kennedy, J. (1991). Policy issues affecting the Medicaid personal care services optional benefit. Oakland, Calif.: Research and Training Center on Public Policy in Independent Living at the World Institute on Disability.

Mahoney, C. W., Estes, C. L., and Heumann, J. E. (1986). *Toward a Unified Agenda: Proceedings of a National Conference on Disability and Aging*. San Francisco: Institute for Health and Aging, University of California, pp. 125–27.

Mandershein, R. W., and Sonnenschein, M. A., eds. (1992). *Mental Health U.S. 1992*. DHHS pub. no. (SMA) 92–1942. Washington, D.C.: Center for Mental Health Services and the National Institute of Mental Health.

Mann, J. (1991). Essay: AIDS and the next pandemic. *Scientific American* (March): 126.

Max, W., and Rice, D. P. (1993). Shooting in the dark: Estimating the cost of firearm injuries. *Health Affairs* 12 (4): 171–85.

Menter, R. R., Whiteneck, G. G., Charlifue, S. W., Gerhart, K., Solnick, S. J., Brooks, C. A., and Hughes, L. (1991). Impairment, disability, handicap, and medical expenses of persons aging with spinal cord injuries. *Paraplegia* 29 (9): 613–19.

Merzel, C., Crystal, S., Sambamoorthi, U., Karus, D., and Kurland, C. (1992). New Jersey's Medicaid waiver for acquired immunodeficiency syndrome. *Health Care Financing Review* 13 (3): 27–44.

Miller, N. A. (1992). Medicaid 2176 home and community-based care waivers: The first ten years. *Health Affairs* 11 (4): 162–71.

Minkler, M. (1990). Aging and disability: Behind and beyond the stereotypes. *Journal of Aging Studies* 4 (3): 245–60.

Mor, V., Piette, J., and Fleishman, J. (1989). Community-based management for persons with AIDS. *Health Affairs* 8 (4): 139–53.

National Spinal Cord Injury Association (1992). Spinal cord injury statistical information. Fact sheet no. 2. Woburn, Mass.: National Spinal Cord Injury Association.

Newcomer, R. J., and Benjamin, A. E. (1995). *Perspectives on the Monitoring of Chronic Conditions and Community Responsiveness*. Report to the Robert Wood Johnson Foundation. San Francisco: University of California, Institute for Health and Aging.

Nosek, M. A., Roth, P. L., and Zhu, Y. (1990). Independent living programs: The impact of program age, consumer control, and budget on program operation. *Journal of Rehabilitation* 56 (4): 28–35.

O'Dell, M. W., Crawford, A., Bohi, E., and Bonner, F. J. (1991). Disability in persons hospitalized with AIDS. *American Journal of Physical Medicine and Rehabilitation* 70 (2): 91–95.

Riley, M. W., Ory, M. G., and Zablotsky, D., eds. (1989). *AIDS in an Aging Society*. New York: Springer Publishing.

Simon-Rusinowitz, L., and Hofland, B. F. (1993). Adopting a disability approach to home care services for older adults. *Gerontologist* 33 (2): 159–67.

Sims, B., Manley, S., and Richardson, G. N. (1993). A model of lifetime services. In G. Whiteneck et al., eds. *Aging with Spinal Cord Injury* (pp. 353–60). New York: Demos Publications.

Stein, R. E. K., ed. (1989). *Caring for Children with Chronic Illness*. New York: Springer Publishing.

Swan, J. H., and Benjamin, A. E. (1993). IV drug use, dementia, and nursing home care for PWAs. *Journal of Health and Social Policy* 4 (3): 79–91.

Thornton, C. (1990). *Characteristics of Persons with Developmental Disabilities: Evidence from the Survey of Income and Program Participation*. Princeton: Mathematica Policy Research.

Torres-Gil, F., and Pynoos, J. (1986). Long-term care policy and interest group struggles. *Gerontologist* 488–95.

Trieschmann, R. B. (1987). *Aging with a Disability*. New York: Demos Publications.

Trieschmann, R. B. (1988). *Spinal Cord Injuries: Psychological, Social, and Vocational Rehabilitation*. New York: Demos Publications.

U.S. Centers for Disease Control and Prevention (1993). *HIV/AIDS Surveillance Report*. Mid-year ed. Vol 7., no.1.

U.S. Congress (1990). House and Senate Bipartisan Commission on Comprehensive Health Care (Pepper Commission). *A Call for Action*. Washington, D.C.: U.S. Government Printing Office.

Vladeck, B. C. (1980). *Unloving Care: The Nursing Home Tragedy*. New York: Basic Books.

White House Domestic Policy Council (1993). *The President's Health Security Plan*. New York: Times Books, Random House.

Yarkony, G. M., Roth, E. J., Meyer, P. R., Lovell, L., Heinemann, A. W., and Betts, H. B. (1990). Spinal cord injury care system: Fifteen-year experience at the Rehabilitation Institute of Chicago. *Paraplegia* 28 (5): 321–29.

Zola, I. K. (1988). Policies and programs concerning aging and disability: Toward a unifying agenda. In S. Sullivan and M. Ein Lewin, eds. *The Economics and Ethics of Long-Term Care and Disability* (pp. 90–130). Washington, D.C.: American Enterprise Institute for Public Policy Research.

5

The Role of Technology in Long-Term Care

Leighton E. Cluff, M.D., M.A.C.P.

Health care technology and improved socioeconomic conditions are significant contributors to increased life expectancy. These changes have also prolonged the lives of many with chronic disabilities. Essential and growing parts of long-term care for those with various functional limitations are supportive and assistive technologies. Further improvement in long-term care and in the lives of the disabled, irrespective of their age, will be determined largely by the availability and appropriate use of current and new technology. The essentiality of the long-term assistance and support provided by skilled and compassionate personal attendants, however, cannot be overemphasized.

It has been estimated that 36 to 42 million people in the United States have disabilities severe enough to interfere with their ability to work or perform activities of daily living, often necessitating long-term care. Activities of daily living encompass the basic abilities to eat, bathe, dress, ambulate, and control excretory functions, along with the more complex tasks needed to prepare meals, shop for groceries, do household chores, drive motor vehicles, and so forth (University of California, San Francisco, 1989; U.S. Department of Education, 1991).

Planners and providers of long-term care must consider the degree to which persons with disabilities require technologic assistance, the clinical condition requiring medical attention, and the extent to which these circumstances vary with an individual's age (LaPlante, 1991). Physical disabilities vary, and the technologies that contribute to impaired persons' functional effectiveness and, at times, their continued survival range from the simple and inexpensive ("low tech") to the more complex and costly ("high tech"). Such technology makes it possible for physically disabled persons to care for themselves, walk, move from place to place, drive automobiles, graduate from college, marry and have children, assume responsibilities, and carry out many tasks formerly considered impossible for disabled individuals.

Thus, people with functional limitations, impairments, or disabilities, if properly assisted and cared for, can enjoy productive lives and personal fulfillment. Although those not afflicted may view physically disabled persons as unhealthy or leading a life of diminished quality, technology and long-term supportive care can help affected persons see themselves as healthy and the quality of their lives as good. In fact, some who are severely disabled accept their condition as a challenge and are motivated to maximize their function. With the assistance of technology and supportive care, they can make significant contributions to their own lives, the lives of others, and their communities.

Applications of Technologies

Health care "definitive technologies," those used to prevent and cure diseases and disorders, have had a profound impact on patient survival from ailments and afflictions that were once fatal. However, supportive or assistive ("half-way") technologies, which do not prevent or cure disease, have shaped, changed, and increased the need and demand for long-term care. Lives have been prolonged for many infants, children, adolescents, adults, and elderly persons suffering from acute and chronic illnesses, congenital and acquired abnormalities, and injuries secondary to trauma or violence. These survivors often experience physical disabilities and functional losses of varying severity that can be permanent and/or progressive. Supportive or assistive technologies have been designed to help restore and maintain patient function; enhance mobility, accessibility, communication, and employment; and assist body functions.

Although there have been important advances in the development of definitive technologies, there has been less investment in the development of the supportive or assistive technologies essential to long-term care. Important contributions have resulted, however, in response to individual impairments and disabilities resulting from military conflicts. In recent years such technologies have also been stimulated by the aging of America's population due to the increase in life expectancy and because people are surviving previously fatal medical conditions. A major goal of long-term care today is to accelerate the development of new technology, to provide patients not just a longer life but a better life.

Technologies for assisting in activities of daily living are many. Their importance to long-term care and to the lives of the disabled is best conveyed by case studies, three of which follow.

A child with cystic fibrosis and respiratory insufficiency, cared for at home by his mother, periodically requires respiratory technology to assist breathing and bronchial suction to remove inspissated secretions, because he is subject to recurrent pulmonary infections. Constant attention is necessary, placing enormous demands on the mother, father, and siblings. Employment of a nurse or other health professional to care for the youngster is prohibitively expensive and, except for the very affluent, is not possible. Episodic home visits by a professional may be available to provide instruction and guidance and to monitor care; but most of the attention needed by the patient must be provided by the mother or other family members. Respite is not easily provided because of the technologic requirements. The patient's father works outside the home and can provide some assistance at night and on weekends, but the mother bears most of the responsibility. The siblings may be neglected because of demands placed upon the parents in caring for the patient. In the absence of definitive technology to prevent or cure the youngster's cystic fibrosis, but with the availability of supportive technology, he may live with his disability for many years. Clearly, technology is necessary to maintain the patient's life, delay the onset of pulmonary infections, slow progression of the disease, and maintain some level of normal daily activity.

In 1952, before the availability of polio vaccine, this patient acquired poliomyelitis, as a teenager. He developed paralysis of both upper and lower extremities and, in the beginning, an electrical (and mechanical) respirator (ventilator) was breathing for him. After his initial hospitalization, he was cared for by his mother at home, where he was confined to the respirator. His excretory functions and bathing (including skin care) had to be carried out while in the respirator. He could speak only during respirator-controlled exhalations. The commitment of the mother to his care contributed to his ability in adapting to his disability and becoming motivated to overcome the limitations imposed by his impairments. With advances in technology he was provided with a positive pressure portable respirator, and with a plastic tube attached to the respirator and placed in his mouth he learned how to inflate his lungs. This enabled him to speak as his chest involuntarily forced air out of his lungs. After the development of electronic instrumentation, he obtained a wheelchair that could be operated with limited hand motion. He entered the University of California at Berkeley, where he had an important role in establishing the Center for Independent Living, to serve disabled persons. He was the first quadriplegic to graduate from the University of California. Today, some 40 years later, still respirator dependent and confined to a wheelchair, he requires an attendant to assist in meeting his personal needs. Over several years he became a champion for the disabled, influencing development of federal legislation to remove discrimination and to provide financial assistance and health insurance coverage for the disabled. He was married and fathered a child. He had a major role in establishing the World Institute on Disability, was honored by the presidents of the United States and France, and received many awards to assist him in his work. Technology saved his life when he was a teenager; with newer technology he was able to be very productive; and he believes he has had a good life.

An 85-year-old woman began to have cognitive impairment with forgetfulness and intermittent inability to remember where she was. One afternoon, when walking in her neighborhood, she fell and broke her hip. While hospitalized she developed a cardiac arrhythmia and heart failure, which was controlled by digitalis and diuretics, after which her hip joint was replaced by a prosthesis. She was discharged from the hospital within five days to a skilled nursing home, where she received physical therapy and assistance in regaining muscle strength and learning to use a walker. On returning home after two months, she was noted by family members that the acuity of her hearing and vision had deteriorated further, possibly contributing to greater cognitive impairment. A hearing aid helped compensate for the hearing loss, but she was found to have a retinal hemorrhage, and her visual acuity could not be fully restored. She was unable to read. A telephone with large numbers and a loud ring made it possible for her to speak to others, but she also made inappropriate and expensive calls to distant places. Television became her principal contact with the outside world. An elevated commode was placed in her lavatory to aid excretory function. She was dependent on a walker to get about her apartment. She often stumbled, however, because of a foot-drop and shag carpet, which had to be replaced with a smooth carpet over which she could ambulate without falling. She became progressively more confused and unable to care for herself, but she remained at home alone, depending upon visits by her aging daughters, home health aides, meals-on-wheels, a physiotherapist, and a podiatrist. One night she awoke to go to the lava-

tory next to her bedroom, fell, and was unable to reach her telephone or rise. In the morning a neighbor went to visit and, getting no response to her knock, called 911 for the emergency response system. On entering the apartment, they found the woman lying on the floor in shock. She was rehospitalized. While in the hospital she suffered a pulmonary embolus and was found to be anemic for which she received blood transfusions. After seven days in the hospital she was readmitted to a nursing home. She developed bedsores, requiring dressings and frequent turning. Her level of cognition deteriorated, which was probably attributable, in part, to the many medications she was receiving. Restrained by guard rails while in bed, when out of bed she was confined to a wheelchair, strapped in to prevent her from attempting to rise and walk. The four years following her hip fracture included two hospitalizations and two nursing home admissions, surgery, blood transfusions, use of a walker, modification of her apartment, physiotherapy, a podiatrist to clip her toe nails, modification of her telephone, provision of a hearing aid, use of an emergency response system, treatment of bedsores, and medication for heart failure and cardiac arrhythmia, as well as for disturbed cognition and behavior requiring restraints. She died in the nursing home.

These cases illustrate that sophisticated, complex, and supportive technologies can prevent death, enable a productive life, place demands and burdens on families and friends, contribute to improved function, but also result in progressive impairment. The growth of simple, complex, and costly technologies in the past several years has been phenomenal, encouraged by their effectiveness and by reimbursement or payment policies (Arras, 1995).

A list of technologies that have become important in long term-care would be extensive. Too often, however, some available technologies are not put to use in long-term care. For this reason, a running examination of both low-level and sophisticated technology is described, to emphasize the extent to which modifications of residential conditions, supportive, and complex technologies all contribute to long-term care.

Showers and lavatories can be equipped with technologically simple devices to help prevent persons from falling. Kitchens can be modified so that physically impaired or disabled persons can prepare their own meals. Special flooring can be placed that will reduce slipping or stumbling. Ramps can be installed for those confined to wheelchairs. Lifts can be placed so that a disabled person can rise from a chair or be transported to a second-story bedroom.

Electronic devices enable persons to communicate with response systems in the event of emergencies. Telephones can be modified for those with hearing or visual impairments. Computer technology enables homebound persons to maintain contact with others and to engage in educational and other productive activities.

Robotic aids, dogs, and even lower primates, can be used to assist with tasks that are difficult or impossible for physically impaired and disabled persons to accomplish on their own (Reardon, 1990; Regalbuto, Krouskop, and Cheatham, 1992). Wheelchairs, computers, and other electronic and mechanical devices are designed to perform specific tasks on command by the user. Control and use of these devices can be customized, to be operated, for example, by joystick, mouthstick, vocal command, or modified keyboard, to meet the particular limitations of the user. On command, these technologies can assist disabled people in performing various activities of daily living.

Prostheses for the upper extremity (above or below the elbow) are relatively well developed. These prostheses can be powered either by remaining, or residual, muscle and skeletal function, or by myoelectric hand and arm devices. Prostheses for the lower extremity (above or below the knee) assist in walking and stance control. Many of these devices now can be manipulated by electronic microprocessors. Various orthoses, such as braces, mobile arm supports, and powered upper and lower extremity devices (including electrically stimulated mechanisms), are particularly important to individuals with neuromuscular, as well as skeletal and articular, impairments. Replacement of dysfunctional or diseased hip, knee, ankle, shoulder, elbow, wrist, and finger joints with artificial prostheses is becoming commonplace.

Wheelchairs may be either hand operated or motorized and controlled by hand, eye, or head movement. Private cars and vans can be customized with wheelchair lifts, and special driver control modifications make it possible for some disabled persons to drive automobiles. Public transport systems are being modified so that wheelchair-bound disabled persons are able to use them. Curbing of walkways can be modified so that persons using wheelchairs or canes are not impeded. Elevators can be adapted for the blind and deaf so that they can identify and signal the floor desired.

Removal of architectural barriers to improve accessibility to houses, public and private buildings, hospitals, nursing homes, and other facilities often is necessary to accommodate the impairments of disabled persons. Desks, chairs, beds, and other furniture can be modified to meet the needs of the disabled. Retirement communities and health-care facilities must be designed to accommodate persons in wheelchairs, with doors that are wider than usual, ramps, elevators, directional signs, and other aids. Rehabilitation facilities must be designed to meet the needs of those with a variety of impairments, as well as providing the modalities needed for treating and training both the disabled and their caregivers.

Increasingly, theaters, auditoriums, and churches are being equipped with sound systems for the hearing impaired, and directional signs in public places are being modified so that visually impaired persons can read them.

Perhaps in no other area have there been such remarkable advances as in computer technology. In addition to the famous example of the noted physicist Stephen Hawking, other persons unable or barely able to speak can communicate by activating a computer or other electronic device, by head motion or with their eyes, which produces understandable language. Even though Hawking's body is confined to a wheelchair because of amyotrophic lateral sclerosis (ALS), his disability has not stood in the way of his making some of the most important scientific accomplishments of this century. Some have even argued that this very confinement of his body has actually been instrumental in allowing his mind to travel where others have never been.

Job-station modifications (machine tools and office equipment adaptations) and specialized assistive devices to enhance job performance make it possible for many physically impaired and disabled persons to be employed and do productive work. Technology can help the blind to see, the deaf to hear, the paraplegic and quadriplegic to write, teach, compose music. Computers have revolutionized the employment of disabled persons, including those with intellectual impairments (Hunt and Berkowitz, 1992).

Various impairments of even vital functions of the body are now amenable to advanced, sophisticated long-term health-care interventions. These include mechanical and electrical devices to assist or maintain respiratory function, pacemakers to control normal cardiac rhythm, hemodialysis for those with chronic and life-threatening kidney impairment, parenteral alimentation for administration of nutrients and medications, devices to assist persons with micturition and defecation control, and copulation aids that have enabled some with profound neuromuscular dysfunction to conceive children.

These are some of the many technologies that are important to the long-term care of many disabled persons, irrespective of age.

The Use of Technology in Different Settings

Home-Based Care

Technologies once available only in hospitals or nursing homes are now available in the home for the long-term care of severely impaired persons. As important as this technologic support is to long-term care in the home, to be truly helpful it must be used correctly. It is essential, therefore, that trained health-care professionals supervise the in-home use of low-tech as well as high-tech long-term care aids. Both the persons dependent on the technology and their caregivers must be helped to manage the complexities of such home care (McInerny, 1988).

Nursing Home Care

Hospitalized patients are being discharged more quickly, often to nursing homes (see Chapter 7). The severity of the illness and disability of the nursing home population is therefore increasing. In addition, when caregivers are unable to manage long-term care at home, their patients usually are admitted to nursing homes (R. L. Kane, 1988). These individuals often require extensive high and low technologic support and professional attention.

To provide this additional care, nursing home personnel must be properly trained to use the technology that is and will become available for the care of their more disabled and ill residents. The number of nursing homes serving as teaching institutions, where physicians, nurses, and other health-care professionals gain experiences in up-to-date nursing home settings, needs to be expanded. Otherwise, provision of necessary skilled care and supervision will not be regularly available.

The Long-Term Acute Care Hospital

Increases in the number of children and adults who are ventilator dependent present enormous problems for acute care hospitals, for nursing homes, and for families. Changes in health care reimbursement have substantially reduced the availability of conventional long-term care options for these individuals. In response, hospitals have developed facilities and services to provide "long-term acute care." Several such institutions have been established nationwide. As long as reimbursement systems provide adequate financing, facilities and programs providing alternatives to acute care hospitals and nursing homes for persons dependent upon critical life-sustaining technology are likely to be established (Lundberg and Nole, 1990).

Rehabilitation Medicine and Physical Therapy

Physical medicine and rehabilitation (PM&R) activities in hospitals, specialized centers, and other institutions, have become important to long-term care. They address aspects of functional limitations and elements of the physical and social environments that preclude participation by impaired individuals in "normal" activities. These services, generally, are provided to improve the quality of life by restoring function to the maximum level possible or by delaying the progression of functional loss (Kottke and Lehman, 1990). The optimal function these services are designed to restore is not only medical but also psychological, social, and vocational. In the past few decades, the traditional belief that rest was the cure for most everything that ailed a patient has become outdated and has been replaced by the realization that mobilization and aggressive rehabilitation provide most patients the best opportunity to return to a full life.

Physical medicine and rehabilitation began in the 1930s as a subspecialty of internal medicine, to address musculoskeletal and neurological problems. During World War II, the field expanded its scope considerably, as thousands of military veterans returned to the United States with significant disabilities. This led to a new direction for the field; that of helping to restore the veterans to productive lives. The civilian medical community soon began to recognize the inherent value of rehabilitative medicine, and in 1947 PM&R was approved as a specialty of medicine dealing with the functional concerns of disability. Since then, allied professional disciplines, such as physical and occupational therapy, have been established to assist the disabled to function beyond the boundaries of their limitations.

The technology of PM&R has expanded greatly during the past 50 years, and the services provided are now extensive. Rehabilitation involves the integration of many procedures and technologies to restore individuals to their optimal functional status at home and in the community. Using a variety of procedures and technical measurements, physiatrists can make functional, vocational, and psychosocial assessments of disabled persons. They also have a wide variety of treatment modalities available, including heat and cold therapies, electrotherapies, massage, biofeedback, traction, therapeutic exercises, mobility devices, extremity prostheses and orthoses, management of chronic pain, training for home-making activities, and procedures and technologies applied in the management of functional loss caused by specific health problems.

Social, political, and medical emphasis on acute health care has limited the use and availability of rehabilitation programs, even though, today, patients with chronic diseases and disabilities constitute the majority of persons needing rehabilitation as well as acute and long-term medical care. In addition, health insurance programs limit the potential establishment, provision, and use of rehabilitation facilities and services. Nevertheless, hospitals, nursing homes, extended-care facilities, and other institutions are establishing rehabilitation components, but there are not enough qualified health professionals to provide the comprehensive evaluation, treatment, and supervision needed to ensure the most effective care.

Other Settings

The increase in the numbers of physically impaired and severely demented elderly persons has led to development of special residential and day-care facilities tailored to these groups' functional abilities. Residential settings designed specifically for those who are demented can provide the assistive technology and architectural design that make it possible for individuals with different levels of dementia and incapacity to function maximally, and be in a protective and supportive environment.

Foster home arrangements have been useful in providing assistance for disabled and technology-dependent children and, to a limited extent, for disabled elderly persons requiring a limited amount of assistance. Similarly, congregate living facilities for frail elderly persons are available but, generally, are not suitable for those who are technology dependent.

Intermediate-care institutions (i.e., assisted living facilities that fall between family home and skilled nursing home) are useful in caring for disabled elderly persons who need some assistance but do not require extensive technologic support and whose circumstances preclude their remaining at home.

Long-Term Care Needs of Specific Age Groups

Long-term care of the young, employed, elderly, and other population groups with chronic disabilities who are technology dependent has some common elements; but often the requirements, methods of financing, and impact upon caregivers, families, and society differ.

Infants, Children, and Adolescents

In the United States, approximately 4 percent of persons under the age of 21 requiring long-term care have one or more developmental disabilities, such as cerebral palsy, mental retardation, hearing or vision impairments, autism, or structural birth defects (e.g., spina bifida) requiring long-term, generally lifelong, care. These disabilities affect about 80,000 additional children each year (Pope and Tarlov, 1991).

Minimizing these impairments and disabilities requires aggressive intervention through education, life-style changes, and treatment, even before a child is conceived. Physicians, midwives, nurses, pharmacists, and other health professionals have a responsibility to assist child-bearing women in avoiding hazardous substances and events, to reduce acquired developmental disabilities in their offspring.

The consequences of lifelong disabilities, whether inherited, acquired during pregnancy, or acquired at birth, combined with growing interest in genetic and perinatal interventions, pose dilemmas for parents and challenges to service delivery systems and social and public policy (Fullerton et al., 1994). Technology that can identify possible genetic and developmental abnormalities, as well as genetic counseling, must be accessible from each community. Detection of fetal and genetic abnormalities can generate parental dilemmas regarding termination of pregnancy or ability to care for a disabled person. This also influences social and policy issues related to abortion and to society's responsibility to provide and finance the long-term care of disabled infants and children, some of whom will be dependent during a long life on costly technologic and supportive care. Society must be informed and have an opportunity to debate, and participate in developing, policies that are responsive to the nation's social diversity, values, and principles, but society must also face the financial obligations it may have to assume.

Despite the potential benefits of prenatal care and other preventive measures, the number of very low birthweight infants who survive with physical and mental impairments requiring long-term care is likely to increase in the decades ahead. Previously, these young persons might have died or been placed in publicly supported facilities. Now, many of these disabled infants survive to become children and adults and are cared for by their families. A survey in New York State, however, revealed that a significant proportion of technology-dependent children were retained "inappropriately" in acute care hospitals, primarily because of a shortage of nursing services in the community as well as of beds in appropriate skilled nursing facilities, and because of family problems that prevented long-term care in the home (O'Connor, Vander-Plaats, and Betz, 1992).

Traffic injuries and violence, often associated with alcohol and drug abuse, are major causes of disability, particularly among teenagers. However, the wearing of automobile seatbelts has been increasing, and supplemental restraint systems (airbags) are being installed in newer automobiles. These factors and improved technology should help decrease the incidence of disability and the need for long-term care resulting from vehicular accidents.

Increasing numbers of children dependent on assistive and supportive technology are being cared for in their family homes (Farrell and Fost, 1989). Yet, long-term care in the home can present many difficulties for parents and siblings. Constant attention is required by children who are dependent on parenteral nutrition or ventilators, who need assistance in bathing, dressing, or eating, or who are confined to bed or wheelchair. Many parents, especially mothers, commit their lives to caring for their impaired and disabled children. As a result, siblings may be neglected and a needed second income may be lost. Respite for family caregivers is not always possible, and persons willing and able to share responsibilities frequently are not available. A study in California revealed that failure of parents to request financial assistance and inadequate reinbursement presented major problems in providing respite services to needy families (O'Connor, Vander-Plaats, and Betz, 1992). As a result, family members frequently experience economic, social, and emotional ordeals that can lead to separation and divorce, which places even further stress on the parent left with care of the disabled child.

The efforts of family caregivers providing long-term care for technology-dependent children can be complemented by help from relatives, friends, fellow church members, and volunteers. Properly trained or experienced retired persons and others in the community can provide significant support and respite for family caregivers. Community professional services may be available but they are costly, and private insurance often provides only limited coverage for necessary services. Federal and state programs may cover some of these services, particularly for the poor, but middle-class Americans often face financial difficulties. Better integration and coordination between social programs and long-term health care, and more appropriate financing methods, are necessary if the services and technology required by physically impaired and disabled children are to become more universally available.

Systematic planning is also necessary for technology-dependent disabled children and adolescents in their educational settings. Appropriate training of all school personnel is important. Data as to the long-term care requirements and performance of disabled and nondisabled children should be provided to health and school authorities on a regular basis to ensure that the children's needs are appropriately met. Federal legislation that "mainstreams" disabled children into regular classrooms can present difficulties. Teachers, administrators, and health care providers should be given assistance as they accommodate technology-dependent children in classrooms. A program in Massachusetts provides schools with the consultation of health professionals and educators with experience in integrating disabled children into conventional educational institutions (Palfrey et al., 1992).

Impaired infants and children may remain technology dependent their entire lives. They may be dependent on ventilator assistance, confined to a wheelchair, have limited if any upper or lower extremity function, or require personal assistance for bathing, eating, or excretory function. Some may have persistent paralysis of the lower extremities, requiring the use of crutches for mobility. Also, as illustrated by those who had poliomyelitis and are now older, long-term use of various assistive or supportive technologies can result in adverse consequences. Disabled persons who have to use crutches throughout their lives can suffer deterioration of shoulder function and other difficulties.

Adults

In 1987, 17 million American workers suffered work-related disabilities, and the number has not varied significantly in the past several years. The incidence of work-related disability is greater in the older work population. Those affected by job-related injuries or environmental hazards usually require either short-term or long-term care at home, depending on the nature and severity of the disability. People who are disabled because of significant skeletal, muscular, or neurological impairments secondary to injury can be permanently dependent on supportive technology.

Courageous efforts by affected persons and family members have helped many disabled workers return to productive lives. Fortunately, federal and state programs provide assistance and support for the health care and technologic needs of disabled workers, and Workers' Compensation also provides financial assistance to those with work-related disabilities. Workers' Compensation programs, though, have become a financial burden for many employers, particularly in industries and businesses where hazards are the greatest. In addition, services provided by Workers' Compensation for work-related disabilities have contributed significantly to the nation's rising health care costs.

Military veterans with service-connected disabilities receive considerable support from the Department of Veterans Affairs, which provides them with needed technologies (e.g., wheelchairs, specially designed vehicles for transportation, ventilators), rehabilitation services, financial support, and personal assistants. The families of disabled veterans are provided with respite services in VA medical centers and hospitals, services that are not readily available for disabled workers and their families. Thus, as universal health-care coverage is developed, it is important to consider ways in which all disabled adults can have access to services that assist them and their families.

Elderly Persons

The elderly population, particularly those 85 years of age and older, is growing in number; and, with advancing age, physical disabilities become increasingly common. Those over the age of 75 are more likely to suffer multiple, chronic health problems. These chronic conditions limit daily activities and the ability to care for oneself. Thus, those over 75 years of age, more than any other age group, depend on assistive and supportive technology.

Appropriate use of health-care technology in managing the medical problems and disabilities of elderly persons is essential for preventing or minimizing the progression of their disabilities (Rusin, 1990; Solomon et al., 1988). Health professionals need to be better trained in providing the long-term care, support, and guidance necessitated by the myriad acute and chronic health problems that elderly persons experience. A geriatric assessment, to accurately identify the health problems, type and level of disability, housing circumstances, and care and technology needed for the person to maintain functional effectiveness is essential to avoiding unnecessary institutional care. Because most disabled elderly persons are cared for in their homes or the homes of family members, usually their children, family members should be involved in any decisions regarding the use of long-term care technology in the home.

Disabled persons with no family and those who live alone must rely on themselves or on community or professional services to manage medications, move about, bathe, dress, eat, and so forth. Because frail elderly persons often are afraid of falling, it may be necessary to modify furniture, carpets, bathrooms, and kitchens in the home to prevent injuries that can cause disability. When alone at home, impaired elders also fear being in a situation where they are in desperate need of assistance. Electronic devices that provide immediate contact with a response system and are worn on the person can be of inestimable value in these circumstances (Millner, 1991). A variety of devices can also provide a more secure living environment; these include door locks, security alarms, and bars on windows. Such technology is provided in many communities and needs to become more widely available.

When community services and members of the community are not able to provide respite and assistance, a caregiver's life can be compromised (Kjellstrand, 1988). Elderly persons, in contrast to children, are more likely to be admitted to nursing homes when home care becomes exceedingly burdensome or difficult (Goldberg, 1988). Day care and hospice programs, however, could provide support for persistently disabled older persons and their families, as they do for the terminally ill.

Estimates indicate that almost 50 percent of nursing home residents are demented, with most of those probably having Alzheimer disease. Although the care of these patients may not demand complex technology, individuals with progressive dementia have specific needs that require special attention. Much can be done to enable demented persons to maintain self-sufficiency and effectiveness. Early on, most of those affected require little more than assistance in carrying out simple daily activities, but as the dementia becomes more severe, the necessary support and the setting where they live require continuing adjustment.

Proper care in the home can avert unnecessary or premature admission of demented persons to nursing homes. Adult day care centers can assist those with early dementia, utilizing simple techniques to enhance mental function and independence. Later, as the dementia progresses, greater supervision will be necessary to prevent persons from becoming lost or injured. Nursing homes and other institutions caring for those with advanced dementia should provide facilities that accommodate the affected person's level of functional ability.

Social and Policy Issues

Economic Issues

Definitive technologies that prevent or cure disease and other disorders can reduce the need for long-term care and result in savings in health-care costs and personnel requirements. Even with such technologic advances, however, the number of elderly infirm and others with chronic and progressive disabilities will persist and probably grow. The need for long-term care technologies, therefore, will increase. Governmental and private investments in the development of definitive and long-term care technologies and prolong the functional effectiveness of those who are disabled are therefore very much in the public's interest and should be expanded and encouraged.

Care and support of disabled persons imposes considerable financial responsibility on families, communities, and the nation. Approximately 15 percent of the noninstitutionalized population that is limited in activity due to chronic conditions make about 30 percent of the visits to physicians and account for approximately 40 percent of hospitalizations. Persons with activity limitations make twice as many physician visits per person than persons with no activity limitations (Pope and Tarlov, 1991). Medicare, which supports health care for the elderly and disabled, has used a standard of "medical necessity" in financing the use of technology, and assistive technologies may be dismissed as not medical and considered only as convenience items. Thus, coverage has been denied for technology such as bathroom grab bars that can reduce the occurrence of falls and hip fractures (Pope and Tarlov, 1991). The federal administration and the U.S. Congress should address these issues and establish policies that assist in financing the assistive technology that enables safer and more independent living, improves the health and well-being of the disabled, and reduces untoward consequences that result in costly medical care.

Technologies such as hemodialysis, ventilators, and structural modifications of homes and institutions are expensive. For example, the cost to the Medicare program for hemodialysis and kidney transplant services in 1990 was more than $5 billion (Green, 1992). Analyses indicate that health care technology is an important contributor to rising health care costs (Lee, Soffel, and Luft, 1992), and its use is at times inappropriate. Policies should be developed that assist health professionals to use only long-term care technologies that will have beneficial effects on the function and well-being of the disabled person.

Although some new technologies allow even the most severely impaired to live productive lives, these advances often require the complementary involvement of health care professionals, delivery systems, and social services in the home, hospital, nursing home, or school (Fitzgerald et al., 1993; Pope and Tarlov, 1991). At the same time, the cost effectiveness of assistive and supportive technology is diminished by the significant number of those affected who stop using or never use the technology after it is provided (Rusin, 1990). Health care delivery systems still are designed primarily to provide acute care, and better systems must be developed to address the needs of those who are chronically disabled and require long-term care, including the use of simple and complex technology.

The cost of nursing home care, averaging $37,000 per annum, is beyond the means of most Americans. Approximately 50 percent of total cost for nursing home care is shouldered by state and federal Medicaid funds. The remainder is covered largely from personal assets (see Chapters 1 and 9). Yet, nursing home costs are increasing as these institutions are required to provide more skilled and more technologically based health care services for more severely impaired persons being discharged earlier from hospitals.

Expenditures from Medicaid for nursing home care are increasing and are creating burdensome problems for state and federal governments (see Chapter 10). Current discussions regarding national health care reform, including proposals to increase home care, might reduce the need for nursing homes. But this could cause a rise in the severity of illness and disability found in the population remaining in nursing homes, further exacerbating the cost and complexity of nursing home care. It is uncertain whether or not provision of more home care would be more cost effective. If home care services are expanded, and more severely impaired persons are at home, it will be necessary to ensure that home care providers have the skills to use long-term care technology.

Despite the obvious costs of long-term care, advances in technology contribute to improving people's lives and productivity, and technology that restores and maintains function of the disabled can also reduce health care dependency and costs. Assessment of long-term care technologies helps identify those technologies that are safe and effective and eliminate those that are unsafe and ineffective. This improves the quality of care and serves to reduce costs (Katz et al., 1992).

Ethical Issues

The survival of more and more technology-dependent children forces us to examine whether medicine is doing what is truly in their best interest, not merely what is possible with the sophisticated tools we have on hand (Carr, 1989; Harms and Giordano, 1990; Kjellstrand, 1988). Children requiring technologic support to survive (e.g., mechanical ventilation) present legal and ethical issues (see Chapter 11). Prolonged use of survival technology, as opposed to withholding or terminating its use, increases the likelihood of persistent technology dependency.

Should the infant be allowed to die without technologic intervention, or should every available technology be applied and continued? Parents and health care providers must jointly decide the course of action to be taken (Groeger et al., 1993; R. W. Hunt, 1993). These decisions, however, cannot always be conclusive. If an infant's condition changes, decisions may need to be revised. Ever-changing questions must be dealt with. The time has come, though, to establish societal positions that consider the limits of using ever more sophisticated technology to sustain a possibly meaningless existence (Avery and Rotch, 1991).

This dilemma was brought to the forefront in an article in the September 24, 1993, issue of the *New York Times*, which reported:

> A hospital in suburban Virginia is appealing a Federal District Court's ruling that it must continue to provide life-sustaining treatment for a baby born there 11 months ago with most of her brain missing. The condition, a congenital defect known as anencephaly, is incurable and quickly fatal without medical interventions. An anencephalic baby has a brain stem, which keeps the heart and other organs working for a time. The baby does not meet the legal definition of brain death. Lacking a cortex, it is permanently unconscious, without sensation or cognitive function. The mother in this case, acting out of a "firm Christian faith that all life should be protected," as the court's opinion described her position, has insisted that everything be done to keep the baby alive.

Conceivably, sustaining the infant's life could lead to a vegetative life and prolonged long-term technologic support.

Ethical concerns regarding the appropriate use of technology also apply to the elderly. Because today's life-sustaining technologies can delay the moment of death for almost anyone, never before in human history have the timing and circumstances of death become more a matter of deliberate choice than an accepted act of nature (Logue, 1991). The ability, or power, to defer death, however, can lead to continuation of a life wholly dependent on technology.

The proliferation of life-sustaining technologies that do not maintain or restore a level of functional effectiveness consistent with a reasonable quality of life presents problems for decisionmakers, including families and physicians. A lack of sufficient information to accurately prognosticate patient outcome further compounds our ability to make appropriate decisions under these circumstances.

Sometimes, life-sustaining technologies can make dying a cruel spectacle. Persons over the age of 70 usually have multiple health care problems, while younger persons usually do not. "Heroic" efforts to keep persons alive in the face of probable fatal outcomes, therefore, make the survivors "victims" of such technology. The use, or misuse, of technology to prolong the life of very old, functionless persons also can have a profound detrimental impact on the patients' families.

Many, though, believe the goal of medicine is to conquer death (as if it were the "enemy," rather than part of the natural course of human life) and to prolong life by any means available, regardless of the person's age or quality of life. Life and death decisions, however, must be based on both personal and societal ethical positions. Institutional committees charged to assist in resolving these issues in individual cases may be helpful, but many such situations are being dealt with in the legal and judicial system. Ultimately, society will have to come to grips with these dilemmas.

The Employment of Disabled Persons

Federal legislation eliminating discrimination against the disabled and opening opportunities for the disabled to be employed has expanded tremendously their ability to live productive and personally satisfying lives. Many examples can be cited to show the extraordinary potential of long-term care technologies as applied to employment of disabled persons. But this is not enough. It is just as important to reduce nontechnologic barriers to employment of the disabled, so that they can enter and make progress in the job market.

Attitudinal barriers continue to impede the employment of physically impaired and disabled persons who are employable. It is necessary for employers to recognize that these individuals can be trained and prepared to do more than menial labor. Without such attitudes, technology is of little help in opening up employment opportunities for the many disabled persons who can perform meaningful and productive work.

Training programs that provide technologic assistance and support for those requiring long-term care are essential if the physically impaired and disabled are to acquire the skills and abilities necessary to obtain appropriate employment. Many such programs exist that are commendable, but there remain significant lags and omissions. It is foolish to train disabled persons for occupations that are declining in importance. Linking training programs to the needs of businesses and employers prepares the disabled for more available job opportunities and facilitates their being employed.

However, much of the technology necessary to improve the functional effectiveness required for certain types of employment is expensive. If the United States is to continue improving employment opportunity for the disabled, better funding mechanisms will be needed for the necessary technology and training. Businesses and employers must recognize the important contributions disabled employees can make, and make funding available to adapt workstations and facilities and provide the technology needed so the disabled can work.

In addition, manufacturers, scientists, and engineers should be encouraged and provided with incentives to develop new technologies that could further assist the disabled and improve their opportunities for employment. In fact, many new assistive and supportive long-term care technologies have been created *by* those who are disabled. Advances in computer and information technologies have been important, but much more can be done to develop electronic methods that expand and enhance the employability of many disabled persons.

As stated succinctly by Hunt and Berkowitz (1992), newly available technologies

> introduce relatively new phenomena, which are just evolving. We should not be surprised to learn that we have not solved all problems of training, access, or employment. What we have learned is tantalizing. Obviously, some disabled persons who would, in an earlier era, have been effectively banned from employment can now lead productive lives. Since the possibility exists, it would be a disgrace if we were not able to master the technology and to muster the will to bring the advantages of new technology to those disabled persons who would profit by them. (p. 162)

Assessing the Effectiveness of Long-Term Care Technologies

Until now, assessment of the effectiveness of long-term care technologies under realistic settings and ordinary living circumstances has been inadequate (Kane and Kane, 1988). Although serious efforts are being made to evaluate acute-care technology, not enough attention has been given to assessing long-term care technologies.

Evaluating the effectiveness of long-term care technology, however, differs from assessing acute-care technology. The prolonged employment of long-term care technology and its use in a variety of different settings (e.g., family homes, nursing homes, intermediate-care facilities, schools, workplaces, entertainment facilities) contrasts sharply with the case of acute-care technology, which is used on a short-term basis within a hospital or other acute-care setting.

Although the effectiveness of long-term care technology itself is critical in terms of its being able to work properly, it is just as important to take into account the setting in which the technology is used, in order to optimize its effectiveness in individuals' care. Moreover, the quality of long-term care depends not only on the reliability and effectiveness of available technologies but also on how well health care professionals and other caregivers perform their tasks, and how well impaired and disabled persons accept and use available services and technology.

Most important, technology should be assessed as to its effect on patient outcome, including restoration and maintenance of function and contribution to quality of life (Kane and Kane, 1988). Understanding, of course, that quality of life cannot be based on any normative standards, but instead must take into consideration the particular perceptions, as well as the functional abilities, of impaired and disabled persons.

Conclusions

Technological developments and advances during the past few decades have forever changed acute medical care, preventing death and prolonging the lives of many. Less well appreciated, but almost as dramatic, have been technological developments that improve and make more functional the lives of many who are disabled because of disease, injury, premature birth, environmental hazards, and other causes.

Nothing in recent times has been more dramatic and impressive than the developments and advances in computer-based technology. The microchip and computer have revolutionized warfare, science, communication, instrumentation, manufacturing, education, financial transactions, medical care, long-term care, and even children's toys. It has been said that the impact of computer technology on all aspects of society and culture can be equated with development of the printing press.

Long-term care technology, from the simple to the complex, has made it possible for disabled children, young and older adults, and elderly individuals to have more productive and effective lives than otherwise would have been possible. The application of computer technology to the lives of the disabled, however, may be only in its infancy.

Unquestionably, long-term care technology is "half-way" technology, in that it compensates for problems that someday might be prevented or cured. It is certain, however, that disabilities will continue to present problems for many persons of every age, but particularly the very old.

Compassion and caring, adequate financing, and being in appropriate settings are necessary for the care of the disabled who require long-term care. Yet, further improvement in the lives of the disabled and infirm will be determined as much by further developments in long-term care technology. Human beings must provide compassion and caring. Society must develop ways to finance long-term care to avoid unnecessary persistence and exaggeration of disability, premature death, and personal impoverishment. Government, industry, research, and evaluation must create the further technological advances and discoveries that will make the lives of the chronically ill and disabled more productive and fulfilling. Encouragement and enhancement of these efforts are dependent upon enlightened social and public policy.

References

Arras, J. D., ed., (1995). *Bringing the Hospital Home.* Baltimore: Johns Hopkins University Press.

Avery, M. E., and Rotch, T. M. (1991). The care of infants and children. *Acta Paediatrica Hungaria* 31 (2): 149–58.

Carr, M. W. (1989). To treat or not to treat: The controversy of handicapped newborns. *Critical Care Nurse* 9 (8): 73–78.

Farrell, P. M., and Fost, N. C. (1989). Long-term mechanical ventilation in pediatric respiratory failure: Medical and ethical considerations. *American Review of Respiratory Disease* 140 (2): 336-40.

Fitzgerald, J., Freund, D. A., Hughett, B., and McHugh, G. J. (1993). Influence of organizational components on the delivery of asthma care. *Medical Care* 31 (suppl. 3):MS 61–73.

Fullerton, J. E., Holtzman, N., Andrews, L. B., and Motulski, A. D., eds. (1994). *Assessing Genetic Risks: Implications for Health and Social Policy.* Washington, D.C.: National Academy Press.

Goldberg, A. I. (1988). Life-sustaining technology and the elderly: Prolonged mechanical ventilation factors influencing the treatment decision. *Chest* 94 (6): 1277–82.

Green, J. (1992). End stage renal disease. *Health Care Financing Review,* ann. suppl.

Groeger, J. S., Guntupalli, K. K., Strosberg, M., Halpern, N., Raphaely, R. C., Cerra, F., and Kaye, W. (1993). Descriptive analysis of critical care units in the United States: Patient characteristics and intensive care unit utilization. *Critical Care Medicine* 21 (2): 279–91.

Harms, D. L., and Giordano, J. (1990). Ethical issues in high-risk infant care. *Issues in Comprehensive Pediatric Nursing* 13 (1): 1–14.

Hunt, H. A., and Berkowitz, M., eds. (1992). *New Technologies and the Employment of Disabled Persons.* Geneva: International Labour Office.

Hunt, R. W. (1993). The critique of using age to ration health care. *Journal of Medical Ethics* 19 (1): 19–27.

Kane, R. L. (1988). Beyond caring: The challenge to geriatrics. *Journal of the American Geriatric Society* 36 (5): 467–72.

Kane, R. A., and Kane, R. L. (1988). Long-term care: Variations on a quality assurance theme. *Inquiry* 25 (1): 132–46.

Katz, R. T., Haig, A. J., Clark, B. S., and DiPaola, R. J. (1992). Long-term survival, prognosis, and life-care planning for patients with chronic lock-in syndrome. *Archives of Physical Medicine and Rehabilitation* 73 (5): 403–8.

Kjellstrand, C. M. (1988). Giving life-giving death: Ethical problems of high technology medicine. *Acta Medica Scandinavica Supplement* 725:1–88.

Kottke, F. J., and Lehmann, J. F., eds. (1990). *Handbook of Physical Medicine and Rehabilitation.* 4th ed. Philadelphia: W. B. Saunders.

LaPlante, M. P. (1991). *Disability in Basic Life Activities across the Life Span: Disability Statistics Report.* San Francisco: University of California, Institute for Health and Aging, 1:1–42.

Lee, P. R., Soffel, D., and Luft, H. S. (1992). Costs and coverage: Pressures toward health care reform. *Western Journal of Medicine* 157 (5): 576–83.

Logue, B. J. (1991). Taking charge: Death control as an emergent women's issue. *Women and Health* 17 (4): 97–121.

Lundberg, J. A., and Nole, M. L. (1990). The long-term acute care hospital: A new option for ventilator-dependent individuals. *Clinical Issues in Critical Care Nursing* 1 (2): 280–88

McInerny, T. K. (1988). The general pediatrician as care coordinator for children with chronic illness. *Pediatrician* 15 (1–2): 102–7.

Millner, B. N. (1991). Physically handicapped children's program: New York State Department of Health, *Bulletin of the New York Academy of Medicine* 7 (2): 1310–14.

O'Connor, P., Vander-Plaats, S., and Betz, C. L. (1992). Respite care services to caretakers of chronically ill children in California. *Journal of Pediatric Nursing* 7 (4): 269–75.

Palfrey, J. S., Haynie, M., Porter, S., Bierle, T., Cooperman, P., and Lowcook, J. (1992). Project school care: Integrating children assisted by medical technology into educational settings. *Journal of School Health* 62 (2): 50–54.

Pope, A. M., and Tarlov, A. R., eds. (1991). *Disability in America: Toward a National Agenda for Prevention.* Washington, D.C.: National Academy Press.

Reardon, K. K. (1990). Psycho-social care for the chronically ill adolescent: Challenges and opportunities. *Health Social Work* 15 (4): 272–82.

Regalbuto, M. S., Krouskop, T. A., and Cheatham, J. B. (1992). Toward a practical mobile robotic aid system for people with severe physical disability. *Journal of Rehabilitation Research and Development* 29 (1): 19–26.

Rusin, M. J. (1990). Stroke rehabilitation: A geropsychological perspective. *Archives of Physical Medicine and Rehabilitation* 71 (11): 914–22.

Solomon, D. H., Judd, H. L., Sier, H. C., Rubenstein, L. Z., and Morley, J. E. (1988). New issues in geriatric care. *Annals of Internal Medicine* 108 (5): 718–32.

University of California, San Francisco. (1989). Disability risks of chronic illnesses and impairments. *Disability Statistical Bulletin* 2:1–7.

U.S. Department of Education. (1991). *Thirteenth Annual Report on Implementation of the Individuals with Disabilities Education Act.* Washington, D.C.: U.S. Government Printing Office.

6

Challenges in Providing Care for Persons with Complex Chronic Illness

Mathy D. Mezey, Ed.D., R.N., F.A.A.N.

In this era of uncertainty over most aspects of health care delivery, there is surprising agreement that persons with complex chronic illness represent the future population of consumers of long-term services (Adams and Benson, 1991; National Center for Health Statistics, 1993; Shaughnessy and Kramer, 1990). This population comprises those persons with continuing multiple health and medical care needs that persist beyond six months, with episodes of remission and exacerbation, each of which leaves the patients with disabilities that are increasingly disabling, that exceed the patients' ability to manage their own self-care, and that, to varying degrees, inhibit personal independence (Diamond, 1983; Guralnik and Simonsick, 1993; Strauss and Glaser, 1975). The lives of people with complex chronic illness are characterized by (1) continuing care needs; (2) periods of functional stability; (3) repeated episodes of the chronic illness; (4) episodes of complicating, intercurrent acute illnesses; and (5) inevitable decline in health. The needs for long-term care of people afflicted with complex, chronic illness inevitably reverberate throughout their immediate families and the larger social system, causing personal distress and economic disruption.

Over the past forty years, health services in developed countries have attempted to adjust to the paradigm shift away from acute care toward long-term care for people with chronic illness. Until relatively recently, the time of physicians and nurses was devoted primarily to providing care and comfort to persons over a short duration of illness. The need for long-term care, while recognized, had only minimal impact on how providers spent their time, and it consumed little of the country's health care resources. Patients with chronic diseases such as diabetes, heart disease, cancer, and asthma succumbed to an acute episode of illness early in the course of their disease.

Changes in health care management and delivery have markedly increased the numbers of people who live into old age with several, overlapping chronic medical conditions. Over 75 percent of ambulatory care for older people and 41 percent of ambulatory care for persons under 45 revolves around visits for chronic illness (Lawrence and Gauss, 1983), this despite the fact that, in 1986, close to 20 percent of people with a chronic illness failed to see a doctor (Freeman et al., 1990). The overwhelming majority of nursing home residents have five or more chronic illnesses (Guralnik and Simonsick, 1993) and almost half of persons 65 or older can expect to spend some time in a nursing home (Kemper and Murtaugh, 1991). The over 1.2 million patients who receive home health care on any given day (National Center for Health Statistics, 1993) have a mean of 10 overlapping nursing problems (SD = 6.0), the most common being physical activity impairment (79 percent), neuromusculoskeletal impairment (63 percent), and circulatory impairment (47 percent) (Helberg, 1993). Over 50 percent of expenditures for ambulatory care, 62 percent of acute care expenditures, and over 85 percent of nursing home expenditures are attributed to care of patients with chronic illness (Lawrence and Gaus, 1983; Rice and Laplante, 1992). Persons with three or more activity of daily living (ADL) deficits also incur substantially higher catastrophic health care costs (Liu, Perozek, and Manton, 1993).

Unfortunately, the consequences of increased survival are such that, while medical aspects of chronic illness may respond to treatment, the consequent physical and functional disabilities often severely limit people's ability to live independently (Guralnik and Simonsick, 1993). As the illness progresses, it is often not the chronic disease, per say, that causes people to use health care services. Those who most tax the skills of primary care providers, and the country's long-term care resources, are persons whose multiple chronic condition(s) grossly interfere with their everyday life. The most pressing need within health care, then, is to develop a delivery system for persons with chronic illness.

Focusing on chronic illness challenges health care providers' and institutions' basic assumptions about health care delivery. In acute care, each symptom is treated as a "new" health problem. Management of chronic illness, on the other hand, requires a system of care that encompasses a full episode of illness. Rather than responding to symptoms as if they were sequential episodes of separate acute illness, chronic illness requires providers of primary, home, acute, and long-term care to configure services for people whose symptoms are primarily sequelae of one or two ongoing illness. While the rate of progression may be somewhat unpredictable, the morbidity associated with chronic illness is not random. Rather than responding with surprise when a patient with diabetes is readmitted to the hospital for cataract surgery, peripheral vascular disease, and metabolic imbalance, the health care system needs to plan for such expected occurrences.

This chapter explores the long-term care needs of persons with complex chronic illness. Specifically, the chapter examines the need for long-term care services, emerging models of health care delivery, and the need to increase manpower among professional and nonprofessional providers of long-term care.

Multiple Perspectives on the Need for Services

One impediment to developing a rational system for managing patients with complex, chronic illness has been the failure to arrive at a universally accepted definition of this population of patients. The elements of chronicity have been well described (Diamond, 1983; Strauss and Glaser, 1975). The most commonly found definitions of chronicity revolve around the concept of physical and functional disability and frailty. Physical disability is defined in terms of limits on peoples' capacity to perform activities of daily living (personal care tasks) or more complex tasks necessary to live independently in the community (instrumental activities of daily living) (Guralnik and Simonsick, 1993). Physical frailty describes persons whose severely impaired strength, mobility, balance and endurance interfere with their ability to conduct activities of daily living (Hadley et al., 1993). (In the interest of space, this chapter excludes from consideration persons whose long-term care needs are primarily related to changes in mental health.)

Lacking a standard definition of disability, the population for whom disability poses a substantial burden varies from study to study. Estimates from the National Health Interview Survey (Adams and Benson, 1991) are that 14 percent of persons have activity limitations due to chronic conditions and 5 percent have limitations in the amount or kind of major activity. Verbrugge (1990) estimated that more than 20 percent of middle-aged adults and close to 45 percent of older adults have a major-activity limitation. Guralnik and Simonsick (1993) estimated that, of people 65 or older, 2.25 million (16% of women and 12% of men) living alone require the assistance of another person. For people 85 or over the number who require assistance rises to 25 percent of women and 15 percent of men (Schneider and Guralnik, 1990).

The consensus among providers (Mezey and Lynaugh, 1994) is that the health care resources needed to meet progressive functional declines do indeed transcend individual chronic medical conditions. Consequences of many different, and multiple chronic diseases appear to evoke similar functional care deficits and long-term service needs. When interviewed, chronically ill patients identify common symptoms and responses associated with different chronic illnesses and similar long-term service needs irrespective of the particular medical condition (Arras and Dubler, 1994). Nurses, social workers, and physicians confirm that the health, functional, social, and financial concerns faced by persons with complex, chronic illness transcend specific disease diagnoses. Obtaining personal hygiene care at home, problems stemming from polypharmacy, pain and immobility, inability to travel to medical treatment, and getting answers to medical and functional health questions — all are major issues for these medically and technologically fragile patients and their caregivers. Because they occur irrespective of the underlying condition, these care needs confirm the wisdom of taking a noncategorical approach to the long-term care needs of patients with complex, chronic illness.

The costs of providing services specifically related to functional needs of persons with complex chronic illness are also reasonably well known. In nursing homes, for example, case mix indexes based almost exclusively on functional ability are used to calculate nursing aide staffing levels (Mezey and Knapp, 1993; Spector et al., 1988). Yet definitions that rely primarily on functional decline as the defining factor of chronicity fail to capture the full scope of the illness, its effects on patients and families, and their need for long-term care. While acknowledging similarities, patients (Arras and Dubler, 1994) and providers (Mezey and Lynaugh, 1994) also emphasize burdens, outside of function limitations, that are associated with a specific illness. Some studies suggest that functional ability explains only a small portion of the variance between total acute care utilization and long-term service utilization for community-residing patients with multiple chronic illness (Helberg, 1993; Mezey and Knapp, 1993; Spector, 1989).

In analysis of nursing home care, for example, there are reasons to question how well functional status depicts the initial health status or changes in health status of residents, how accurately ADLs correlate with utilization of other health care resources, such as hospitalizations, and how useful ADLs are in predicting professional as opposed to nonprofessional staffing for residents with complex chronic illness. Nursing homes rely heavily on functional status to characterize residents' health status, allocate nursing personnel, and assign reimbursement (Institute of Medicine, 1986; Solomon, 1988; Spector, 1989), even though functional status of long-term nursing home residents remains remarkably stable over time (Spector, 1989) and does not correlate consistently with other measures of acuity, such as clinical complexity, diagnoses, complications, changes in physical and mental health status, or hospitalization (Kearnsk, 1989; Mitty, 1989; Spector, 1989).

Focusing primarily on medical conditions, on the other hand, also fails to capture the complexity of long-term care needs of people with chronic illness. Research, in fact, suggests that medical conditions add little in explaining the service needs associated with chronic illness (Spector, 1989). Rather, it is the combination of chronic conditions and personal characteristics that best captures the true complexity of chronic illness.

The preceding discussion underscores the need for a uniformly agreed on definition that describes the chronic illness trajectory in terms of a person's function, acute and chronic medical condition, and psychosocial status. Development of such a definition has been hampered by the lack of studies that accurately depict the use and cost of ambulatory, acute, and long-term services of the complex chronically ill.

The mechanisms for reimbursing primary, home, and acute care and institutional long-term care have impeded the ability to carry out the type of analysis needed to provide such data. Available cost data are segmented into long-term institutional care and home care. Utilization of primary and acute care are rarely included in calculations of the full cost of care for the complex, chronically ill. While a few studies (Zimmer et al., 1988; Van Buren, 1981) have attempted to extrapolate costs from existing data resources, the true cost of care for a full episode of illness for the complex, chronically ill remains obscure.

Challenges of Providing Appropriate Services

Conceptually, what constitutes "good care" for persons with complex chronic illness is well described in the literature. In a good care system, services are: accessible, flexible, and continuous; considerate of physical, functional, psychological, and social needs; integrated as to primary, acute, and long-term care; responsive to and as much as possible controlled by the individual; and family oriented rather than patient oriented.

The major challenge lies not in characterizing quality care but in translating that definition into actual practice. As but one of many examples as to the paucity of programs serving this population, interviews with health care providers (Mezey and Lynaugh, 1994) yielded only three programs in New York City designed specifically to deliver long-term care to children with complex chronic illness. Together, at any one time, these programs served a total of only 450 children.

Despite a consensus as to the needs of those with complex chronic illness, and a few existing and evolving models (Mezey and Lawrence, 1995; Stone, 1993), current attempts at service delivery continue to fall short of their intended goals. Identified gaps in services, the most important of which are highlighted below, include: fragmentation, duplication, and lack of articulation among ambulatory, acute, and long-term care; a service delivery system that is unresponsive to individual needs; funding streams that make access to such services virtually impossible; and unavailable and/or unprepared personnel (Diamond, 1983; Stone, 1993).

Absence of Primary Care Services and Difficulty Coordinating Specialist Care

Two major problems in the delivery of care to persons with complex chronic illness are the lack of primary care services and the difficulty in coordinating quality specialist care. The programs serving people living in the community and the health care services in nursing homes often address a specific chronic illness; patient needs, however, do not easily fit into such defined categories.

Because building familiarity and trust is crucial to the successful delivery of long-term primary care services for this population, continuity of the primary care provider is essential. Yet, programs serving community-residing patients who are geographically dispersed often cannot overcome severe barriers to the delivery of optimal primary care services. Some programs designed specifically to serve persons with complex chronic illness residing in the community require people to receive their primary care in a centralized location. While this provides good control over some primary care services, it interferes with the provider's ability to develop a comprehensive ongoing relationship. It makes knowing the patient's environment and neighborhood impossible, and thus severely impedes the efficient and effective coordination of primary care services. Other agencies serving persons with complex chronic illnesses who are geographically dispersed contract with existing clinics and providers for primary care. Even agencies, such as long-term care facilities, that provide both primary and specialist care acknowledge that their disease-focused service sometimes overwhelms the ability to provide good primary care.

In addition to having deficiencies in their provision of primary care, both community agencies and long-term care facilities serving this population have difficulty in identifying specialists, including rehabilitation and psychiatric specialists, sympathetic to the needs of their clients and they have difficulty in coordinating specialist care. Agencies providing long-term care to these patients use a variety of strategies for assuring that patients are seen by specialists. Some have specialists on staff to whom they refer patients. Some have relationships with specialists in private practice. Still other programs relate to specialists in several clinics dispersed throughout a geographical area, a system that makes coordination of care difficult.

Absence of Linkages across Institutions and Separation of Social and Health Resources

Delivering care to persons with complex chronic illness is severely hindered by the arbitrary separation of the social and health resources and of primary, acute, and long-term care services. The literature (Estes, 1993; Kane, in press) and providers (Mezey and Lynaugh, 1994) stress the need for coordination between social services, such as housing and transportation, and health services, such as personal care and treatments, if community-based programs are to succeed. Yet funding and service delivery mechanisms mitigate against creating linkages between these service components. Funding from child welfare agencies in New York City, for example, does not reimburse for health care or nursing time. New Alternatives for Children, an organization that keeps children with complex chronic illness in their own homes or places them in foster care, pays the nurse clinicians who oversee care for its very sick children through fundraising (Mezey and Lynaugh, 1994). In Oregon, even though legislation has fostered the development of small, family-style long-term care settings, insufficient regulatory oversight and restrictions regarding on-site health supervision have led to concern as to the quality of care in these settings (Kane and Wilson, 1993).

A similar, although somewhat different set of constraints limits consideration of how best to apportion care for this population between long-term institutional and acute care. In contrast to only a few years ago, only the sickest of people now gain admission to long-term care facilities. Persons in nursing homes are increasingly sicker in comparison to community residents. This is due primarily to restrictions in long-term care bed capacity (National Center for Health Statistics, 1987), to increases in the population 85 years of age and older who are proportionally higher users of nursing facilities and have more complex chronic illness, and to substitution of a stay in nursing facility for posthospital care either for recuperation or for terminal care (Lewis et al., 1987; Spector, 1989).

While direct Medicare payments to nursing homes remain small (less than 5 percent of nursing home care), Medicare policy influences much of the health care of the elderly with complex chronic illness who reside in nursing homes, and, in actuality, Medicare pays for almost all of this care. Medicare's prospective reimbursement to hospitals and unwillingness to reimburse for care delivered in the nursing home encourages both early discharge of patients from hospitals to nursing facilities and discharge of nursing home residents back to acute care settings for the slightest change in health status. Thus, health problems beyond the most routine result in the resident's transfer from the nursing facility to a physician's office, emergency room, or hospital. This continuous "ping-ponging" of patients between the nursing facility and hospital (Lewis et al., 1987) contributes to this population's receiving its care in emergency rooms, and it deters consideration as to whether care for such persons might not be better provided in the more familiar and controlled environment of the nursing home.

Several studies have documented that close to one-third of hospital admissions generated by skilled nursing facilities could be avoided by improving health care coverage in the nursing home (Holmes et al., 1991; Shaughnessy, Kramer, Hittle, and Steiner, 1995; Van Buren, 1981). Moreover, increasing numbers of nursing facilities are able to care for such residents in a manner that maintains quality (Garrard et al., 1990; Mezey and Lynaugh, 1992; Shaughnessy, Kramer, Hittle, and Steiner, 1995; Small and Walsh, 1988).

Unfortunately, data to substantiate the potential cost savings that might accrue if the acute illnesses of persons with complex chronic illness were managed in long-term care facilities as opposed to hospitals are hard to obtain. Actual calculation of the total charges to Medicare Parts A and B for all health care encounters of nursing facility residents over a period of time are largely unavailable. A 1981 Health Care Financing Administration study of nursing facility residents eligible for both Medicare and Medicaid in four states (HCFA, 1985) estimated that these residents each used $2,909 of hospital care and $1,183 of physician care. Using these figures as a guide, Medicare Parts A and B costs for all nursing facility residents would be in the billions of dollars (Mezey and Scanlon, 1988). A study of hospital readmissions in the Medicare population suggested that in 1984, Medicare spent close to $8 billion dollars on readmissions to hospitals (Anderson and Steinberg, 1984). Several studies have imputed Medicare costs savings of between $3,000 and $4,000 per resident to preventing inappropriate hospitalizations of nursing home residents (Holmes et al., 1991; Van Buren, 1981; Zimmer et al., 1988). Firmer cost data would allow a more reasoned reconsideration of how best to apportion ambulatory, long-term, and acute care services for those with complex chronic illness.

The Need for Programs to Support Caregivers

Both patients and providers emphasize the importance of organizing services to assure assistance to the sick person's caregiver. Caregivers of residents receiving both community and institutional long-term care require ongoing support (Zarit, 1992), although the type of support needed may differ between the two groups. Family members and friends of the community-residing chronically ill become exhausted and demoralized careening from crisis to crisis in the present fragmented system. Errors in care, premature or unnecessary institutionalization, and needless suffering are often the result. Planned support and respite for caregivers is as fundamental to home care of the chronically ill as professional staffing is in hospitals and nursing homes.

The ability of caregivers to fulfill their own health and social needs directly affects their ability to sustain care for the dependent patient. A key strategy in the care of community-residing persons with chronic illness is home visiting, which provides the opportunity to assess and educate patients and caregivers, provide preventative care, and respond appropriately to acute crisis or emergent complications. Some home care agencies and day hospitals have instituted "exit" groups for caregivers, both to assist them with caregiving tasks and to prepare them for the time when services may be diminished or discontinued.

Caregiving can be equally burdensome whether the family member is caring for a person at home or in an institution (Zarit, 1992; Arras and Dubler, 1994). Family members of the institutionalized need professional help in meeting their ongoing need to care for the patient, in dealing with the consequences of caregiving, and in meeting their own health needs.

One caveat about supporting family caregivers is worth noting. Recent attention has focused on the potential that care needs over the course of an illness will exceed the ability of family caregivers, and long-term care facilities, to provide adequate care to persons with chronic complex illness. Arras and Dubler (1994) alluded to the limits of family members to provide long-term high-tech home care. In nursing homes there is an emerging appreciation that the level of resident need may exceed the facilities' capability and place residents at risk for receiving inadequate care (Sager, 1989). Munro (1990), for example, found that as the number of residents requiring complex nursing care exceeded the number of knowledgeable and skilled nursing personnel, quality of care declined.

Promising Models of Long-Term Health Care Delivery

There is mounting evidence that the choice of model for long-term care delivery can profoundly influence outcomes for persons with complex chronic illness. How care is delivered influences whether persons with similar disabilities will be able to live independently in the community or require institutionalization. Guralnik and Simonsick (1993), for example, attributed the greater ability of elderly Bostonians with a high prevalence of disability to continue to reside in the community, as opposed to a similar population in Iowa, to an active home care program for Boston's very frail elderly.

While much is known about this population, many issues of service delivery, including those of definition and scope of service, remain unresolved. Nevertheless, several past and ongoing demonstration projects have shown promise in improving care to persons with complex chronic illness. Practitioners (Mezey and Lynaugh, 1994) confirm that the models described below have the potential to substantially improve long-term care to patients with complex chronic illness and their families. These models represent approaches that have been tried episodically or piecemeal but not on a sufficiently broad scale to test their true effectiveness, and/or have proven effective but require replication in relationship to the long-term care needs of patients. Among the most important common elements of these programs are that they: (1) are community based, (2) provide comprehensive services, (3) utilize teams of professional providers, and (4) effectively utilize nonprofessional providers from the community.

Partnerships between Professional and Nonprofessional Staff

Large-scale federal, state, and foundation-funded demonstration projects (Freund, 1993; U.S. Congress, 1986), including the original and replication of the ON LOK model (Kane, Illston, and Miller, 1992; A. P. Mezey and Lawrence, 1995), have confirmed the effectiveness of nurse practitioner (NP) long-term management of patients with chronic illness in ambulatory settings; three large demonstration projects have confirmed NP effectiveness in nursing homes (Garrard et al., 1990). Community Nursing Organizations (CNOs, 1993) are testing nursing models for long-term management of elderly patients with differing levels of complexity. One site funded under the Primary Care Physician Program, sponsored by the John A. Hartford Foundation of New York City, places nurse practitioners as case managers in physicians' offices to improve long-term outcomes for patients, many of whom have complex chronic illnesses (Czerenda and Best, 1994).

While delegation of function from professional to nonprofessional provider is the hallmark of community and institutional long-term care, very few models of care have attempted to create true partnerships between professional and nonprofessional staff. Such a community model would, for example, link a nurse practitioner with a nonprofessional paid provider from the sick person's community. The nonprofessional provider would be cross-trained to perform services such as (1) direct personal care, (2) facilitation of instrumental activities of daily living (shopping, cooking, laundry, etc.), (3) accompanying the patient and family to health care appointments to facilitate the visit and reinforce the plan of care on the patient's return home, and (4) administering treatments and medications under the NP's supervision.

Knowledge of the local community, cross-training, and flexibility in the use of time are key to the role of the community worker. Knowledge of the community allows the worker to act as a facilitator in arranging services. Cross-training allows the worker to perform a range of tasks necessary to maintaining the person in the community and encourages agencies to rethink what activities can safely be performed by a community worker under nursing supervision. Flexibility of time allows one worker to care for a cluster of patients in a circumscribed geographical area. For example, the worker might make "rounds" each morning to get patients out of bed and prepare breakfast, accompany someone to an office visit, then make "rounds" again to help people back to bed in the evening.

In this model, the NP performs the following functions: (1) assesses each person's and family member's overall health and illness needs, (2) provides nursing and medical care, (3) coordinates all ambulatory and inpatient services with the help of the nonprofessional provider, (4) helps the patient and family sort out normal from abnormal symptomatology and advises and oversees appropriate action, and (5) tracks patients over time.

This model expands on the "block nurse" (Jamieson, 1990) by establishing a system of community based long-term care. It also builds on the case-management model currently being tested in hospitals, in which NPs are assigned to care for the most complex patients (Cesta and Cohen, 1993; Naylor et al., 1994). Clusters of chronically ill persons who would benefit from this model of care are found in urban and rural neighborhoods and in boarding houses, retirement communities, and parishes, all of which could be termed "naturally occurring retirement communities." Crucial to the integrity of the model is the coordinating role of the NP who directs care in collaboration with the patient and family and assures that essential services are provided in a timely manner.

Measurable proofs of the effectiveness of this professional-nonprofessional approach might include (1) decreased patient use of emergency rooms, (2) improved compliance with the treatment regimen, (3) prevention or delay of complications, (4) lowered admissions to nursing homes, and (5) caregiver or family stability. Evidence of effectiveness of the community worker might include (1) low turnover and absenteeism, (2) job satisfaction, and (3) pursuit of educational advancement.

Team Case Management

The disappointing results from the Channeling Project (Mathematica Policy Research, 1987) dampened enthusiasm for community-based long-term case management, especially for elderly patients. The Channeling Project was deficient, however, in that it used poorly trained (and poorly paid) personnel to modify what were frequently medically complex plans of care.

Persons with complex chronic illness in all likelihood require a more robust case management model, in which experienced social workers and nurse practitioners, working in teams, have wide latitude to order, change, and oversee health services (including admitting and prescriptive privileges) and social services for a caseload of patients. The model is analogous to the practice of placing all the services of a hospital unit (i.e., nursing, dietary, physical and occupational therapy, housekeeping) under the direction of an experienced clinician.

The progression of complex, chronic illness is such that at times there is a need to "saturate" the patient's environment with services, while at other times, when the patient (and family) are more stable, services can be diminished or withdrawn. Appropriate deployment of services over time requires professionals who know the patient and family well and who have the authority to quickly reconfigure the service package. An experienced social worker or NP model meets these criteria (Capitman, MacAdam, and Abrahams, 1993).

Patients needing care under this model have many medical problems that reduce mobility and require multiple services; at the same time, family support is often missing or unstable. For many elderly living alone, this model could serve as an alternative to institutionalization. Several programs have used a variation of this model with some success (Cesta and Cohen, 1993; Kane and Wilson, 1993; Stone, 1993), although staff still often lack the latitude to quickly change the plan of care. In this model, physicians are consultants to the social worker-NP team and serve as the access route for specialist care. The goal is to sustain safe care outside of institutions as long as possible or permanently. Measurable outcomes for this model include (1) prevention or shortening of the length of hospitalization and long-term institutionalization; (2) decreasing morbidity such as infection, incontinence, immobility, and mental incapacity (all of which lead to institutionalization); and (3) decreasing the costs of service delivery.

Improving Rehabilitative and Mental Health Services

Rehabilitative services are extremely difficult to obtain for adults and children with complex chronic illness either at home or in institutions. Personnel are often not available, are unwilling to make home or nursing home visits, especially in certain urban and rural areas, or lack a rehabilitation and long-term care perspective. Similarly, there is a paucity of basic psychiatric services to this population. People with complex chronic illness often need mental health assessment, management of stress, help in complying with complex treatment regimens, in overcoming isolation and stigmatization, and in developing a meaningful life.

Given the current shortage of physical therapists and the lack of certainty as to future funding of mental health services, a prudent approach would be to assure that all nurses working with this population have a basic proficiency in concepts of rehabilitation and mental health, while preparing a small number of specialists in rehabilitation and psychiatric long-term care. Such a model has been successfully tried by the Visiting Nurse Service of New York in delivering psychiatric services in their home care program for patients with HIV/AIDS (Visiting Nurse Service, 1993).

This model would require the development and evaluation of educational modules in rehabilitation and mental health for use in associate and baccalaureate nursing programs, and the development of master's programs to increase the number of physical therapy, nursing, social work, and psychology specialists in rehabilitation and mental health focused specifically on the needs of people with complex chronic illness. A similar model, used to train nursing faculty and clinicians in the area of alcohol and substance abuse, was developed by the Division of Nursing at New York University under a grant from the Division of Alcohol and Substance Abuse of the U.S. Department of Health and Human Services. It included development of faculty fellowship programs and development and dissemination of a model curriculum (Naegle, 1993). Follow-up on actual practice patterns of personnel completing such training would validate such an investment.

Care of the Chronically Critically Ill

Twentieth-century medical innovations have created a new form of chronic illness — the adult or child who survives treatment and can be maintained alive, but who does not recover health. Examples of chronically critically ill persons are those who only partially recover after surgery, low birthweight infants who remain ventilator dependent and need constant care, and persons who survive incapacitating trauma or neurological afflictions (Arras and Dubler, 1994). These people make up a disability population with complex functional problems and often difficult pain management and life-support needs. They require complex multidisciplinary, collaborative long-term care systems. In some hospitals and nursing homes, special units have been established for these patients (Daly et al., 1993).

The chronically critically ill cannot be cared for on general nursing care units, yet they do not improve under intensive care. Many suffer from one or more of the following problems: incomplete recovery from coronary by-pass procedures (CABG), chronic obstructive lung disease (COPD), end stage congestive heart failure, sepsis, cerebral vascular accident (CVA), and ventilator dependency. Survival may be up to one year, with total dependence throughout that time. About half may leave the hospital for long-term institutional or home care.

Long-term care units that have been established for these chronically critically ill persons in hospitals and nursing homes are often nurse managed and staffed by a combination of expert critical care nurses, nurse technicians, doctors, support staff, and secretaries. A crucial aspect of care is a team approach that involves helping patients and families understand the current and future illness situation. The nurse case manager oversees the patient's transfer to the unit, orients and tours the family around the unit, takes a history, and initiates a plan of care, including resuscitation status and goals. Patient care protocols guide ventilator weaning, nutrition, and emergency situations. Similar patterns of care have been implemented at home (Daly et al., 1993).

In addition to providing high-quality care, the central focus of programs for the chronically critically ill is to facilitate decisionmaking about further treatment. Experienced, mature nurses and social workers engage patients and families in conversations about choice of treatment. Persons with prior complicating medical conditions such as COPD or diabetes may experience a failed CABG procedure or incur complications due to their prior condition. Such patients and families often are confronting the question of terminating life-sustaining treatment after an arduous course of illness.

An innovative project conducted by the Ohio Lung Association approaches this issue at an earlier point in the continuum of illness (Daly et al., 1993). In this project, nurses help patients think through treatment options in the face of very high odds against a successful outcome. In particular, these nurses work with COPD patients, whose fear of suffocation dominates their thinking when considering treatment choices.

New Models of Hospice Care

Many clinicians believe that with detailed, up-front assessment and care by a well-coordinated, multidisciplinary team they can predict and plan an effective program of care for patients with complex, chronic illness through the course of illness until death (Strahan, 1993). A team approach is thought to be less costly and more humane than the usual practice of each discipline's taking on an individual medical or social problem. Such a model is based on the assumption that enough is known to identify the service needs of patients at each successive stage of certain complex chronic illnesses.

Essential to the extension of the hospice model to the care of persons with protracted illnesses is a philosophical and social commitment to home based or "cottage" care. The severe financial burden now associated with care of the severely chronically ill is linked with hospitalization, medical and surgical interventions, and drug therapy. If the base site for care were the home (or possibly nursing home), then resources would be committed to care there, as is the case with home-based hospice care under Medicare.

As an example, a person with insulin-dependent diabetes who has had a CVA suffers from incapacitating peripheral vascular changes and, unable to ambulate alone, is likely to need continuous assistance. In the current system, these very impaired people receive rehabilitation after their CVA and then are discharged from care. At home without physical therapy they rapidly become deconditioned, lose earlier gains, and become progressively more dependent on family caregivers. To be reimbursed under Medicare for physical therapy or other eligible care, it is necessary for patients to be rehospitalized. Medical and social services are often denied because patients are unable to travel or because improvement is not an obtainable goal (Siegler, 1994).

At present, persons with chronic illness only qualify for reimbursed home care for specified periods of time — usually a few weeks after hospitalization. Then patient and family are left on their own until the next problem occurs, when they are once again hospitalized, and the cycle repeats itself until death. For patients nearing the end of their illness trajectory but not near enough death to qualify for hospice, the current hospital, office-based care system is a poor fit.

A life time plan of continuous home-based care, punctuated as needed by intermittent nursing home placement and medical consultation, might curtail use of emergency and hospital services and alleviate much distress for the patient and family. Nursing care systems organized around a prepaid, capitated design could provide long-term care in a flexible manner more closely attuned to the day-to-day care requirements of such patients.

Educating Providers in the Principles of Long-Term Care

Physicians and Nurses

To date, the major problem in imparting knowledge about long-term care to medical and nursing students has been the lack of a place in the curriculum to teach long-term care and the unavailability of appropriate clinical sites where students can learn about long-term care and actually deliver care for persons with chronic illness. Overexposure to hospital patients experiencing acute exacerbations of chronic illness, and underexposure to ambulatory settings where students can see the health care fluctuations associated with chronic illness have had two serious negative consequences: (1) students lack experience and guidance in helping individuals and families cope with the profound long-term events associated with chronic illness; and (2) students learn a model that is highly dependent on specialists for delivery of care (Siegler, 1994).

The paucity of clinical sites offering continuous care for complex chronic illness means that integrated, extrainstitutional models of care will remain an abstract ideal for many students in the primary care professions. Nevertheless, the increasing attractiveness of home-based and community-based care as clinical sites bodes well for the education of medical and nursing students. These are settings where the patient population overwhelmingly reflects the problems of chronic illness. As these sites expand, students will gain broader insights into the problems of the chronically ill. The expansion of case management models will provide further opportunities for students to follow patients during a full episode of illness (Kane, Illston, and Miller, 1992; Kane and Wilson, 1993; A. P. Mezey and Lawrence, 1995; Naylor et al., 1994).

The long-term care of persons with complex chronic illness would be substantially enhanced by curriculum revisions in basic and advanced nursing and medical education which would (1) provide greater balance between content on individual chronic illnesses and a broader conceptualization of the generalities across chronic illness; (2) shift the emphasis of content away from acute, episodic care toward long-term, continuous care; and (3) include additional content on concepts related to rehabilitation. In addition, there is a strong need to increase the preparation of nurse and physician faculty skilled in care for complex chronic illness. Faculty development must include expansion of the number of model practices that provide long-term care to this population and can serve as clinical sites for undergraduate and graduate students.

Nurse Practitioners

Since the early 1970s, studies have strongly supported the effectiveness of nurse practitioners in providing long-term care to patients with complex chronic illnesses in ambulatory settings (U.S. Congress, 1986), hospitals (Naylor et al., 1994), and nursing homes (Garrard et al., 1990; Kane et al., 1989; Mezey and Lynaugh, 1992; Shaughnessy, Kramer, Hittle, and Steiner, 1995). Nurse practitioners are especially adept at managing patients with complex, chronic, but stable conditions and predictable acute conditions. Students in NP programs are taught to create linkages between patients and their families and the health care system, to provide direct care, and to oversee care provided by nonprofessional and other professional staff. There are, at present, about 13,500 students enrolled in masters-level programs preparing this kind of advanced clinician; 4,500 graduate annually. About 80 percent of all nurses with the MSN are engaged in clinical practice (Fulmer and Mezey, 1994).

The high demand for NPs generally may limit their recruitment for work with this population. There is a tendency in American culture to veer away from investing manpower development in populations viewed as nonproductive. Unless we support systems of long-term care at a level sufficient to attract and retain providers, they will be unable to compete with acute care settings for well-trained NPs and physicians (Mezey et al., 1994).

Full use of NPs to care for persons with complex chronic illness is further constrained by barriers to full practice that many states have placed on NPs. Such restrictions include physician supervision clauses, restrictive reimbursement relative to nursing services, liability issues, and problems in obtaining hospital privileges, all of which impair the effective and innovative use of NPs (Boullough, 1993).

Nursing Assistants and Attendants

Nonprofessionals learn on the job or through agency-based educational programs. Nursing assistants working in nursing homes certified by Medicare and Medicaid are now required to undergo a prescribed course of training, which states and individual nursing homes are free to supplement (Survey of State Implementation of OBRA Requirements, 1992). Home health aides have highly variable preparation, depending on the agency where they work. Some states, Maryland for example, regulate home health aide training; most do not. On the other hand, home health aides are often self-taught and may have an invaluable wealth of clinical know-how and local knowledge (Mitty, 1989).

Larger agencies with high standards expend considerable resources on recruitment, training, and oversight of aides. In organized home care, the home health aide is the backbone of intense service to the chronically ill. Unfortunately, little is known about how nurse aide training affects patient outcomes (Mitty, 1989). Without such data, government and voluntary agencies will be reluctant to commit additional resources in this direction.

Conclusion

Unfortunately, despite recent advances, the overwhelming evidence continues to suggest that persons with complex chronic illness remain at the margin of health care, functioning at the periphery of public consciousness and isolated from the mainstream of health care. The challenges of treating chronic illness force us to confront the imperative need for protracted care. As gerontological nursing pioneer Doris Schwartz so powerfully phrased it over 40 years ago, "Patients who get better are said to do a great service to their caretakers." Most of the time, the chronically ill fail to do us that service, and they pay heavily for the omission because they conflict with our enormous need to be successful, to be responsible for a dramatic recovery.

Much remains to be done to improve care for persons with complex chronic illness. Lack of a uniform definition hinders our ability to fully understand the service needs of this population. Current health care financing continues to impede full development of appropriate clinical models of care, and stifles innovations which require a relaxation of the arbitrary distinctions between health and social services. Absence of a population-based approach hinders our ability to assess the supply, demand, and distribution of practitioners needed to care for persons with complex chronic illness.

Yet, in reflecting on the care provided to these persons, the good news is in the number and variety of innovative health care models currently being tested. Capitated managed care offers an opportunity to reconfigure ambulatory and long-term services to be more in keeping with patients' desire to exert control over their lives. The increasing array of long-term care options has the potential of maintaining people in the community and possibly of making institutional care more flexible and homelike. As a result of greater emphasis on primary care in nursing and medical education, increasing numbers of health care students will be exposed to faculty and clinical practice sites that deliver exemplary ambulatory and long-term care services. As these and other models bring persons with chronic illness more consistently into our range of vision, their care needs can become the cornerstone for restructuring of the health care system.

Acknowledgments

This work was partially supported by a grant from the Robert Wood Johnson Foundation.

References

Adams, P. F., and Benson, V. (1991). Current estimates from the National Health Interview Survey. *National Center for Health Statistics, Vital Health Statistics* 10:181–89.

Anderson, G., and Steinberg, E. (1984). Hospital readmissions in the Medicare population. *New England Journal of Medicine* 311:1349–53.

Arras, J., and Dubler, N. N. (1994). Bringing the hospital home: Ethical and social implications of high-tech home care. *Hastings Center Report, Special Supplement* S19–28.

Boullough, B. (1993). In M. Mezey and D. O. McGivern, eds., *Nurses, Nurse Practitioners: Evolution to Advanced Practice* (pp. 267–80). New York: Springer Publishing.

Capitman, J. A., MacAdam, M. S., and Abrahams, R. (1993). Case management roles in emergent approaches to long-term care. In P. Katz, R. Kane, and M. Mezey, eds., *Advances in Long-Term Care I* (pp. 124–46). New York: Springer Publishing.

Cesta, T., and Cohen, E. L. (1993). *Nursing Case Management.* St. Louis: C. V. Mosby.

Community Nursing Organizations (1993). *American Nurses Association Cost-effective Primary and Managed Care Models Using Nurses.* Washington, D.C.: American Nurses Association.

Czerenda, J., and Best, L. (1994). System case management: Internists and advanced practice nurses, partners in system-wide case management. *Gerontologist* 34 (special iss.): xiii.

Daly, B. J., Rudy, E. B., Thompson, K. S., and Happ, M. B. (1993). Development of a special unit for chronically critically ill patients. *Heart and Lung* 20 (1): 45–51.

Diamond, M. (1983). Social adaptation of the chronically ill. In D. Mechanic, ed., *Handbook of Health, Health Care, and the Health Professions* (pp. 636–54). New York: Free Press.

Estes, C. L. (1993). The aging enterprise revisited. *Gerontologist* 33:292–98.

Freeman, H. E., Blendon, R. J., Aiken, L. H., Sudman, S., Mullinex, C. F., and Corey, C. R. (1990). Americans report on their access to health care. In P. H. Lee and C. L. Estes, eds., *The Nation's Health*, 3rd ed. (pp. 309–19). Boston: Jones and Bartlett.

Freund, C. (1993). Research as to the role of nurse practitioners. In M. Mezey and D. O. McGivern, eds., *Nurses, Nurse Practitioners: Evolution to Advanced Practice* (pp. 59–87). New York: Springer Publishing.

Fulmer, M., and Mezey, M. (1994). Contemporary geriatric nursing. In W. R. Hazzard, E. L. Bierman, J. P. Blass, W. H. Ettinger, J. Halter, eds., *Principles of Geriatric Medicine and Gerontology* (pp. 249–58). New York: McGraw-Hill.

Garrard, J., Kane, R., Ratner, E., and Buchanan, J. (1990). The impact of nurse clinicians on the care of nursing home residents. In P. Katz, R. Kane, and M. Mezey, eds., *Advances in Long-term Care I* (pp. 169–85). New York: Springer Publishing.

Guralnik, J. M., and Simonsick, E. M. (1993). Physical disability in older Americans. *Journals of Gerontology* 48:3–10.

Hadley, E., Ory, M., Suzman, R., and Weindruch, R. (1993). Forward. *Journal of the American Geriatrics Society* 48:vii

Health Care Financing Administration (1985). Unpublished data.

Health Care Financing Administration (1992). Unpublished data.

Helberg, J. L. (1993). Factors influencing home care nursing problems and nursing care. *Research in Nursing and Health* 16:363–70.

Holmes, D., Bloom, H., Teresi, J., Monaco, C., and Rosen, S. (1991). An examination of nursing home transfers to hospitals: Final report. New York: United Hospital Fund.

Inglis, A. D., and Kjervik, D. (1993). Empowerment of advanced practice nurses: Regulation reform needed to increase access to care. *Journal of Law, Medicine and Ethics* 21 (2): 193–205.

Institute of Medicine (1986). *Improving the Quality of Care in Nursing Homes.* Washington, D.C.: National Academy Press.

Jamieson, M. P. (1990). Block nursing: Practicing autonomous professional nursing in the community. *Nursing and Health Care* 11:44–49.

Kane, R. A. (in press). The elusive definition of home: An imperative for rethinking home care. *Milbank Quarterly.*

Kane, R. A., and Wilson, K. B. (1993). Assisted living in the United States: A new paradigm for residential care for frail older persons. Washington, D.C.: American Association of Retired Persons.

Kane, R. L., Garrard, J., Skay, C. L., et al. (1989). Effects of a geriatric nurse practitioner on process and outcome of nursing home care. *American Journal of Public Health* 79 (9): 1271–77.

Kane, R. L., Illston, L. H., and Miller, N. A. (1992). Qualitative analysis of the program of all-inclusive care for the elderly (PACE). *Gerontologist* 32:771–80.

Kearnsk, J. M. (1989). Report of the 1989 Panel of Experts meeting to review and update the criteria for the criteria-based model. U.S. Department of Health and Human Services, Bureau of Health Manpower.

Kemper, P., and Murtaugh, C. M. (1991). Lifetime use of nursing home care. *New England Journal of Medicine* 324:595–600.

Lawrence, D. B., and Gaus, C. R. (1983). Long-term care: Financing and policy issues. In D. Mechanic, ed., *Handbook of Health, Health Care, and the Health Professions* (pp. 365–78). New York: Free Press.

Lewis, A., Leake, B., Leal-Sotelo, M., and Clark, V. (1987). The initial effects of the prospective payment system on nursing home patients. *American Journal of Public Health* 77:819–22.

Liu, K., Perozek, M., and Manton K. (1993). Catastrophic acute and long-term care costs: Risks faced by disabled elderly persons. *Gerontologist* 33:299–307.

McDermott, S., Arnold, S., and Kepferle, L. (1989). Effect of a geriatric nurse practitioner on the process and outcomes of nursing home care. *American Journal of Public Health* 79:1271–77.

Mathematica Policy Research. (1987). *The Evaluation of the National Long-Term Care Demonstration: Final Report.* Princeton, N.J.: Mathematica Policy Research.

Mezey, A. P., and Lawrence, R. S. (1995). Ambulatory care. In T. R. Kovner, ed., *Health Care Delivery in the United States* (pp. 122–61). New York: Springer Publishing.

Mezey, M., Dougherty, M., Wade, P., and Mersman, C. (1994). Nurse practitioners, certified nurse midwives, and nurse anesthetists: Changing care in acute care hospitals in New York City. *Journal of the New York State Nurses Association* 25:13–17.

Mezey, M., and Knapp, M. (1993). Nurse staffing in nursing homes: Implications for achieving quality of care. In P. Katz, ed., *Advances in Long Term Care* (vol. 2, pp. 130–51). New York: Springer Publishing.

Mezey, M., and Lynaugh, J. (1992). Care in nursing homes: Patients' needs; nursing's response. In L. Aiken and C. Fagin, eds., *Charting Nursing's Future: Agenda for the '90s* (pp. 198–215). Philadelphia: Lippincott.

Mezey, M., and Lynaugh, J. (1994). The role of nursing professionals and non-professionals in the care of patients with complex and chronic illness. Paper prepared for the Robert Wood Johnson Foundation.

Mezey, M., and Scanlon, W. (1988). Registered nurses in nursing homes. Paper prepared for the Secretary's Commission on Nursing. Washington, D.C.: Department of Health and Human Services.

Mitty, E. (1989). Response to institutional care: Caregivers and quality. *Indices of Quality in Long-Term Care Research and Practice*. New York: National League for Nursing.

Mullan, F., Rivo, M., and Politzer, R. (1993). Doctors, dollars, and determination: Making physician work-force policy. *Health Affairs* suppl.:138–51.

Munro, D. (1990). The influence of registered nurse staffing on quality of nursing home care. *Research in Nursing and Health* 13:263-70.

Naegle, M. A., ed. (1993). *Substance Abuse Education in Nursing,* vols. 1–3. New York: National League for Nursing.

National Center for Health Statistics (1987). Nursing home characteristics: Preliminary data from the 1985 National Nursing Home Survey. Advance Data from Vital and Health Statistics, no. 131 (DHHS pub. no. 87-1250). Hyattsville, Md.: U.S. Public Health Service.

National Center for Health Statistics (1993). *Health United States, 1992.* Hyattsville, Md.: U.S. Public Health Service.

Naylor, M., Brooten, D., Jones, R., Lavizzo-Mourey, R., Mezey, M., and Pauly, M. (1994). Comprehensive discharge planning for the hospitalized elderly. *Annals of Internal Medicine* 120:999–1006.

Rice, D. P., and Laplante, M. P. (1992). Medical expenditures for disability and disabling comorbidity. *American Journal of Public Health* 82 (5): 739–41.

Sager, A., Pendleton, S., Lees-Low, C., Dennis, D., and Hoffman, V. (1989). *Living at Home: The Roles of Public and Informal Supports in Sustaining Disabled Older Americans.* Waltham, Mass.: Brandeis University.

Schneider, E., and Guralnik, J. M. (1990). The aging of America: Impact on health care costs. *Journal of the American Medical Association* 263:2335–40.

Shaughnessy, P., and Kramer A. (1990). The increased needs of patients in nursing homes and patients receiving home health care. *New England Journal of Medicine* 322:21–27.

Shaughnessy, P., Kramer, A., and Hittle, D. (1990). The teaching nursing home experiment: Its effects and implications. Study paper 6. Denver: Center for Health Services Research, University of Colorado.

Shaughnessy, P. W., Kramer, A. M., Hittle, D. F., and Steiner, J. F. (1995). Quality of care in teaching nursing homes: Findings and implications. *Health Care Financing Review* 16 (4): 55–83.

Siegler, E. (1994). A collaborative geriatric rehabilitation practice concept for noninstitutionalized elderly post-stroke patients. In E. Siegler and F. Whitney, eds., *Team Training in the Health Professions* (pp. 87–100). New York: Springer Publishing.

Small, N., and Walsh, M., eds. (1988). *Teaching Nursing Homes: The Nursing Perspective*. Owings Mills, Md.: National Health Publishing.

Solomon, P. (1988). Geriatric assessment: Methods for clinical decision making. *Journal of the American Medical Association* 259:24-50.

Spector, W. D. (1989). Reforming nursing home quality regulation: Impact on cited deficiencies and nursing home outcomes. *Medical Care* 8:789–801.

Spector, W. D., Kapp, M., Eichan, A., Tucker, R., Rosenstein, R., and Katz, S. (1988). Case-mix outcomes and resource use in nursing homes. Providence, R.I.: Center for Gerontology and Health Care Research, Brown University.

Stone, R. I. (1993). Integration of home and community-based services: Issues for the 1990s. Prepared for the Visiting Nurse Service of New York and the Milbank Memorial Fund Home-based Care for a New Century Project, New York.

Strahan, G. W. (1993). Overview of home health and hospice care patients: Preliminary data from the 1992 National Home and Hospice Care Survey. *Advance Data from Vital and Health Statistics*, no. 235. Hyattsville, Md.: National Center for Health Statistics.

Strauss, A., and Glaser, B. 1975. *Chronic Illness and the Quality of Life*. St. Louis: C. V. Mosby.

Survey of state implementation of OBRA requirements for the nurse aide training and competency evaluation program. Vol. 1: Introduction and summary. Washington, D.C.: National Citizens' Coalition for Nursing Home Reform.

U.S. Congress (1986). Office of Technology Assessment. *Nurse Practitioners, Physician Assistants, and Certified Nurse-Midwives: A Policy Analysis* (Health Technology Case Study 37, OTA-HCS-37). Washington, D.C.: Government Printing Office.

Van Buren, C. B. (1981). The acute hospitalization of residents of skilled nursing facilities in Monroe County, N.Y. Rochester, N.Y.: Masters thesis. Department of Preventive Medicine and Rehabilitation, University of Rochester.

Verbrugge, L. M. (1990). Longer life but worsening health? In P. H. Lee and C. L. Estes, eds. *The Nation's Health*, 3rd ed. (pp. 14–34). Boston: Jones and Bartlett.

Visiting Nurse Service of New York (1993). A psychiatric nurse consultation service for patients with HIV-AIDS. New York: Visiting Nurse Service.

Zarit, S. H. (1992). Measures in family caregiving research. In B. Bauer, ed., *Conceptual and Methodological Issues in Family Caregiving Research*. Proceedings of the invitational conference on Family Caregiving Research. Toronto, Ontario: University of Toronto.

Zimmer, J., Eggert, G., Treat, A., and Brodows, B. (1988). Nursing homes as acute care providers. *Journal of the American Geriatric Society* 36:124–29.

III

EXPLORING THE FUTURE OF SETTINGS FOR CARE

7

The Evolution of the American Nursing Home

Robert L. Kane, M.D.

The nursing home is the product of a mixed lineage, none of which is especially attractive. It is the offspring of the almshouse and the boarding house, and the step-child of the hospital (see Chapter 2).* Although there is no specific date of birth, private nursing homes were fostered by the passage of the Social Security Act in 1935, which specifically prohibited coverage for patients in publicly funded institutions run by cities and counties (Dunlop, 1979), and they became an industry with the establishment of Medicaid and Medicare in 1965.

In the intervening 30 years since these laws were passed, much has changed with regard to nursing home care. During this period the nursing home has been shaped by external forces, primarily governmental regulations and payment. Spurred in part by Social Security's prohibition against paying for persons in publicly funded institutions, nursing homes have emerged as largely private institutions heavily financed by public funds. Over half the revenues for nursing home care come from governmental sources (Helbing and Cornelius, 1993). Nursing homes have become very adept at adapting to the regulatory environment and have established a tradition of reaction rather than initiative. Because innovation raises threats of regulatory response or failure to pay, the nursing homes have developed a risk-averse posture.

*It is not a coincidence that when nursing homes were covered under Medicare and life safety requirements were established, the model used was the blueprint for the small rural hospitals built with support from the Hill-Burton program. Hence, there is a whole generation of nursing homes built in the later 1960s and early 1970s that look just like small hospitals.

Inasmuch as the majority of public funding for nursing home care comes from a welfare program, Medicaid, the status of care in nursing homes has been further diminished. The nursing home has been viewed as the refuge of last resort, avoided by potential residents and health care professionals alike. Medicaid reimbursement rates have generally been set as low as possible; hence nursing homes have been operated on a complicated minimalist philosophy, pressed to contain costs on the one hand and pushed to provide an acceptable level of care on the other. Because many nursing home clients are cognitively impaired and almost all are quite frail, public attitudes have favored a severe regulatory approach designed to protect these vulnerable persons from mistreatment or underservice. This perspective was greatly reenforced in the early 1970s by a series of scandals that uncovered examples of terrible neglect (Moss and Halamandaris, 1977) and by periodic episodes since (Long, 1987).

A series of regulatory reforms has shaped the industry in terms of both its structure and its practice. The most comprehensive were included in the 1987 Omnibus Budget Reconciliation Act, which carried out many of the recommendations of an earlier Institute of Medicine committee report (Institute of Medicine, 1986).

Despite its flawed image, the nursing home has served as the touchstone of long-term care. Programs have been proffered as "alternatives" to nursing home care. Repeated efforts have been made to create other types of programs, interestingly referred to as "community-based," as if nursing homes were not in the community. Different modes of institutional care are possible and care in the community may often overlap with that given in one of these institutions. It has taken almost 20 years of research, however, to appreciate that community care should not be viewed as a simple substitute for institutional care (Weissert, Cready, and Pawelak, 1989). The next logical step is to recognize that the marriage represented by the term *nursing home* need not be consummated as it has been. Newer combinations of lodging and services are possible.

In addition to the changing demographics of an aging society (see Chapter 3), at least eight major, but often interrelated, themes will affect the shape of nursing home care over the next decade: managed care, role diversification, acute and chronic care linkage, uncoupling nursing home care, information technology, changing ethics, accountability, and changing payment.

Managed Care

Managed care refers to efforts to contain the costs of care by holding the providers of that care responsible for some share of the financial risks of providing it. The purest form of managed care is capitation, a practice in which an entity agrees to provide a given set of services (or benefits) for a fixed price per person, thereby assuming the entire financial risk. Because health insurance can fill a similar role, managed care has come to mean health insurance with some form of active oversight, such as case management or special contracts with providers. Usually case management is directed towards those at greatest risk of being heavy users of care. One such group is frail older persons. At present, managed care is largely focused on acute care, but as the boundaries between acute and chronic care become less clear, nursing homes will be affected. Already nursing homes are being used by some managed care corporations to provide services previously provided more expensively in hospitals.

Several factors combine to make managed care attractive to political forces. At a time of growing concern about the costs of medical care, managed care offers a way to cap expenditures by setting a total price on a set of services. Because working within a budget cap will necessitate some sort of rationing or controlled distribution, contracting out that care to some external agency distances political figures from the responsibility of making the difficult decisions.

Managed care has the advantage of permitting greater degrees of innovation. Because the method of providing care is no longer influenced by what is reimbursable, newer forms of care, such as geriatric nurse practitioners (Kane et al., 1991, 1989), can be used to provide care in various settings, including nursing homes. Indeed, the whole philosophy of care is turned on its ear. Moving from fee-for-service to capitated reimbursement changes the fundamental rules of the game. What were formerly revenue-generating activities now become cost centers, and all incentives point to finding more efficient ways to deliver services.

Although managed care has been established primarily with respect to acute care, it is already extending into chronic care in several respects. Under the pressure of both managed care and Medicare's prospective hospital payment scheme, hospital lengths of stay are falling. As hospital stays become ever shorter, much of the slack is picked up by nursing homes, which are being called upon to treat patients who would formerly have been hospital patients. Many managed care patients, including some who require nursing home care, also have chronic conditions. Some managed care programs are being established specifically to deal with this sub-group of chronically disabled persons. In these cases considerable money can be saved not only by shortening hospital stays but also by preventing them altogether. Closer attention to primary care and a greater willingness to treat problems in the nursing home can avoid the need for hospitalization in many cases.

It seems very likely that models providing managed care to the chronically ill will be established. Under the 1982 Tax Equity and Fiscal Responsibility Act (TEFRA), Medicare established a mechanism for paying a capitated rate that would be equivalent to the average costs for Medicare beneficiaries in a given geographic area. Many of these so-called TEFRA HMOs, which cater specifically to Medicare beneficiaries, have not adopted many geriatrically oriented practices (Friedman and Kane, 1993). However, a few examples of managed care programs attend to the disabled older population. The On Lok program, which began in San Francisco's Chinatown, has been replicated in a number of places across the country. It specifically targets frail older persons and has developed a program designed to reduce the use of all institutions, hospitals and nursing homes (Kane, Illston, and Miller, 1992). To do this, the program relies heavily on day health care, but dissatisfaction among some clients with that particular mode of care has prompted other approaches as well.

The social health maintenance organization (S/HMO) was established as a way to combine acute and broadly defined long-term care for older persons by adding a payment for long-term care coverage to a capitated fee that covers the basic Medicare benefit package (Leutz et al., 1985). Its four demonstration sites offer a modest long-term care package on top of a standard TEFRA Medicare HMO contract. By combining these resources, the programs have the ability to create innovative ways to meet the complex and interactive demands of such patients. To control the costs of such a program, the S/HMOs have restricted their enrollees to a group whose fraction of disabled members is proportionate to that in the general older population. The evaluation of the original demonstrations suggests that the results of such care are not very different from those obtained from more typical Medicare HMOs (Newcomer, Harrington, and Friedlob, 1990).

In the early 1990s the Medicare HMO model was specifically extended to cover persons who were already in nursing homes. Under a program called EverCare, nursing home patients are enrolled in HMOs which cover the cost of all acute care but not the cost of nursing homes. EverCare's developers believed that they could make a profit serving this frail group by giving more attention to preventing expensive problems through more active primary care. The underlying theory, which appears to work, is that more intensive primary care can alleviate the need for expensive hospital care in enough cases to more than offset its cost (Malone, Chase, and Bayard, 1993).

Several states are addressing the portion of the Medicare population also covered by Medicaid primarily by developing other models of care that include the costs of both acute and long-term care. The extent of the coverage varies with the model. Some include all long-term and acute care; others cover only some of the nursing home care. However, with the move to some form of universal health insurance, Medicaid is likely to be eliminated, as the responsibility for such care is folded into the general care system, and new programs will have to find ways to provide a broader set of coverage.

Role Diversification

The nursing home has been shaped largely by external forces. For example, as the pattern of acute care has changed, the nursing home has been caught in the current. The impetus for paying hospitals on the basis of diagnosis-related groups and the trend toward "quicker and sicker" discharges from hospitals (Kahn et al., 1990) have left the nursing home caring for a group of patients it was ill-equipped to handle, although just such a role had in fact been envisioned by the framers of Medicare.

Some years ago, Bruce Vladeck suggested that nursing home patients be divided into three groups. The recuperating and the terminally ill needed hospital care. The chronically ill and the socially isolated who were not entirely helpless could be cared for in the community. Those who suffered from moderate to severe senility or other psychiatric or physical disability were the only group who needed nursing home care (Vladeck, 1980). Today's nursing home is being asked to play even more roles in caring for a heterogeneous group of patients. At least five distinct subgroups can be identified:

— Those needing recuperation and perhaps rehabilitation from acute care episodes
— The terminally ill
— The chronically physically disabled but alert
— The severely demented
— Those in permanent vegetative states

Each of these subgroups needs a different type of care. The future of nursing homes will see great role diversification to meet these varied needs.

The variety of the patients' needs implies different social contracts. While those who are being treated for a condition that is expected to improve may be willing, as is the case in hospitals, to trade the loss of autonomy and individual identity for the expected benefits of care, for those who do not harbor such hopes of recovery, the treatment is, in effect, an end in itself. The therapeutic milieu is the patients' living environment. The benefits are as likely to be measured in terms of quality of life as in reduced morbidity and mortality.

In the context of ever-shorter hospital stays and even trends toward completely avoiding hospitalization, many patients still need technologically sophisticated care. The nursing home is one potential vehicle for such care. Patients discharged from hospital to recuperate from their illnesses in skilled nursing facilities resemble those who would still have been in hospitals in earlier times. However, many nursing homes may not have the staffing levels to be able to provide this level of care. Indeed, it is conceivable that patients today can be too sick for nursing home care and instead need to be sent home with active home health care. Some degree of discomfort may be tolerable if it leads to quicker or surer recovery. The format of care in these situations may more closely resemble the logistics of hospital care. The critical question for such cases is how effective the care in these settings is at restoring the patients' health status to what it was prior to the acute event. Little solid evidence is yet available to answer this important question, but preliminary data from a study of the outcomes of post-hospital care for selected conditions suggests that patients discharged to nursing homes fare less well than comparable patients sent to other settings, even going home without formal care. If confirmed, such a finding suggests the need for substantial reforms in nursing home care if it is to continue to fill this role. A new form of nursing home care, subacute care, which will be discussed below, is being promoted to respond to this market opportunity. It purports to offer a new approach to nursing home care.

Nursing homes are also used as hospices. Here the goals of care are quite different. By definition, no hope of cure or recovery is offered. Instead, attention is focused on comfort. Care is palliative. Rules are few and opportunities are created for patients to achieve as much pleasure as their condition and remaining days permit. Although most hospice care will likely continue to be provided in patients' homes, there should continue to be a need for providing some of this care in settings like nursing homes. The more immediate question is, Why is it possible to create more benign environments for dying persons but apparently to feel justified in not offering such a service to the living? Ought not some of the lessons of the hospice movement be applied more widely, to create environmental changes that will enhance the quality of life for all nursing home residents?

Many patients are in nursing homes because they suffer from chronic problems that limit their ability to care for themselves. For those who are physically impaired but mentally alert, the nature of their environment can greatly affect the quality of their lives and the likelihood of their preserving their remaining function. False concepts of efficiency, designed to minimize staff time, may encourage staff to perform tasks for such patients rather than have them try to do the tasks themselves. Because patients are often limited in the ability to leave the institution, their environment is shaped by the persons around them. Being forced to share their living space with strangers, especially persons who may behave in inappropriate ways, can greatly reduce the few pleasures available to them.

While it is not clear that cognitively impaired patients profit from being treated in facilities where patients are segregated according to their behavioral status, the mentally alert assuredly benefit enormously from not having to share their quarters with such people. Few of us would willingly endure such cohabitation with persons whose disease destroyed their inhibitions to the point where their behavior became socially inappropriate. Having other people wander into your room or go through your things destroys any sense of privacy and personhood. Although there is currently work under way to test the benefits of so-called special care units for the cognitively impaired, there is no question that segregating them from the alert physically impaired patients will improve the quality of life for the latter. Much of the work to be done lies in determining how care for the mentally impaired can be delivered separately and efficiently. It is not clear that separate facilities must inevitably be more expensive (Grant, Kane, and Stark, 1994).

A smaller set of nursing home patients are in permanent (at least expected to be permanent) vegetative states as the consequence of trauma, stroke, or end-stage dementia. These cases raise painful ethical issues about whether the quality of lives (which is impossible to determine) justifies sustaining their care (see Chapter 11). Side-stepping the ethical land mine of passive euthanasia, there is still a question of what proportion of the long-term care resources should be devoted to the care of such patients. More efficient means of caring for this group of unfortunate individuals must be found. This care is directed toward avoiding the secondary consequences of their conditions, problems like decubitus ulcers, dehydration, and starvation. At present, such care is resource intensive (U.S. Congress, 1987).

The Linkage between Acute Care and Chronic Care

The distinction between acute and chronic care has always been vague and is becoming ever vaguer. Many episodes of long-term care begin with an acute event, often a hospitalization. This trend has been amplified by the changes in Medicare's reimbursement of hospitals, which encourage shorter stays and hence greater use of other types of care. Designating a person as an acute care or long-term care patient becomes an artificial exercise determined more by payment source than clinical need.

From the opposite perspective, being in long-term care does not abrogate the need for acute care. Just the opposite, in fact; long-term care patients use more acute care than those less disabled. For example, in establishing a capitation rate for Medicare coverage, the current system, the average adjusted per capita cost (AAPCC) allows a substantial upward adjustment above the base rate for persons in nursing homes. Indeed, chronic care patients need active primary medical care. At least one organization, EverCare, has demonstrated the effectiveness of more attentive primary care. They offer a capitated program of care for nursing home patients and have proven profitable by reducing hospital use. In essence, they have shown that an investment in aggressive primary care for nursing home residents can more than pay for itself through savings in more expensive acute institutional care. This philosophy of investment is also the underpinning for a series of geriatric assessment and treatment programs that have been successful in reducing mortality and morbidity and lowering the rate of nursing home use among older persons discharged from hospitals and even for some who were living in the community (Stuck et al., 1993).

Subacute Care

As noted above, the changing pattern of hospital care has created intense demands for post-hospital care to replace care that was formerly provided in hospitals. A new form of specialized nursing home care has sprung up to meet this market opportunity, subacute care. In effect, this care provides approximately the same intensity of care offered in the general wards of hospitals but without all the overhead that is a major part of the modern hospital. For example, there are usually no on-site laboratory or x-ray facilities. Administrative overhead is much lower.

There are good reasons to believe that this sort of care will expand in the future. Indeed, the hospital of tomorrow may consist of only intensive care units, with all other care being delivered in subacute care facilities. Important questions are thus raised about the basis for providing this emerging type of care. One does not want to relive the history of hospital care with a variety of marginal facilities that require time and effort to bring into line. At present not enough is known about the factors that are associated with effective subacute care to become overly dogmatic about the structural characteristics that should be required. However, the proliferation of such units motivates an urgent need for just such information and appropriate regulatory action.

Because these units are currently considered nursing homes, they are subject to much more stringent regulation than they would face as hospitals, which have a more established tradition of self-regulation. Given the growing trend toward reducing hospital bed supply, it is not clear whether the subacute units of the future will emerge from nursing homes or will be reclaimed by the hospital industry. As hospitals continue to reduce their bed complement, they will invariably rediscover these very same patients they discharged and develop special care units at a lower level of intensity to address this subacute care population. Thus, it is unclear under which historical mandate they will operate. There is good reason to question whether hospitals can master the art of operating as efficiently as have nursing homes. It may prove easier for nursing homes to trade up than for hospitals to trade down.

The competition between hospital and nursing homes for the subacute care business may take another turn, namely through mergers and acquisitions. There is already evidence of hospitals entering into various types of ownership and cooperative arrangements with nursing homes. In some cases they are owned by a larger corporate entity; in others they develop joint ventures; in still others they have developed special contractual relationships. From this a new hybrid may emerge that will include elements of both, with perhaps more emphasis on rehabilitation.

Rural Issues

Long-term care and its relationship to acute care are somewhat different in rural areas. The populations of rural areas are older on average, because of out-migration of younger persons. Because they are less densely populated, rural travel distances are longer, and programs such as home care become more logistically difficult. At the same time, rural institutions often display more flexibility than their urban counterparts in such matters as staffing patterns in response to changing occupancy and greater role interchangeability.

As hospital occupancy has been declining, rural nursing homes have become more important as sources of both care and revenue. Over 20 years ago, in recognition of the problems of low hospital occupancy and a shortage of nursing home beds in rural areas, Medicare regulations were changed to permit the use of "swing beds" in rural hospitals. In effect, a patient could be discharged from acute coverage and enter Medicare supported skilled nursing home care without leaving his bed. By most accounts the program has been a great success (Shaughnessy, 1991).

Uncoupling

For those nursing home patients who have retained the ability to appreciate their environment, today's nursing home represents a special paradox. It offers little of either nursing or home. A more appropriate way to meet the needs of this group may lie in recombining the roles represented by the nursing home. It is feasible to provide people with a place to live and to bring to that dwelling a package of services tailored to each individual. Brody's "Procrustean bed" model of the nursing home (Brody, 1973) can be replaced with one more tailored to individual needs and abilities.

The heart of this concept, often referred to as "assisted living" (Kane and Wilson, 1993), is affording each person a separate living situation. This may be nothing more than the equivalent of a studio apartment, using little more area than is currently required under nursing home regulations, but it includes the provision of the minimum necessities for self-care: living and sleeping space, some sort of cooking and food storage facility, and a bathroom.

A key element of this arrangement is that the individual is first and foremost a tenant with property rights. In effect, the fundamental social contract that pertains in a nursing home is altered. The dweller has the right to privacy. Services are provided with that person's permission. Entrance is possible only with the person's consent. Under such a situation, the relationship with service providers takes on a new cast. The patient retains much more control. Care plans must be negotiated and agreed to. The situation is closely akin to that encountered in home care.

While there is growing enthusiasm for the principles of assisted living, there remains active debate as to how the care should be offered and to whom. Some stop short of providing recipients with all the amenities of independent living, especially cooking facilities, often claiming that such equipment is not safe for many frail older persons. In practice, those residents who are too confused to be trusted with equipment for heating food can have it disconnected. Some assisted living operations have shared bathrooms on the grounds of cost-savings, but most believe that in the long run, independent facilities will prove cheaper and easier to manage.

The question of for whom assisted living is suitable is still open to active debate. Experience continues to show that even quite frail persons can flourish in such an environment. Even those who have proved actively disruptive in more traditional settings often adjust well to this environment. Those who require large amounts of frequent care may not be appropriately cared for here, but those who need only intermittent, if skilled, attention can receive it well in this setting. Indeed, assisted living is compatible with visiting nursing services.

In effect, by redefining nursing home care in this way, the distinction between community-based care and institutional care is vitiated. The basic approach to care is the same in both situations. The difference lies in the need to provide housing. This need may occur for several reasons. Some people need housing because they have no housing or because their current housing cannot support their level of disability. In other cases, the decision to relocate to assisted living may be based on grounds of efficiency. The relative cost of professionals' travel time may approach, or even exceed, the cost of the service itself. In such cases, providing care may require that recipients live in some form of congregate housing where services can be offered efficiently.

This kind of reconceptualization of the relationship between housing and services permits a reexamination of financial coverage. While services should be provided on a universal entitlement basis, housing can reasonably remain the responsibility of the individual. In some cases, people may not be able to afford housing and will require income supplementation or subsidization, but many older people can afford to pay for their housing. Indeed, one of the rewards of prudent living and saving should be the opportunity to live better in one's old age. Uncoupling housing and services payment provides a motivation to save, even perhaps a reason to purchase some form of long-term care insurance that would underwrite the cost of better housing. The Clinton administration's plan for health reform included a provision quite compatible with this concept. It proposed covering community-based care universally but specifically excluded from this coverage any payment for room and board.

Many see in the idea of assisted living the opportunity to redevelop the nursing home as it should be. As assisted living emerges as the blueprint for institutional care in the future, it will provide greater flexibility and hopefully be free of the historical burdens that have been used to justify the heavy regulatory hand laid on nursing homes. The enemy of assisted living is demands for a "level playing field." Nursing homes have been shaped by regulations. If those regulations are likewise applied to assisted living situations, they will transform these establishments into traditional nursing homes.

At a minimum, the model of single rooms and a shift in the relative power between recipients and providers of care should stand as essential building blocks for any reconceptualization of the nursing home. In whatever form they emerge, nursing homes need to provide a more homelike environment and to offer services to clients rather than require the residents to adapt to the dictates of the institution.

Information Technology

Although the role of technology in improving care for older persons in general is discussed in Chapter 8, some observations regarding nursing homes, in particular, are in order here. The future of nursing home care will be improved by the use of modern information technology. The ability to collect and display information on patients' status can improve care by offering early indications of change in patients' clinical courses and stimulating timely interventions. It is now feasible to use graphic presentations to display a great deal of information in easily comprehensible formats.

Electronic information has the advantage that it can be shared without loss of the original. The problems of making medical records available to providers geographically distant without giving up the original set can be readily overcome. Updated information can be provided to home care workers, primary care providers, nursing home personnel, and hospitals to ensure that everyone is working with current data.

Computers can be harnessed to guide care. Protocols can be established to provide workers with the best information available about appropriate care. Reminders can be programmed to foster timely attention to problems of importance. Special warnings can be developed to alert providers about potential interactions and risk factors. Assessments can be targeted at problems of particular interest, and changes in status can be immediately noted.

One simple technology with great potential is laser-read bar coding that allows a great deal of information to be stored in a few lines. Inexpensive hand-held devices are now available and better technology is certain to come. Comparing the bar code identifier for each patient and the identifier on single-dose packaged drugs, can virtually eliminate medication errors. Specific activities, such as timed toileting, can be monitored using these devices (Schnelle, 1990). Data gathered several times each day can be graphed and displayed readily, to show incidents and progress, and the results compared with other care providers or previously established targets. Bar coding can offer a foolproof way to assure that the home caregiver is present for the time committed and can be used to monitor checking of routine functions.

Changing Ethics

The current pressures for age-based rationing of services (Callahan, 1987) are likely to become more intense. While many question the premise of using age as the basis for allocation decisions, there is more support for relying on other measures, such as functioning or quality of life. One group that would become more highlighted under such different measures is the population in nursing homes. Ironically, the most aggressive advocates of age-based rationing are very willing to trade more and better long-term care for less acute care, but this focus will likely change as mores change. The current emphasis on advance directives, written in statements in which patients express their desires regarding treatment at a future date, is probably an overture to a broad examination of the desirability of active treatment efforts on behalf of those who have lost the capacity to enjoy their environment. Already, passive euthanasia by the withdrawal or discontinuance of life support measures is becoming increasingly feasible. It is not a big step from there to withholding other forms of supportive care, and even to accelerating the demise of those already far gone and in permanent vegetative states.

For many, such a step will reawaken legitimate concerns about eugenics (eliminating those deemed unfit), although in this case reproduction is not an issue. Specific procedures will need to be developed to assure impartial review of all cases. Persons not immediately involved in the care of such persons will have to play a central role in any final determinations of appropriate steps. Ethicists will debate actively the premise of redistributing public support from those least likely to benefit to those more able to gain from it.

At a less wrenching level, the growing enthusiasm for advance directives can be viewed as part of a wave of support for greater patient control in all aspects of health services. The older models of doctor-patient relationships, in which paternalism and beneficence played a great role (Szasz and Hollander, 1956), have given way to a new power relationship, in which the patient has much more to say about what happens.

In the case of persons viewed as vulnerable, this empowerment has come more slowly. Ironically, an emergent political alliance in the arena of long-term care, which joined the causes of frail older persons and disabled adults, has done a lot to catalyze this development (see Chapter 10). The younger disabled refuse to accept a passive recipient role and insist that they should retain control of their services rather than have them directed by some form of case manager. As with other persons their age, they express a strong eagerness to accept the consequences of their choices and demand the right to make their own decisions. Some have suggested that the social goals of younger and older disabled persons are quite different, but the younger advocates argue that older persons, including many of those in nursing homes, need to be educated to recognize a potential for self-determination.

Today's older persons, perhaps because they are perceived as vulnerable and perhaps because of the socialization experienced by their birth cohort, have accepted a more passive role. That situation is likely to change. If the current cohort of younger adults, the so-called "baby boomers," retains its commitment to self-improvement and active consumerism, they will emerge as very different older persons than those now filling today's nursing homes. As the distinction between community care and institutional care is reduced, and even eliminated, the right of patients to take risks will become more apparent. Older persons will be offered (and may demand) more choices about both the nature of the care provided to them and the vendors who provide it. They will live with what may be thought of as "managed risk," the recognition that some care options carry greater risks, usually as a trade-off for greater autonomy. Some older persons may opt for a safer, more confining environment; whereas others will choose freedom over safety.

Having recognized the right of older persons to make such choices, society must also fairly attribute the risk. Care providers can no longer be held to a risk-free standard of care. Rather, accountability must come to be based on reasonable, and statistically sound, expectations of outcomes, including adverse events.

Accountability

People in nursing homes are viewed, almost by definition, as vulnerable adults. The combination of this vulnerable status and the early history of extensive abuse of the system by unprincipled providers has led to a strong tradition of aggressive federal and state regulation of nursing homes. As in other areas, the need for regulation has outstripped the knowledge base of what constitutes good care and how to promote it. Much of the effort in quality assessment is spent on detecting problems, and much less is devoted to assessing (and acknowledging) good care. Much more effort goes into finding problems than solving them. Rules are promulgated on the basis of expert opinion rather than empirical observation. To maintain some distance between the regulator and the industry, to preserve a sense of objectivity, the regulators are proscribed from offering suggestions for improvement. The situation has degenerated into a game of "gotcha" claims and counterclaims with extensive litigation.

There is no question about the need for accountability in nursing home care, but there is great room for debate about how to operationalize this need. The 1986 Institute of Medicine report on nursing homes called for greater emphasis on the outcomes of care and less stringent demands for adherence to rules based on the process and structure of care, especially where the relationship between these two and outcomes was poorly established (Institute of Medicine, 1986). For nursing home care, this relationship is especially weak. There is little correlation between most of the regulatory dictates and their effects on care outcomes.

Discussions of the accountability for long-term care are often couched in terms of quality of care and quality of life, as though these were mutually exclusive. They need not be. Good long-term care should address both; the price of obtaining one should not be the loss of the other.

When what is done in the way of care is not strongly associated with results, it makes more sense to shift attention to the outcomes of care, where these outcomes are expressed, so as to recognize the importance of comparing actual and expected outcomes. In effect, one wants to adjust any judgment about outcomes to take cognizance of potential differences in case mix and baseline states.

A focus on outcomes raises several important questions. A critical issue is the marginal effect of care. In contrast with recipients of acute care, much of the fate of nursing home patients may lie with the nature of the patient. Care may play only a modest role in improving the patient's clinical trajectory, although poor care can create a host of iatrogenic problems. Before entertaining any serious discussion about how to measure the effects of care on outcomes, one must first decide what are the relevant outcomes.

Nursing home care addresses much more than simply medical concerns. It deals with a broad array of issues. There is generally good consensus about the domains addressed by such care. They include:

— physiological function (e.g., blood pressure, blood sugar, edema)
— function (usually described in terms of activities of daily living [ADLs] and instrumental activities of daily living [IADLs])
— pain and discomfort
— cognition
— affect
— meaningful social activities
— interpersonal contact
— satisfaction

Measures are available for each of these constructs, and techniques have been developed to contrast expected with actual outcomes (Kane et al., 1983a, 1983b).

Several principles must be borne in mind when using outcomes for establishing accountability. Outcomes are meaningful only for grouped observations where the rate of performance, appropriately adjusted for case mix differences, can be described. Because outcomes are the result of several factors, much of their interpretation is directed toward identifying the contribution that can be fairly assigned to the treatment given. In effect, outcomes can be thought of as the product of clients' baseline status, their sociodemographic factors (including such things as age, education, and gender, as well as the strength of social support), clinical factors (including both current and historical information), and treatment. Case-mix correction, which statistically adjusts for differences in relevant sociodemographic and clinical elements, is needed to assure that valid comparisons of outcomes are made.

It is worth noting that, while most nursing home residents have a trajectory of decline, such deterioration is not universal or inevitable. Some patients show improvement (Siu et al., 1993) and others are capable of improving with aggressive care (Fiatarone et al., 1994).

The availability of meaningful outcomes data can improve care directly, as well as through regulation. It can be used to motivate line workers who need a better sense of the effects of their care. Facing patients whose general trajectory is decline can have a numbing effect. Difficulty in discerning the difference care makes can lead to discouragement. Giving them evidence that contrasts the patients' actual course with what would otherwise have occurred with ordinary care can improve caregivers' morale and performance.

Meaningful outcomes data can also enlarge the role of patients and families in determining the quality of care. Patients and their families can be effective as both informants and judges. For example, they can tell us a lot about what was done and what happened as a result. It is impossible to think about obtaining functional data without getting it from patients, either directly or second hand. Patients have also been shown effective in describing what was done during a clinical encounter (Davies and Ware, 1988). Patients and their families are the best source of information on satisfaction with the way they were treated, including problems with access.

On the other hand, they are not able to judge accurately the correctness of diagnoses or treatments. Too often patients assume that their caregivers have basic technical competence when the opposite may be true. Patient input into quality assessments needs to be carefully designed to inquire about those aspects of care for which the patient can serve as a competent judge. Asking them to make global judgments about the quality of care they receive may undermine this essential function.

Developing Comparable Expectations

Collecting data on outcomes and relating it to actions taken can create an empirical basis for improving nursing home care. Outcomes are basically the result of several factors: baseline status, elements of care, patient factors (both clinical and demographic), and environment. Analyses can separate the impact of these several components and help to isolate the role of specific care elements, to determine what types of care are most effective with different sets of patients. The same information base can also be used to compare the performance of different providers and different care settings.

Leveling the Playing Field

As indicated above, in the name of equity, some have called for a leveling of the playing field, that the same criteria and standards used to measure nursing home care should be applied to care delivered in innovative settings such as assisted living. Such an approach is fair if the emphasis is on outcomes, but if structural and process criteria are used, the fundamental nature of the assisted living innovation would be directly threatened. One cannot impose a set of rules developed for one type of operation and expect it to be applicable to another.

Delegation

Moving away from the traditional nursing home model will require re-examining the role and regulation of health professionals. The current trend toward increasing the use of expensive skilled health professionals to provide what are often basic services may impede the creation of more efficient service delivery. Not all services need to be provided by highly trained and certified individuals. For example, family members can provide a range of services, from simple to complex, but strangers giving the same care may need to be specifically certified. Some states have already recognized the incompatibility of more flexible care and rigid professional requirement by passing nursing practice acts that permit delegation of specific tasks (such as giving of injections) to health workers who have been trained by nurses and certified competent to perform the task. Similar steps will be needed to clear the way for a broader range of service mixes and a more varied set of potential providers.

Family members have always been and will likely continue to be the backbone of long-term care. "Family" is really a euphemism for women, who supply the large majority of informal care. Despite the changes in women's roles, as they enter the labor market in increasing numbers (Brody et al., 1992), they will probably continue to provide such care. Although some observers attribute nursing home admissions to families' inability or unwillingness to continue caring for a frail older person, data from repeated studies suggest that, even when adequate formal care is available without a heavy financial burden involved, informal care continues to account for at least 80 percent of all long-term care (Kane, Evans, and Macfadyen, 1990).

The Minimum Data Set

One of the innovations of the 1987 nursing home reforms was the Minimum Data Set (MDS), a standardized assessment tool designed to assure that all nursing patients were appropriately assessed. It includes both a basic evaluation and specific protocols for further exploring a predetermined set of problems.

Unfortunately, because the MDS was introduced as part of a regulatory effort rather than a quality improvement process, it has been viewed as something imposed by government rather than as a basic tool for improving caregiving. Nonetheless, it provides the basis for standardized data collection on nursing home residents at regular intervals. That information can be used as the basis for carrying out the type of outcome analyses described earlier. Yet, because the MDS was not designed primarily for this purpose, it does not cover many outcome parameters as completely as one might wish. Moreover, the providers of care cannot be expected to collect accurate information on some of its topics, such as customer satisfaction.

Even with these caveats, the MDS represents a good beginning. It affords data on ADLs and cognitive functioning and at least the beginnings of information on psychological affect. It can also be used to assess the occurrence of specific untoward events, such as decubiti, falls, and urinary incontinence.

Client Autonomy

As clients are reempowered to choose what sorts of care they will receive, new thinking must be given to questions of accountability. Although holding providers accountable for the outcomes they produce remains the strategy of choice, provisions must be made for a role of the client in making choices. It is unfair to hold providers responsible for choices made by clients. It is equally unrealistic to believe that providers have no responsibility. Just as with home care, they have a role to educate and assist. It will undoubtedly be more difficult to implement an outcomes-based approach to quality assurance as clients gain greater autonomy, but it is not an impossible task. It is very likely that the models will, in fact, come from home care.

Changing Payment

Whether or not the move toward managed care becomes substantially realized, new attention needs to be directed to the way in which nursing homes are paid. The current system requires a basis that reflects the costs of care, but no one seems to understand just what this means. Costs vary widely from state to state, with far more variation than can be attributed to wage differences. In an effort to respond to the federal dictate for cost-based reimbursement under Medicare and Medicaid, many states have opted for some form of case-mix payment. This approach has the dual advantages of meeting federal requirements and avoiding the disincentive against admitting heavy care patients.

The idea behind case-mix payment is that nursing home clientele can be categorized on the basis of indicators of the intensity of care they require. This categorization is usually accomplished by assessing the nursing time spent with a sample of patients with defining characteristics, such as dependencies and specific diagnoses or problems. Such an approach subdivides the nursing home population on the basis the type of care currently being provided, but it says nothing about what type of care should be given to achieve the best results.

Case-mix payments, in fact, create a perverse incentive. Effectively, the more disabled a patient becomes, the greater is the payment. In this regard, case-mix payment is the antithesis of outcomes-based payment, which would provide some sort of reward when patients did better than reasonably expected and a penalty when they did worse. The only way to avoid creating a disincentive for improvement in the case-mix approach would be not to reassess the patient. An outcomes-based approach would create a care climate that would emphasize doing what works rather than what is accepted.

These two payment approaches can find some common meeting ground. A case-mix approach could be used on admission only. Patients who improved and hence required less care should not create a penalty for the institution that contributed to their improved status. Likewise, nursing homes where patients got worse because of negligence should not benefit. If the case-mix system were applied only on admission, one would then be free to add to it an outcomes-payment approach.

Some observers have suggested that the bonuses and penalties associated with outcomes payment would not even be needed if there were an adequate means of reporting the outcomes of care. In a situation where there was free choice of providers and an ample supply of services, consumers who were aware of the performance of different nursing homes could base their decisions about where to go at least in part on these results. The marketing pressures alone might be enough to encourage nursing homes to work hard to encourage better patient outcomes. However, the competitive market conditions do not always apply. For example, in some locations there may be only a single facility. Or people may be forced to choose between geographic convenience and quality. Some nursing homes cater to specific types of clients, identified by religion or ethnicity, further reducing choices. A payment system that recognized outcomes could provide further incentives for delivering more effective care, especially useful in areas where choice among nursing homes is limited.

In managed care situations, choices would also likely be constrained by contracts with specific providers, but the managed care corporations would be at least as likely to use outcomes information to decide with which nursing homes they wanted to contract. Here too, information on outcomes should be made available to potential users as part of their decisionmaking and should be made public as part of required disclosure when alternative managed care plans are competing.

Conclusions

The future of the American nursing home is uncertain, but it is likely to be different from the present. Those who favor a cyclical interpretation of history will note that the pattern of convergence may now yield to one of diversity. An institution that was asked to fill a variety of roles may now have to become more specialized, reconstituting itself in separate institutions or other forms of care that respond to different constituencies.

Historically, the nursing home has largely been shaped by external forces. It has inherited the hospital's cast-offs. It has bent to meet government regulations, and it has responded to the incentives of different approaches to payment. There is no reason to expect that this reactive posture will change dramatically. Thus, the future will be shaped largely by broader influences in the health care arena. A policy like that proposed by the Clinton administration to support only community-based long-term care services would prove a strong stimulus to separating the "nursing" and "home" components of the current package. Even if such a policy is not implemented, the debate about long-term care may well take on a different complexion once the strong demand for more community-based services is appreciated. The challenge will be to present a definition of services that will permit the recognition of the often legitimate need for housing in the context of more individualized services.

The shifting role of hospital care will probably make some type of subacute, or extended, care necessary. Faced with a shrinking bed base, hospitals may make strong efforts to retain such care roles by converting unused bed capacity into skilled nursing units. If managed care becomes the rule, the distinction between hospital and nursing home care will be less important anyway, as both merge into a larger health care corporation. Subacute care under this scenario might emerge as more of a hybrid between a hospital and the traditional nursing home model.

New regulations will be needed to permit greater specialization among nursing homes; it is unrealistic and inefficient to ask all homes to provide all services, if their patients do not need them. The rush toward specialization could lead to another episode of excess orthodoxy, in which unproven requirements are imposed on nursing homes for structures and services that have not been shown to play a definitive role in improving the outcomes of care. Positive pressures to reform nursing home care could then come from a policy that encouraged a payment system that covered only services and offered rewards for better than expected outcomes.

Ironically, although the health care environment has changed a great deal in the past decade and should change even more in the decades to come, the concept of recognizing the diversification of the nursing home clientele by developing more appropriate venues for their care closely follows recommendations offered by Vladeck over a decade ago (Vladeck, 1980). Further, the current enthusiasm for subacute care closely recalls the plans for extended care incorporated into the initial design for Medicare and demonstrates the potential for rediscovering old ideas. Thus, while one can safely predict only that things will change, the cyclical nature of policy rediscovery suggests that many of the answers to tomorrow's challenges to nursing home care will be found in ideas already put forward.

References

Brody, E. M. (1973). A million procrustean beds. *Gerontologist* 13:430–35.

Brody, E. M., Litvin, S. J., Hoffman, C., and Kleban, M. H. (1992). Differential effects of daughters' marital status on their parent care experiences. *Gerontologist* 32 (1): 58–67.

Callahan, D. (1987). *Setting Limits: Medical Goals in an Aging Society.* New York: Simon and Schuster.

Davies, A. R., and Ware, J. E. J. (1988). Involving consumers in quality assessment. *Health Affairs* 7 (1): 33–48.

Dunlop, B. (1979). *The Growth of Nursing Home Care.* Lexington, Mass.: Lexington Books.

Fiatarone, M. A., O'Neill, E. F., Ryan, N. D., Clements, K. M., Solares, G. R., Nelson, M. E., Roberts, S. B., Kehayias, J. J., Lipsitz, L. A., and Evans, W. J. (1994). Exercise training and nutritional supplementation for physical frailty in very elderly people. *New England Journal of Medicine* 330 (25): 1769–75.

Friedman, B., and R. L. Kane (1993). HMO medical directors' perceptions of geriatric practice in Medicare HMOs. *Journal of the American Geriatrics Society* 41:1144–49.

Grant, L. A., Kane, R. A., and Stark, A. J. (1994). Dementia care in and out of special care units: Design of a comprehensive survey of all units in Minnesota's nursing homes. *Alzheimer's Disease and Associated Disorders* 8 (suppl. 1): S106–11.

Helbing, C., and Cornelius, E. S. (1993). Skilled nursing facilities. *Health Care*

Financing Review: Medicare and Medicaid Statistical Supplement. Baltimore: U.S. Department of Health and Human Services.

Institute of Medicine (1986). *Improving the Quality of Care in Nursing Homes.* Washington, D.C.: National Academy Press.

Kahn, K. L., Rubenstein, L. V., Draper, D., Kosecoff, J., Rogers, W. H., Keeler, E. B., and Brook, R. H. (1990). The effects of the DRG-based prospective payment system on quality of care for hospitalized Medicare patients: An introduction to the series. *Journal of the American Medical Association* 264:1953–55.

Kane, R. L., Bell, R., Riegler, S. Z., Wilson, A., and Keeler, E. (1983a). Assessing the outcomes of nursing home patients. *Journal of Gerontology* 38:385–93.

Kane, R. L., Bell, R. M., Riegler, S. Z., Wilson, A., and Keeler, E. (1983b). Predicting the outcomes of nursing-home patients. *Gerontologist* 23 (2): 200–206.

Kane, R. L., Evans, J. G., and Macfadyen, D., eds. (1990). *Improving Health in Older People: A World View.* Oxford: Oxford University Press.

Kane, R. L., Garrard, J., Buchanan, J. L., Rosenfeld, A., Skay, C., and McDermott, S. (1991). Improving primary care in nursing homes. *Journal of the American Geriatrics Society* 39:359–67.

Kane, R. L., Garrard, J., Skay, C. L., Radosevich, D. M., Buchanan, J. L., McDermott, S. M., and Arnold, S. B. (1989). Effects of a geriatric nurse practitioner on the process and outcomes of nursing home care. *American Journal of Public Health* 79:1271–77.

Kane, R. L., Illston, L. H., and Miller, N. A. (1992). Qualitative analysis of the Program of All-inclusive Care for the Elderly (PACE). *Gerontologist* 32:771–80.

Kane, R. A., and Wilson, K. B. (1993). *Assisted Living in the United States: A New Paradigm for Residential Care for Frail Older Persons?* Washington, D.C.: American Association of Retired Persons.

Leutz, W. N., Greenberg, J. N., Abrahams, R., Prottas, J., Diamond, L. M., and Gruenberg, L. (1985). *Changing Health Care for an Aging Society.* Lexington, Mass.: D. C. Heath.

Long, S. (1987). *Death without Dignity.* Austin, Tex.: Texas Monthly Press.

Malone, J., Chase, D., and Bayard, J. (1993). Care for nursing home residents. *Journal of Health Care Benefits* (January/February): 51–54.

Moss, F. E., and Halamandaris, V. J. (1977). *Too Old, Too Sick, Too Bad: Nursing Homes in America.* Germantown, Md.: Aspen Systems.

Newcomer, R. J., Harrington, C., and Friedlob, A. (1990). Social health maintenance organizations: Assessing their initial experience. *Health Services Research* 25 (3): 425–54.

Schnelle, J. F. (1990). Treatment of urinary incontinence in nursing home patients by prompted voiding. *Journal of the American Geriatrics Society* 38:356–60.

Shaughnessy, P. W. (1991). *Shaping Policy for Long-Term Care: Learning from the Effectiveness of Hospital Swing Beds.* Ann Arbor, Mich: Health Administration Press.

Siu, A. L., Ouslander, J. G., Osterweil, D., Reuben, D. B., and Hays, R. D. (1993). Change in self-reported functioning in older persons entering a residential care facility. *Journal of Clinical Epidemiology* 46 (10): 1093–1101.

Stuck, A. E., Siu, A. L., Wieland, G. D., Adams, J., and Rubenstein, L. Z. (1993). Comprehensive geriatric assessment: A meta-analysis of controlled trials. *Lancet* 342:1032–36.

Szasz, T. S., and Hollander, M. H. (1956). A contribution to the philosophy of medicine: The basic models of the doctor-patient relationship. *Archives of Internal Medicine* 97:585–92.

U.S. Congress (1987). Office of Technology Assessment. *Life-Sustaining Technologies and the Elderly*. Washington, D.C.: Government Printing Office.

Vladeck, B. G. (1980). *Unloving Care: The Nursing Home Tragedy*. New York: Basic Books.

Weissert, W. G., C. Matthews Cready, and Pawelak, J. E. (1989). Home and community care: Three decades of findings. In M. D. Peterson and D. L White, eds. *Health Care of the Elderly: An Information Source Book* (pp. 39–126). Newbury Park, Calif.: Sage Publications.

8

Care in the Home and Other Community Settings: Present and Future

James J. Callahan, Jr., Ph.D.

The year 2020 is approximately twenty-five years from now. How much and what kind of change can occur that will affect care for functionally dependent people in the home and community? Twenty-five years is not a long time in the life of a nation. It is not difficult for most of us to recall 1970 — a mere twenty-five years ago. The engines of long-term care services — Medicare and Medicaid — were just beginning to develop momentum. Expenditures for long-term care services were barely visible in federal fiscal reports. Much of the money being spent on institutional services was buried in the categorical public assistance programs of Old Age Assistance and Disability Assistance. There was practically no long-term care insurance, no intermediate care facilities (ICF was not made a designation until 1972), no federal accessible-facilities legislation, a tiny for-profit sector in home health, with most services being provided by visiting nurse associations or public health departments. The idea of the "long-term care system" had barely emerged. Rather, the terminology of the National Commission on Chronic Illness, "care of the long-term patient," was still being used.

Futurists, a cadre of various scientists, professionals, and business-people who attempt to anticipate events that lie ahead, use a number of methods in their craft. They project trends, create likely and unlikely scenarios, conduct polls of experts (such as the Delphi technique used to generate the forecasts reported in the Epilogue to this volume), develop models, and run simulations (World Future Society, 1992). One wonders whether, from the vantage point of 1970, futurists could have predicted that in twenty-five years

— the older population would appear to be more healthy (Manton, Corder, and Stallard, 1993);
— the disability community of young adults and others would have inspired the Americans with Disabilities Act and persuaded the current president to include disability groups of all ages in long-term care reform;
— the health care system, both so-called nonprofit organizations and proprietary health businesses, would be driven by survival and competitive values rather than the value of service to others;
— home health services would be one of the fastest-growing components of the Medicare budget (Bishop and Skwara, 1993); and
— the United States would rank as the number one debtor nation.

Even if some observers had predicted such changes (and I am aware of none who did), would they have been believed? Would their predictions have been institutionalized in policy, or might the predictions themselves have engendered change?

In fact, some predictions made in the mid-1970s that turned out to be wrong did influence policy. The Congressional Budget Office predicted in 1977 that the number of persons in nursing homes would increase from about 1.3 million in 1977 to 2.2 million in 1985 (U.S. Congress, 1977). Such growth would have had a large impact on the federal budget, and policymakers rightly were concerned. This prediction, in part, served as an impetus for the National Long Term Care Demonstration (Channeling), the National Long Term Care Survey, and planning grants to states for long-term care and related initiatives.

By 1985, only 1.5 million persons resided in nursing homes — an increase of 200,000 rather than the expected 900,000 persons. In fact, beds per thousand persons ages 65 and older decreased from 59.7 to 56.9, residents per thousand decreased from 47.9 to 46, and bed occupancy rose from 89 percent to 91.6 percent. The nursing home population became older and more disabled (National Center for Health Statistics, 1987). Instead of significantly more beds being available, the use of beds intensified, with higher occupancy and a greater degree of disability among residents. It is likely that growth was dampened by state requirements for obtaining certificates of need for new nursing home beds, the elimination of certain financial incentives, such as allowing depreciation to be taken more than once in rate-setting formulas, and the high cost of borrowing money during this period. There was, however, significant growth of home health services during this same period. The number of certified home health agencies increased from 2,212 in 1972 to 3,636 by 1982, and 6,012 in 1986 (*Home Health Line,* 1988). In 1974, only 17 persons per thousand Medicare eligibles received home health services, compared to 56 in 1985 (Bishop and Stassen, 1985).

Did the prediction that turned out wrong generate forces, such as regulation, that undermined the growth of nursing homes, or did policymakers overlook "signs of the times" that might have helped anticipate the slower growth in nursing homes and the explosive growth in home care? In this chapter we will search for signs of the times that may help predict the state of home- and community-based care in the year 2020.

The Present State of Home and Community Services

Demand for Services by Persons of All Ages

Presently about 4 percent of the noninstitutionalized U.S. civilian population experiences difficulty in certain basic life activities, often referred to as activities of daily living (ADLs) — bathing, dressing, toileting, feeding oneself, transferring, and mobility — and instrumental activities of daily living (IADLs) — household chores, shopping, handling money, and moving about the community (U.S. Department of Education, 1992). Most people (76.7%) with these difficulties receive supportive help, ranging from 91.3 percent for persons under age 17 to 70 percent for persons aged 55 to 64 (p. 2). Nearly 74 percent of the help is provided only by unpaid informal caregivers, usually family members, and 5.5 percent by formal paid helpers only. Combined care from both paid and unpaid helpers accounts for the remaining 21 percent (Liu, Manton, and Liu, 1985). As a person's levels of disability increase so do levels of help, ranging from 12.1 percent for those with limitations in IADLs only, to 30.4 percent for those with three limitations or more in ADLs.

Persons ages 65 and over constitute the largest cohort with limitations in ADLs and/or IADLs, totaling about 5.6 million, compared to 3.4 million persons under 65. They are also the group with the largest proportion of persons with difficulties — 20.1 percent compared to 1.9 percent (U.S. Department of Education, 1992).

Disabled persons of all ages, however, are service users. "About 15 percent of people with difficulty receive home care, and 21 percent receive community services. Assistance most frequently obtained through home care included housework, bathing, nursing, or medical and meals. The

Table 8.1
National Home Care Usage by Client Age, 1987

Age	U.S. Population (millions)	Number Receiving Home Care (millions)	Average Number of Visits per Home Care User
0–39	153.1	1.7	15.0
40–64	59.7	1.2	37.9
65–74	16.4	1.2	55.7
75–84	8.1	1.2	66.9
84+	2.0	0.6	70.6
All ages	239.4	5.9	44.0

Source: National Association for Home Care (1992).

most frequently used community services include special transportation, goods, or cash from other than family and friends, senior center visits, and meals obtained through a day care center" (p. 3). Data on use of home and community-based services for disabled children and disabled adults under age 65 is sparse, in part because such services have largely not been available through public dollars, and those that have are lumped in with expenditures for all categories of recipient. An exception to this limitation is data for home care. Table 8.1 displays home care service use by all disabled persons. It shows that both the percentage of an age group receiving home care and the average number of visits per user (intensity) increases with age.

Service Use by People Aged 65 or Older

Certain medical and supportive services are important resources for persons ages 65 and over. They provide opportunities for socialization, meals, transportation, and actual assistance with ADL and IADL needs. Figure 8.1 shows the percentage of persons 65 or over who use these formal services. Figure 8.2 breaks out the home care category to show the distribution by type of provider. The bulk of providers are homemakers and home health aides rendering largely unsophisticated but necessary help. Of those persons 65 and older with any difficulty who use services, 61.7 percent receive them only at home, 27.3 percent only in the community, and 11 percent in both settings (Short and Leon 1990).

There is some evidence that users of home health care (visiting nurse or home health aide) are significantly more impaired than users of community services and that community services do not appear to substitute for

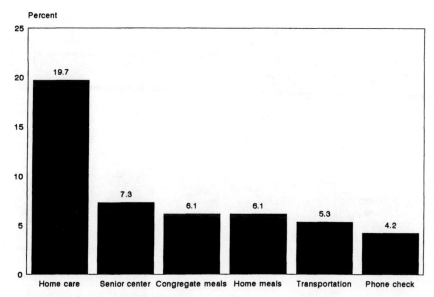

Figure 8.1. The percentage of persons aged 65 or older with any functional difficulty who are using particular services. Reprinted from Short and Leon (1990), p. 5.

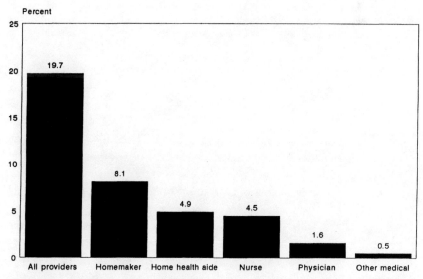

Figure 8.2. The percentage of persons aged 65 or older with any functional difficulty who are receiving services from home-care providers. Reprinted from Short and Leon (1990), p. 7. Note: The total of five services is 19.6 percent, although source showed 19.7 percent.

Table 8.2

Multiple Logistic Regression Results: ADL Limitations and Other
Characteristics Associated with Users of Home Health Care versus
Users of Other Community Services

Variable	Users of Home Health Care versus Users of Other Community Services
Difficulty eating	4.09
Difficulty going outside	3.17
Difficulty dressing	1.94
Difficulty bathing	1.64
Unmarried (versus married)	1.67
Poor health	2.76
Lives with others (versus alone)	2.27

Source: Adapted from Friedman, Droge, and Rabin (1992), p. 645, Table 3.

Table 8.3

Total Average Effects of ADL Disabilities among Persons Ages 65 and
Older on Hours of Care per Week

ADL Disabilities	Formal Care	Visiting Informal Care	Resident Informal Care	Total
Five	9.8	7.7	37.2	54.7
Four	8.0	5.3	30.0	43.3
Three	7.2	3.1	20.8	31.1
Two	5.0	2.9	7.8	15.7
One	4.6	3.1	9.2	16.9

Source: Data from Kemper (1992), p. 439.

home health care in meeting ADL and IADL needs. Table 8.2 shows that
there are differences in characteristics of and service use by the frail elderly
living in the community between those who are using in-home health
services and those using only community services. The in-home service
group is more than twice as likely to be living with others, and over three
times more likely to have difficulty going outside. They are also in poorer
health with a greater likelihood of having ADL problems. This suggests
that amount and type of service use reflects the underlying health of the
older person and that such service use prima facie seems desirable.

Table 8.3 demonstrates that as disability increases both formal and
informal care (resident or visiting) increase. "Moreover, the amount of
informal care received increases with disability at a much greater rate than

does formal care under the same circumstances. This suggests that as care needs increase, family and friends step in to provide the bulk of care" (Kemper, 1992, p. 447).

The formal and informal systems seem to interact well in the case of the very frail because of the integration activities of the informal caregivers. Zarit, Pearlin, and Schaie (1992) noted, "This linking activity becomes part of the complement of tasks carried out by informal caregivers and imposes varying amounts of demand on time and energy. The caregivers' efforts will determine to what extent the systems interface adequately" (p. 304).

Morris and Morris (1993) were optimistic about the future of the informal support system: "Families may be getting smaller, distance may be more of a reality, and female participation in the labor market has undoubtedly increased. Yet, in spite of all these changes, the role and effectiveness of informal support systems have not undergone a significant change" (p. 85). Others, however, raised some cautionary signs on the role of families: "Women and their families will experience increasing conflict as women make choices and compromises in their dual roles as caregivers and breadwinners. Many families will rely upon community services or nursing homes, or be forced to 'make do,' in effect neglecting the needs of their older relatives" (England et al., 1991, p. 239).

The Living Situations of Frail Elders

The United States did not have to create the suburbs after World War II. In 1940, less than 40 percent of housing units were owner occupied, and some authors were arguing against large-scale home ownership because it limited job mobility, saddled families with expensive home repairs, and subjected residents to real estate speculation (Chase, 1938). But build the suburbs we did and they are aging along with their occupants.

Large numbers of people have aged in place in the suburbs, usually in single-family houses. They face problems of transportation, upkeep of the home, and participation in neighborhood life as they lose their ability to drive, undertake heavy chores, and go out after dark. Hare (1993) predicts that suburbs will experience waves of frail elderly aging in place, with the earliest-built suburbs being hit first by the wave. This, he noted, will put demands on communities for home repair and modification programs, improved traffic control, new forms of transportation, and change in zoning laws to accommodate small businesses, and home additions.

Ninety-five percent of all elders live in the community, and 5 percent reside in nursing homes. The frailty characteristics of elders differ by site

Table 8.4
Selected Characteristics of Nursing Home and Community
Residents Ages 65 and Older

Subject	Nursing Home Residents, 1985 (%)	Community Residents, 1984 (%)
Age		
65–74	16.1	61.7
75–84	38.6	30.78
85+	45.3	7.6
Sex		
Men	25.4	40.8
Women	74.6	59.2
Marital Status		
Widowed	67.8	34.1
Married	12.8	54.7
Never married	13.5	4.4
Divorced or separated	5.9	6.3
With living children	63.1	81.3
Assistance required in		
Bathing	91.0	6.0
Dressing	77.6	4.3
Using toilet	63.2	2.2
Transferring	62.6	2.8
Eating	40.3	1.1
N (thousands)	1,318	26,343

Source: Adapted from U.S. Department of Health and Human Services
(1991), Table 5-7.

of residence. Table 8.4 shows how the nursing home population differs
from the community population on selected variables. Elders who live in
nursing homes are older, primarily women, and substantially more disabled than those residing in the community. They have fewer living children than the community population, in part because a higher proportion
of them never married. Table 8.5, which compares *frail* elders (not all
elders) in the community with nursing home residents, shows that the
nursing home population is proportionately far more functionally disabled than the frail elderly population in the community. In absolute numbers, however, slightly more persons with three or more ADLs are in the
community than in nursing homes.

Table 8.6 shows the distributions of frail older people living in the

Table 8.5

Disabled Persons Ages 65 and Older, by Disability and Place of Residence

	Community Residents		Nursing Home Residents	
	in thousands	%	in thousands	%
IADL only	2,301	45	101	8
1–2 ADLs	1,815	36	274	21
3+ ADLs	957	19	940	71
Total	5,073	100	1,315	100

Source: Adapted from Leutz et al. (1992), p. 23, Table 2.1. Data from 1982 Long-Term Care Survey and 1985 National Nursing Home Survey.

Table 8.6

Housing and Household Composition of Community Long-Term Care Populations Ages 65 and Older

	1–3 IADLs, No ADLs (%)	4+ IADLs, No ADLs (%)	1–2 ADLs (%)	3+ ADLs (%)	Totally Impaired (%)
Type of housing					
House	66	71	66	73	68
Duplex	7	6	7	6	7
Apartment	20	14	20	14	19
Room	1	2	0	1	1
Trailer	6	5	6	6	6
Other	0	1	1	0	0
Total	100	99	100	100	101
Household composition					
Live alone	38	18	33	15	31
Married couple	39	36	36	42	38
Two individuals	10	15	12	16	12
3 or more individuals	4	12	7	11	7
Unknown	9	19	11	16	12
Total	100	100	99	100	100

Source: Leutz et al. (1992), p. 26; reprinted with permission of Greenwood Publishing Group, Inc., Westport, Conn. Data from 1982 National Long-Term Care Survey tapes.

community, by type of residence and household composition. Type of housing shows that persons with the highest number of IADLs or ADLs live in a house, not an apartment. Household composition indicates that more severely disabled persons are less likely to live alone and more likely to live with two or more individuals. This suggests that for severely disabled persons to live in the community they need to share a residence with others. It suggests also that the opportunity to live with others enhances the likelihood of remaining in the community as disability increases.

Ethnicity

The location and type of household in which elders live can be related to race or ethnic background. Skinner (1993) reported that older African Americans and other minority elders predominate in inner-city areas, where they may be confined by patterns of residential segregation. They make less use of nursing homes, and a large proportion live with spouses or others. Skinner attributed this to the importance of community to minority elders. Alternatively, such community support may be necessitated by the fact that 45 percent of all elderly African Americans are poor or have incomes of only 125 percent of the poverty line (Hall, 1993).

The changing ethnic composition of the population underscores the importance of understanding the influence of ethnicity on the use of home-based and community services. "The white population has gone from 83.1 percent of the resident population in 1980 to 80.3 percent in 1990. The respective figures for other groups are: Blacks 11 percent to 12.1 percent, Hispanics 6.4 percent to 9.0 percent, Asian 1.5 percent to 2.9 percent, and Native Americans 0.6 percent to 0.8 percent" (Barresi and Stull, 1993, p. 11). Recognition of this mix of population and accompanying cultural values is essential to ensure proper access and appropriate services for older people in the future.

Supply of Formal Service Providers

As noted above, the greatest amount of care is provided by unpaid informal caregivers rather than the formal service system. Nonetheless, the formal system is very important for certain groups of elders; 5.5 percent of frail elders receive formal care exclusively, and 20.6 percent both formal and informal care.

Formal in-home services are provided by nurses, licensed practical nurses, home health aides, physical therapists, occupational therapists, respiratory therapists, speech and hearing specialists, and social workers.

Table 8.7
Employees (Full-Time Equivalents), by Type, Working in
Medicare-certified Home Health Agencies, 1987 and 1990

	1987	1990	Percentage Increase
RNs	40,736	56,867	39.6
LPNs	4,106	7,762	89.0
Physical therapists	6,025	10,822	79.6
Home health aides	27,312	38,265	40.1
Other	29,933	33,242	11.1
Total	108,112	146,958	35.9

Source: Adapted from National Association for Home Care (1992).
Note: This table refers only to Medicare-certified agencies. MacAdam et al.
(1991, pp. 70–71) estimated a total of 223,014 home health aides in all
types of community agencies.

Table 8.7 shows the estimated number and growth of such providers
between 1987 and 1990.

Social and Policy Scenarios

Other chapters in this book treat demographic trends, technology, and
financing. This brief review of disabled persons, generally, and in particular of frail elders, their living situations, and their use of in-home and
community services provides some basis for constructing general scenarios for thinking about the future. The most striking feature of the facts
outlined above is how the present state of home and community services
appears to be what one would expect. The more disabled a person is the
more help he or she receives, even if it may not be considered the best quality of care or the most appropriate. Most of the help and even more of the
responsibility for assuring that there is help comes from those closest to
the frail person — spouse, other household members, family, and friends.
Frail elders therefore are cared for by those who may be presumed to love
them, feel responsible, or at least be in a situation where it is awkward to
deny such help. Very frail individuals without family and friends are more
likely to be found in nursing homes; those with families are often found
living with their families. Persons using home nursing services are more
frail than those who use services out in the community. The system does
not always match need with services, but frailty, site of care, and input of
both formal and informal resources seem to exhibit a logical pattern.

Table 8.8
National Ranking of States by Prevalence of
Disability

	Ages 16–64	Ages 65+
Washington, D.C.	1	11
Mississippi	2	1
Louisiana	3	4
Alabama	4	2
South Carolina	5	9
West Virginia	6	3
New York	7	15
Arkansas	8	7
Kentucky	9	5
Georgia	10	6

Source: U.S. Department of Education (1993), p. 24, Table 3.

While disability is concentrated among older people, it is substantial among nonelderly persons as well. Both groups use formal and informal services. Both ADL and IADL limitations require human care comparable to what nondisabled persons do on their own. It is no surprise that the greatest number of workers serving the disabled are nonspecialized home health aides rather than nurses and therapists.

On the basis of this general picture, one can hazard some predictions about the future of home-based and community-based care between now and 2020.

Prediction 1: Whatever national long-term care program there is in the future, be it a Medicare extension, federal grant in aid program, or private insurance, it is likely to include all age groups. The disability facts — the number of aged and nonaged disabled and their advocacy groups — will drive it. The Clinton long-term care proposal, for example, provided coverage for all persons with three ADLs or with defined levels of cognitive impairment, or with mental retardation, and for technologically dependent children under age 6.

Although these definitions of eligibility move toward meeting equity considerations, it is not clear whether they are a useful basis for designing programs. On the one hand, Callahan (1981) argued for separate systems for specific categories of disabled persons (e.g., children, young adults, elders) since, to a large degree, such systems already exist and can be the focal point for articulate constituent advocacy. On the other hand, some states are moving toward more integrated systems, and the distribution of disability by different age groups among the state would seem to support such an approach.

As shown in Table 8.8, states that have high levels of disability prevalence by some measures among persons under 65 also have high levels of disability among persons over 65. Eight of the top 10 states in prevalence of mobility and self-care problems among persons over 65 were among the top 10 for persons 16 — 64. This suggests continuity of disability from youth into old age and emphasizes the importance of disability prevention and rehabilitation programs to reduce disability. It is possible that the social and economic characteristics of states have a bearing on the prevalence of disability. These findings help the argument for an age-blind disability policy, because intervention early in the life course may allow better handling of lifetime disability.

Prediction 2: Home- and community-based services will no longer be perceived or referred to as alternatives to institutional care but will have importance in their own right. It will have taken a long time to bury the alternative perspective, but success will be achieved. Beginning in the early 1970s, home- and community-based services for the elderly were justified on the basis that they were cheaper than nursing home care. This notion made some sense in the context of trying to limit Medicaid nursing home expenditures. At the same time, however, this argument ran counter to both past and contemporary policies that supported community living. Since the abandonment of the poor house in the late 1800s, significant social legislation has been enacted to provide support and assistance to individuals and families in the community irrespective of the argument that it is cheaper than a nursing home. This legislation included the Vocational Rehabilitation Act of 1920, the Social Security Act of 1935, the Community Mental Health Act of 1963, special education legislation in 1975, the Vocational Rehabilitation Act, 504 accessibility provisions in 1973, the Older Americans Act of 1965, and numerous state home-care programs. All of this legislation supported a policy of community inclusion rather than institutional separation.

The Americans with Disabilities Act of 1990 expands this community inclusion by providing, in a bill of rights, that disabled people should live and work in the community. President Clinton's long-term care plan proposed extending eligibility for home- and community-based services to all individuals with certain degrees of disability, regardless of age, income, or assets. The effect of all of these policies will drive away the notion of the nursing home as the gold standard against which to measure home- and community-based services.

Developments in the home care service industry are also moving toward decoupling services and location. Traditionally, the provision of relatively intensive services has been linked to particular places, and usually those places are licensed to provide those kinds of services. For example, nursing supervision and rehabilitation services are common to nursing homes. Hospitals provide intensive medical and nursing interventions. Recently, however, services formerly provided exclusively in these places have moved into home and community settings. Hospice programs care for many individuals who would have been hospitalized. Short-term stabilization beds are used for mentally ill people who would have been hospitalized. Assisted living services, including meals, medication administration, and therapies, are being delivered to people in group homes, apartments, and their own home. Wheelchair-bound adults live in modified apartments and provide for their own care through the use of personal care attendants. The future, therefore, will be characterized by mobile arrangements and packages of services delivered in a variety of settings. The Clinton administration's long-term care proposal already anticipates this development.

Finally, adding to these pressures is the fact that most older people prefer to remain in their own home and community and strive through a mix of formal and informal help to do so.

Prediction 3: The time-honored ADL and IADL measures of long-term care disability will be supplemented by PDADL and AADL measures. There are 24 hours in the day, and time budgets show that personal time is allocated to a variety of activities — for example, sleep, work, personal care, and leisure (Robinson, 1977). The allocation varies by age, work status, health, and interests, with the time allocation of disabled individuals being affected by the type and degree of disability. Long-term care disability is usually measured by an ability to perform activities of daily living, such as eating, dressing, toileting, and instrumental activities of daily living, such as shopping, cooking, keeping a checkbook. These measures, however, are incomplete in portraying the range of activities that a disabled person undertakes at home and in the community. In the future these measures will need to be supplemented by two additional categories. These are: professionally dictated activities of daily living (PDADLs) and appreciative activities of daily living (AADLs).

PDADLs will be those activities that are required by persons technologically dependent on artificial limbs, wheelchairs, respirators, and similar devices. They include routine maintenance of equipment, ordering of supplies, special skin care, and so forth. Individuals need to devote time and effort to insuring that these artificial extensions are doing their job. (See Chapter 5 for a discussion of the range and type of emergent technologies.)

ADLs, IADLs, and PDADLs are instrumental in the sense that they make a certain standard of life possible. But there is more to a person's life than eating and keeping a checkbook. This is where AADLs come in. They include playing, enjoying, conversing, and dining (not eating) and must be included in the calculation of assessors, case managers, and others who will make it possible for disabled people to "remain in the community." Without including these elements in the calculus, home- and community-based care could become as imprisoning and sterile as any second-class institution. New instruments will be developed to measure these activities, and care plans will incorporate them.

Prediction 4: The family will not collapse as the primary source of responsibility for care of its members, despite many of the structural changes that are occurring. Blood produces strong bonds, and technology will reduce the effect of distance. The distribution of activities between formal and informal services and between government and family may change somewhat but it is difficult at this time to predict even the direction of the changes. Suzman and Manton (see Prediction 5) make an estimate of what these shifts might look like.

In the event that we have a wealthier society, families and individuals may be willing to spend more money on formal services to replace informal caregiving activities. If the effective demand is strong enough, the supply of workers will be forthcoming (see Prediction 5). The expenditure of this wealth, however, could be unevenly distributed, with richer families buying their way out of informal care and poorer families bound to informal care. Wealth as it applies to home and community care could be more evenly distributed if there was a tax-funded government program that derived revenue based on income and distributed benefits based on need.

On the other hand, the demands of the global economy, the reduction of our economic power, continued budget deficits, and possible negative effects of the General Agreement on Tariffs and Trade and the North American Free Trade Agreement on social benefits may affect how much public and private wealth will be available for caretaking. In either case, however, there will be more expenditures for home- and community-based services, even if that means cutting back on fancy cars and VCRs.

Prediction 5: There will be a greater need for home and community care workers, and they will be there if people are willing to pay what it takes to attract them. This is a function of wealth, necessity, and desire to use formal services. For some individuals, formal care will be a survival necessity and will be purchased with private or public dollars. For most, use of formal care will be a lifestyle choice affected by income and desire.

Based on current predictions, the number of care workers required in the future will be relatively small compared to the estimated future labor force of 120–150 million. Suzman and Manton (1992), assuming medium mortality and 50 percent increase in families switching from informal to formal care, estimate a need for about 500,000 home health aides in the year 2020. In 1985 they estimated that number to be about 200,000.

The supply of more technically trained practitioners may or may not be adequate, there being a limited number of training programs. MacAdam et al. (1991, p. 75) cited problems in the supply of physical therapists, which is constrained by the capacity of schools of physical therapy. They asserted that current shortages of certain health personnel are likely to continue unless steps are taken to change this situation.

Prediction 6: The struggle over medical versus nonmedical control of home- and community-based services will continue. Old age and disability are seen frequently as medical problems. Elderly and disabled people have more frequent physician visits, greater utilization of hospitals, longer lengths of stay, and greater prevalence of disease. This usually translates into service needs met or overseen by physicians and the medical system. Public policy has supported innovations (see Chapter 4) which link the medical orientation of care more closely to persons with disabilities.

There is, however, resistance to what some regard as overreaching medicalization. George Maddox (1993) noted: "We are not, however, talking frankly yet about attacking what I call the 'strangleholds' [on policy thinking]. This notion that 'aging' belongs to welfare, and 'care' belongs to medicine. We haven't heard much yet today about a battle that is impending. It is about who owns care? Where are the dollars going to go?" (p. 48).

Sarah Matthews (1993) argued that, in the context of family and community life, old people are not medical problems but rather individuals with full lives and some medical problems. Levesque (1993), after examining home care services in the Province of Quebec, warned that their autonomy and orientation toward the community were vulnerable to the strong hospitals which were absorbing funds for their priority clients. Added to this was a limited availability of home-based services, which further undercut the credibility of the home care community option.

The medicalization of the care of older people is fueled in part by the belief that the rising costs of health care are the result of the aging of the population. In this view, more medical control is required, because this demographic imperative will lead to much larger portions of the GNP being spent on health care, much of it in the last years of life. Disabilities (read "the disabled") are a threat to the good of the community. This, however, is not an accurate picture.

True, there will be more older and disabled persons in our society. It is true also that older folks have greater ADL and IADL needs. It is true that they use services. They use physicians at the rate of about 9 visits per year, compared to 5.4 for all age groups (U.S. Department of Commerce, 1991, Table 4-9). They use hospitals at the rate of 350 discharges per 1000 per year compared to 138.2 for all ages (U.S. Department of Commerce, 1991, Table 4-7).

All of this utilization by older persons, however, does not account for the high cost of care in the United States. The correlation between the percent of GNP being spent on health care and the percent of aged in a population is not very significant. Using cross-national comparisons, Binstock (1993) concluded, "Simple cross-national comparisons of expenditures and selected aspects of population aging suggest that little if any direct relationship exists between these factors" (p. 38). Getzen (1992) reached a similar conclusion. Evans (1985) attributed the cost problems of health care delivery to the health system itself: "They are generated, not by external forces — demographic shifts, technological evolution, culturally determined moral imperatives — but by the way in which the health care system responds to these and other forces" (p. 464). Alan Schick (1989) wrote that most economic explanations of the problem — large public expenditures, lack of cost sharing, overcapacity of facilities and providers, and excess utilization — fail to explain U.S. expenditures when compared to other industrial democracies. Rather, he sees the problem in the conflict of U.S. values of equality and enterprise: "Through much of its history, however, the United States had mitigated conflict between [equality and enterprise] by conceiving of enterprise as the primary way to expand equality" (p. 52).

Conclusion

The past is no longer. The future is not yet. We live and make decisions in the present. These decisions, however, are constrained by history on one side and by vision on the other. What emerges may be the triumph of vision over inertia or possibilities crushed by tradition and vested interests. For home- and community-based services the vision of a better life is clear — a vision of care with dignity, in familiar surroundings, and with the greatest degree of autonomy possible. It is seen in the advocacy movements of both elders and younger disabled persons, in a cadre of policymakers committed to this vision, and in the hearts of millions of families. The threats from investors in institutions, budget deficits, and global economies are real but will not be overwhelming. A better community life for all will emerge.

References

Barresi, C. M., and Stull, D. E. (1993). Ethnicity and long term care: An overview. In C. M. Barresi and D. E. Stull, eds., *Ethnic Elderly and Long Term Care* (pp. 3021). New York: Springer Publishing.

Binstock, R. H. (1993). Healthcare costs around the world: Is aging a fiscal 'black hole'? *Generations* 17 (4): 37–42.

Bishop, C., and Skwara, K. C. (1993). Recent growth of Medicare home health. *Health Affairs* (fall): 95–110.

Bishop, C., and Stassen, M. (1985). Prospective reimbursement for home health care. *Pride Institute Journal* 5 (1): 17–27.

Callahan, J. J., Jr. (1981). Delivery of services to persons with long term care needs. In Judith Meltzer et al., eds., *Policy Options in Long Term Care* (pp. 148–81). Chicago: University of Chicago Press.

Chase, C. (1938). The case against home ownership. *Survey Graphic* 27 (5): 261–67.

England, S. E., Keigher, S. M., Miller, B., and Linsk, N. L. (1991). Community care policies and gender justice. In M. Minkler and C. L. Estes, eds., *Critical Perspectives on Aging: The Political and Moral Economy of Growing Old* (pp. 227–44). Amityville, N.Y.: Baywood.

Evans, R. G. (1985). Illusions of necessity: Evading responsibility for choice in health care. *Journal of Health Politics, Policy, and Law* 10 (3): 439–67.

Friedman, L., Droge, J. A., and Rabin, D. L. (1992). Functional limitations among home health care users in the National Health Interview Survey Supplement on Aging. *Gerontologist* 32 (5): 641–46.

Getzen, T. E. (1992). Population aging and the growth of health expenditures. *Journal of Gerontology* 47 (3): S98–104.

Hall, C. (1993). Long term care and the minority elderly. *Pride Institute Journal* 12 (4): 3–8.

Hare, P. H. (1993). Frail elders and the suburbs. In J. J. Callahan, Jr., ed., *Aging in Place* (pp. 61–71). Amityville, N.Y.: Baywood.

Home Health Line (1988). Vol. 13, May 16, p. 186.

Kemper, P. (1992). The use of formal and informal home care by the disabled. *Health Services Research* 27 (4): 421–51.

Leutz, W. N., Capitman, J. A., MacAdam, M., and Abrahams, R. (1992). *Care for Frail Elders*. Westport, Conn.: Auburn House.

Levesque, L. (1993). Quebec Home-Care Services: A program at the local county level. In S. E. Zarit, L. I. Pearlin, and K. W. Schaie, eds., *Caregiving Systems* (pp. 217–32). Hillsdale, N.J.: Lawrence Erlbaum Associates.

Liu, K., Manton, K., and Liu, B. M. (1985). Home care expenses for the disabled elderly. *Health Care Financing Review* 7 (2):51–58.

MacAdam, M., Howard, A., Pendleton, S., and Sadowsky, E. (1991). *Work Force to Serve the Vulnerable Elderly*. Waltham, Mass.: National Aging Resource Center: Long Term Care, Brandeis University.

Maddox, G. (1993). Remarks. *Supportive Services Programs in Senior Housing: Marking Them Work*. Waltham, Mass.: Policy Center on Aging, Brandeis University.

Manton, K., Corder, L., and Stallard, E. (1993). Estimates of change in chronic disability and institutional incidence and prevalence rates in the U.S. elderly population from the 1982, 1984, and 1989 National Long Term Care Survey. *Journal of Gerontology* 48: S153–66.

Matthews, S. (1993). Undermining stereotypes of old through social policy analysis: Tempering macro- with micro-level perspectives. In J. Hendricks and C. J. Rosenthal, eds., *The Remainder of Their Days* (pp. 105–18). New York: Garland.

Morris, J. N., and Morris, S. A. (1993). The role of formal human services. In J. J. Callahan, Jr., ed., *Aging in Place* (pp. 73–88). Amityville, N.Y.: Baywood.

Mutschler, P. H. (1992). Where elders live. In J. J. Callahan, Jr., ed., *Aging in Place* (pp. 5–18). Amityville, N.Y.: Baywood.

National Association for Home Care (1992). *Basic Statistics about Home Care, 1992*. Washington, D.C.: National Association for Home Care.

National Center for Health Statistics (1987). Advance Data Report No. 131, March, p. 27.

The Regulation of Board and Care Homes (1993). Washington, D.C.: American Association of Retired Persons.

Robinson, J. P. (1977). *How Americans Use Time*. New York: Praeger.

Schick, A. (1989). Health policy: Spending more and protecting less. In M. E. Lewin and S. Sullivan, eds., *The Care of Tomorrow's Elderly* (pp. 29–52). Washington, D.C.: American Enterprise Institute for Public Policy Research.

Short, P. F., and Leon, J. (1990). Use of home and community services by persons age 65 and older with functional difficulties. National Medical Expenditures

Survey. Research Findings 5, U.S. Department of Health and Human Services. Washington, D.C.: U.S. Government Printing Office.

Skinner, J. (1993). Aging in place: The experience of African American and other minority elders. In J. J. Callahan, Jr., ed., *Aging in Place* (pp. 89–95). Amityville, N.Y.: Baywood.

Suzman, R., and Manton, K. (1992). Forecasting health and functioning in aging societies. In M. G. Ory, R. P. Abeles, and P. D. Lipman, eds., *Aging, Health and Behavior* (pp. 327–57). Newbury Park, Calif.: Sage Publications.

U.S. Congress (1977). Congressional Budget Office. *Long Term Care for the Elderly and Disabled*. Washington, D.C.: U.S. Government Printing Office.

U.S. Department of Commerce, Bureau of the Census (1993). *Sixty-Five Plus in America*. Washington, D.C.: U.S. Government Printing Office.

U.S. Department of Education, National Institute on Disability and Rehabilitation Research (1992). *Disability Statistics Abstract*, no. 3. Washington, D.C.: U.S. Government Printing Office.

U.S. Department of Education, National Institute on Disability and Rehabilitation Research (1993). *Disability Statistics Report*, no. 3, State estimates of disability in America. Washington, D.C.: U.S. Government Printing Office.

U.S. Department of Health and Human Services (1991). *Aging America*. Washington, D.C.: U.S. Government Printing Office.

World Future Society (1992). *The Art of Forecasting*. Bethesda, Md.: World Future Society.

Zarit, S. H., Pearlin, L. I., and Schaie, K. W. (1992). Family caregiving: Integrating informal and formal systems of care. In Zarit, S. H., Pearlin, L. I., and Schaie, K. W., eds., *Caregiving Systems: Formal and Informal Helpers*. Hillsdale, N.J.: Lawrence Erlbaum.

IV

SOCIAL AND POLICY ISSUES

9

The Financing and Organization of Long-Term Care

Mark R. Meiners, Ph.D.

What the future of long-term care financing and organization will be is an ongoing debate. Current indications are that there will be more emphasis on home and community care, greater federal support for state and local initiative, and advances in private market options. The last will take the form of improved long-term care insurance with more managed care applications and more attention to geriatric subacute services.

Though financing and organization are clearly intertwined, experience suggests that form follows finance, and we have yet to resolve how to pay for long-term care. That is a debate in progress, which by its very nature has made consensus difficult to achieve.

Three Basic Reform Strategies

There are three basic approaches to consider in framing the debate. There is the social insurance model, in which participation is mandatory, everybody is covered (at least all those in select groups, such as the elderly or disabled), benefits are mandated, and the financial burden is spread through taxes on the general population. Social Security and Medicare are the best examples of this public policy approach. There is the means-tested model, in which benefits are limited to those who are poor or nearly poor. Medicaid and most of our welfare programs are examples of this approach. Somewhere between these is the public-private partnership, recognized alternately as the long-term care system we already have or the yet to be determined solution to our discontent with that system.

Because the future financing system is likely to build on what we have, it is worth briefly reviewing some of the key issues that have surrounded the debate on long-term care financing. The social insurance program, Medicare, was not designed to cover long-term care. It is basically a health insurance plan covering the elderly mostly for their hospital and physician expenses. While it does pay for some nursing home and home health care, these benefits follow the medical model, providing limited subacute care but not long-term care. This distinction has contributed to some confusion and to the general lack of preparation for the potentially catastrophic financial risk of long-term care. Recent legal challenges have caused a more liberal interpretation of the home health benefit, resulting in dramatic growth in the use and cost of that component. Estimates for 1993 from the Brookings Institution indicate that Medicare covered 14.4 percent of the $107.8 billion cost for all long-term care services (Wiener, 1994). About 70 percent of the Medicare share went for home health care.

Medicaid, on the other hand, does cover significant amounts of long-term care, mostly in nursing homes. It is funded through a federal and state match, with primary administrative responsibilities going to the states under general federal guidelines. The Brookings estimates put the Medicaid share at 40.8 percent of the total long-term care cost in 1993. About 83 percent of the Medicaid expenditures went for institutional care. Eligibility requires impoverishment, either directly or through having spent-down assets and income to poverty levels. Recently, "gaming" Medicaid by divesting or transferring assets to others has become such a commonly discussed way to avoid paying for long-term care (Burwell, 1991) that the rules in the Omnibus Budget Reconciliation Act of 1993 were significantly tightened, to further restrict such practices.

Private out-of-pocket payments comprise the other major source of payment for long-term care. About 36 percent of the 1993 long-term care bill was paid out-of-pocket by individuals and their families, about 77 percent of which went for institutional care (Wiener, 1994). Third-party insurance, a significant source of funds for acute care, is new to long-term care within the past ten years. As yet, it is not a major source of financing, but the market is beginning to grow, and there is considerable interest in its potential and pitfalls. By the beginning of 1993 a total of 2.9 million policies had been sold nationwide, and 135 insurers reported having products (Coronel, 1994).

Without risk pooling, the chances of personal impoverishment from long-term care are great. Estimates suggest that about 25 percent of those admitted to nursing homes as private pay patients spend down to Medicaid (Adams, Meiners, and Burwell, 1993). But the fact that long-term care is now generally recognized as an insurable condition has actually fueled a debate on the merits of public versus private insurance.

These three financing sources (Medicare, Medicaid, and private payment out-of-pocket or through insurance) represent the basic structure of payment that can be viewed as a public-private partnership, because the relative roles are highly dependent on one another. The amount of coverage by Medicare has a direct impact on how much must be spent by consumers on noncovered services, the costliest of which is long-term care. Large private payments increase the risk of impoverishment, which triggers Medicaid eligibility. The problem with this partnership notion is that it is more by default than intent.

Medicaid's Pivotal Role

The risk of catastrophic long-term care expenses, along with the aging of our population, has made the role of Medicaid in long-term care more significant than was originally intended or expected. This in turn has heightened the interest of the states in seeking solutions, because they feel the fiscal pressures very directly and, unlike for the federal government, deficit financing is not an option at the state level. States must maintain their fiscal solvency despite lacking control of the money supply.

States have been experimenting with home and community alternatives to nursing home care. Delivery of care in the home or the community is commonly preferred to institutional care, and there is a strongly held belief that home and community services, once developed, can limit the rapid rise in nursing home costs without an equally large increase in alternative care costs. Through numerous demonstrations and evaluations this belief has been tested and retested, but the results are not encouraging. Home and community benefits tend to be an add-on cost to the system, because they are difficult to target to those who will be able to use them effectively to delay or prevent the need for institutional care.

Three funding strategies for home and community care benefits are available to states under the Medicaid program, beyond the skilled medical home health benefits that are required for any person entitled to nursing facility services under the state's Medicaid plan. Current statutory authority for home care allows states to offer as optional services personal care, day care, private duty nursing, and case management. These benefits must be provided to the entire categorically eligible population, those aged, blind, and disabled who meet income and asset standards on a statewide basis. This broadens the cost and complexity of home care programs beyond what many states feel they are prepared to or interested in providing. There may be inadequate infrastructure and distinct differences in need among Medicaid's long-term care populations (e.g., developmentally disabled, chronically mentally ill, adult disabled, and elderly). Moreover, Medicaid eligibility rules do not allow limiting the availability of selected services to only a subset of the elderly poor population, and there are restrictions on the types of services offered (Etheredge, 1988).

A "2176 waiver" program gets around many of these problems but has had significant limitations. The Omnibus Budget Reconciliation Act of 1981 included a section 2176 (currently section 1915 [c] of Medicaid law) that permits states to apply for special Medicaid waivers, allowing them to pay for nonmedical services selectively if the average cost to Medicaid was no greater than if the person had been placed in a nursing home. Services need not be provided statewide, they can be targeted to selective groups of Medicaid recipients, and income eligibility levels can be the same as those used for determining Medicaid eligibility of nursing home residents. Before this waiver authority, Medicaid services to persons living in the community were generally restricted to being medically related. Under the waiver, services such as case management, respite care, personal care services, home modification, and transportation can be covered.

The implementation of this program by the Federal Health Care Financing Administration (HCFA) has been conservative. States have had to deal with a protracted approval process, strict limits on who will qualify, and close scrutiny of projected cost estimates. A criterion of budget neutrality tied to an already restricted supply of nursing home beds has served to limit participation. In 1987, 37 states had operational 2176 waiver programs, but only about 59,000 elderly were being served (Neuscheler, 1987). By 1991, 40 states were operating 53 waiver programs for elderly or disabled persons, but these accounted for only 32 percent of total waiver spending. In contrast, waiver programs for mentally retarded or developmentally disabled persons accounted for 64 percent of the spending (Congressional Research Service, 1993).

To address some of these problems, a second waiver option was passed (section 1915 [d]), with the target population limited to persons 65 years or older who, without home- and community-based care, would require Medicaid- funded nursing home care. The budget neutral test in this program is not dependent on a state's supply of nursing home beds. States are allowed to increase their long-term care spending as long as the total increase (including nursing homes) does not exceed the greater of 7 percent or a rate calculated on the basis of a formula reflecting the growth in the state's population aged 75 or older, the costs of providing long-term care services, and a 2 percent "intensity factor." To date, only Oregon operates such a waiver program.

To further encourage states to offer home and community care for those who were Medicaid eligible, a third option was enacted in 1991. For persons 65 years or older and unable to perform two of three specified activities of daily living (toileting, transferring, and eating), states could provide a variety of home and community care benefits. Besides defining the eligibility criteria explicitly on the basis of significant disability, this option differs from others in that federal matching payments are capped at specific legislated amounts, starting at $40 million in 1991 and rising to $180 million by 1995. The allocations must take into account the state's share of persons age 65 and the number of elderly persons with low income. The high disability level required and uncertain matching have resulted in only Texas and Rhode Island taking advantage of this option so far.

Besides Medicaid, the federal programs most involved in financing home and community assistance for long-term care are the Older Americans Act, the Social Service Block Grant, and the Supplemental Security Income Program. Each of these programs has different goals, operates under different administrative authority, and has its own focus in terms of service benefits and eligibility. In each program, states have been delegated much of the responsibility for administering the programs, along with substantial flexibility in designing those aspects that can enhance the availability of home and community care benefits. This delegation of authority combined with the significant budgetary constraints of the programs has prompted states to view these programs as only limited opportunities to leverage state revenues for the purpose of long-term care system development.

Despite cost-containment considerations, the preference for home and community care is strongly held, even to the point where some states have developed their own programs without federal support. Three primary factors have typically been involved in the decision to commit state funds to those benefits. State funding allows for flexibility in the design of programs, avoiding the need to meet federal Medicaid requirements; it allows states the use of existing programs and institutions that have grown up outside the Medicaid system with their own practical and political traditions; and it is essential if the programs of home- and community-based services are to be available to the broader constituency of those who are not Medicaid eligible but need similar support (Etheredge, 1988). The importance of the last factor has prompted considerable discussion along three fronts: (1) the need for some kind of universal availability of long-term care programs, (2) the need for improved means-tested programs for long-term care, and (3) the need to encourage more personal responsibility and private sector initiatives to finance long-term care.

The Latest "New" Thinking

The election of President Clinton marked a significant point in the debate on long-term care. A newly elected Democratic president (the first in twelve years) was joining the Democrat-controlled Congress with the promise of accomplishing health care reform that could include long-term care. What transpired from that commitment is highly revealing. The plan details, the approach to implementation, the alternatives rejected, and the reaction to the plan give good insights to our collective thinking about the future of long-term care financing and organization.

At the outset of the planning process, the Clinton team could be characterized as preferring a social insurance approach over means testing. This position was reinforced by strong opposition from the American Association of Retired Persons (AARP) to means testing and their dislike of private long-term care insurance. Nonetheless, four options were suggested to the president as an accommodation to political realities (White House Task Force, 1993a).

Option 1 was characterized as incremental Medicaid reform. Key features included flexibility for states to provide home and community services with long-term care block grants; income and resource protections for nursing home residents; and improved regulation combined with some tax incentives for private insurance. Its price tag for 1994 was estimated at $5 billion.

Option 2 was a new and different federal-state program to replace Medicaid. There would be a new community-based services program for low-income people, the same nursing home protections as in option 1, and a separate block grant for the mentally retarded and developmentally disabled populations. A limited voluntary public insurance program would be offered, along with work incentives for disabled persons; and private insurance would be included, as in option 1. The cost was estimated at $7 billion in 1994.

Option 3 was social insurance for home and community care, covering people with severe disabilities without regard to income and age. However, a federal financing cap would be imposed and co-payments required to control cost growth. Services for the mentally retarded and developmentally disabled populations would be as in option 2, and a liberalized

Medicaid program and private insurance strategies would be as in option 1. The cost was put at $15.4 billion in 1994.

Option 4 was full social insurance, covering nursing home care along with home and community care for severely disabled persons of all ages, to be fully phased in by 2010. It would begin with the means-tested home care program in option 2, with the eligibility level increasing over time until it reached 300 percent of poverty in 2005, at which time nursing home coverage for stays beyond six months would be introduced. Full coverage for nursing home and home care without regard to income would be implemented in 2010. The cost was put at $6 billion in 1994, rising to $126 billion in 2020.

The Clinton Plan

After a process of "toll gate" scrutiny, mixing and matching, further analysis, and trial balloons, the decision was made to go with a version that most closely resembled option three (White House Task Force, 1993b). The Clinton plan encompassed five key components: expanded home and community care, liberalized Medicaid coverage for nursing home care, federal regulation of private long-term care insurance and tax incentives to buy it, tax incentives to help individuals with disabilities to work, and support for demonstration projects that integrate acute and long-term care.

The Clinton team clearly chose something much less than a universal social insurance approach and decided it would be most realistic to seek incremental solutions. Nonetheless, the new long-term care benefits were estimated to cost $80 billion (current dollars) over the five-year phase-in period, 1996–2000. The program was estimated to cost $28 billion a year when fully implemented, with most of the cost ($25 billion in 2000) being for expansion of community and in-home services. The money was to be raised from savings in Medicare and Medicaid brought about through efficiencies associated with health reform and from some tax increases on tobacco products.

The centerpiece of the plan was a new home and community care program. It was designed to accomplish several goals: avoid and offset the current institutional bias; provide state and local flexibility in program design; offer eligibility without regard to age, income, or type of disability; and render more interstate equity in the availability and quality of this type of care. To control costs and stay within a budget, the program specified a "capped entitlement" to states (not individuals). Also, eligibility was restricted to those most disabled (needing assistance in three of five ADLs, or with severe cognitive or mental impairment, or with severe mental retardation, or children under six with chronic disabilities and who would otherwise require hospitalization or institutionalization).

The expected appeal to states of the proposed long-term care program came from a significantly higher federal match than they received under Medicaid, averaging about 28 percentage points more. Resources to help fund the match were expected to come, in part, from savings that would accrue by shifting some needs currently met by Medicaid to the new program and from shifting some state responsibilities for acute care services for the nonelderly to the health alliances under the health care reform plan. None of the Medicaid rules would apply, but every person who received services would have to have an individual assessment and care plan. Besides this, the only mandatory services were personal care services, though it was expected that there would be an ongoing performance review to monitor quality.

Improvements to Medicaid took the form of greater eligibility for nursing home care, produced by requiring that all states have a program for the medically needy, so that individuals with high medical and long-term care expenses would be allowed to spend down to gain access to Medicaid's benefits. Currently some states do not have such a program. In addition, those in nursing homes would be allowed to keep $100 in monthly income (compared to $30 now), and states could allow persons to protect up to $12,000 in assets (compared to $2000 now).

The Clinton plan recognized a role for private long-term care insurance by establishing a grant program to states to assist in educating consumers about long-term care insurance, as well as a grant program to assist in the enforcement of regulations. It also called for federal establishment of minimum regulatory standards and tax clarification so that long-term care insurance would receive treatment similar to that for other health insurance.

The plan reflected support for the disabled of all ages by calling for tax credits of up to 50 percent of costs to a maximum of $15,000 per year for individuals with disabilities who purchase personal care and assistance services so they can work. The integration of acute and long-term care was to be encouraged through demonstration projects.

Early Adjustments

The basic structure of the Clinton administration's long-term care plan reflected a mix of preference, politics, and practicality. It reflected the president's desire to give states flexibility in design and administration, presumably grounded in his years as a governor struggling with Medicaid waiver programs as a way to contain costs. It reflected the feeling that home and community care options must be encouraged as a key element of that struggle. It also clearly reflected a sense of fiscal constraint, by proposing something less than a new entitlement program for all long-term care. At the same time, it rejected the notion of means testing for the new home and community benefits, at least as an opening position. Somewhat revealing of what the Clinton administration faced in developing its proposal were several last minute changes made to accommodate special concerns (Clinton administration, 1993).

The proposed community-based service program originally had an income-related co-insurance that was 10 percent for those between 150 and 249 percent of the federal poverty standard, 25 percent in the 250 to 399 percent of poverty range, and 40 percent for anyone over that, with the option for states to apply a nominal cost-share for those below the 150 percent poverty standard. In response to means testing fears of the AARP, the parameters were changed to 10 percent for those in the 150 to 199 percent of poverty range, 20 percent for those in the 200 to 249 percent of poverty range, and 25 percent for those above this level.

The increased asset protection level of $12,000 was originally proposed as a new expansion of Medicaid. States, fearing that this would significantly increase eligibility (another in a long line of new unfunded liabilities that Congress has imposed on them), lobbied to have the liberalized asset level be a state option. In addition, the proposed monthly allowance was lowered from $100 to $70.

States liked the original plan that gave them the option to combine into a single capped program the new home- and community-based care budget, former Medicaid community care funding, and Medicaid institutional care expenditures for any or all categories of recipients of long-term care, and to create a new program with increased flexibility to set financial or functional eligibility standards. This provision, however, apparently went too far for those who do not trust the states to be the key actors in long-term care, and it was not included in the version that the President ultimately sent to Congress. It is noteworthy in this regard that, while there is interest in seeing integration of acute and long-term care, there was no explicit mention of administrative changes in Medicare to help that to happen.

Partitioning the Risk and Roles

The key features of the Clinton plan were the new home- and community-based benefits and the expected role of private long-term care insurance.

Implicit in the debate on these issues was the preferred partitioning of financial risk between the public and private sectors. Underlying this preference was the issue of means testing.

To some, most notably the AARP, means testing and private insurance are twin devils to be avoided. This point of view is supported by the desire to solve the problems of long-term care finance by having government pay for it, regardless of a patient's financial status, something that can be accomplished only with universal social insurance. Means-tested programs, it is argued, have a history of being poor programs because they lack the political constituency to keep them up. Private insurance is viewed as underdeveloped, too expensive, and fraught with consumer protection problems. Perhaps more important, private insurance is viewed by the AARP as enough of a solution to be a threat to broader program initiatives that could result in a social insurance program.

To others, notably the Health Insurance Association of America (HIAA), scarce public dollars should not be used to supplant any opportunity for private market development of vehicles that might shoulder some of the financing burden. This point of view is supported by high initial cost estimates for public programs, budget deficits and competing priorities, a track record of underestimating future cost growth, general opposition to new taxes, and the recognition that our other social insurance programs, Social Security and Medicare, are themselves in fiscal crisis.

The Clinton administration's "middle of the road" approach was to leave the nursing home component means tested. The underlying premise was that, for those not Medicaid eligible, private long-term care insurance would be better able to fill the need for nursing home coverage than for noninstitutional benefits. Insurance companies have much less experience with covering home and community care. They have tended to view it as difficult to predict and control. For insurers, however, this concern is overshadowed by the realization that consumers prefer to be cared for at home and that the marketing of long-term care insurance can be better accomplished when that option is readily available.

Nonetheless, nursing home care remains a primary catastrophic expense for older persons (Liu, Perozek, and Manton, 1993). Focusing private insurance only on the nursing home part of this risk would make the necessary coverage less expensive, thus encouraging more sales. It is a matter of interpretation whether there was intended to be any gap-filling role for private insurance in the new home and community program. It likely would depend on how the program unfolded in the states.

While it is hard to separate basic philosophical differences from the concerns of threatened vested interests, it is safe to say that alternatives to the Clinton plan have also been shaped by cost concerns. Legislative strategies have ranged from preserving the basic Clinton home care plan through delays in its implementation, to emphasizing a means tested approach as an alternative. Those wanting more than what was offered by the Clinton plan have been muted, because early on they realized the tenuous position of a more generous program in light of cost concerns.

Senators Kennedy and Wofford, for example, recognizing the lack of nursing home financing assistance for the middle class, proposed a self-funded public insurance program for nursing home care that was meant to be complimentary to the Clinton plan (Kennedy and Wofford, 1994). It was to be a voluntary program with a special incentive that protected $30,000 to $90,000 from Medicaid rules, depending on the amount of insurance purchased. The program would have more liberal sign-up rules than private insurance, allowing all comers during an open period at each of ten-year age intervals, beginning at age 35, regardless of preexisting conditions.

Those most vocal in opposition to the Clinton plan predicated their concerns on fear that the program would be ineffective at structuring an improved public-private partnership. The proposed home care program, by not being means tested, had the potential of being misunderstood by consumers, much like Medicare's lack of long-term care protection is misunderstood. HIAA, for example, believed that the large demand generated by the lack of age and income caps, along with the limited funding allocated for the program, would result in states' providing very limited benefits for the severely disabled who were eligible (Garner, 1993). This, combined with not understanding the eligibility limitations, would keep people from adequately preparing for the risk and need for long-term care.

For insurers, the Clinton proposal also represented a difficult challenge, in terms of coordinating private insurance with the public program. Because each state would have the discretion to establish its own benefit packages, insurance carriers would have been faced with ongoing state-specific features around which they would have to wrap their benefits. Furthermore, they feared that the limited nature of the program would create continued pressure for bigger government solutions, which would prolong the argument for a larger public role, which in turn would erode their market.

Because of these concerns, the HIAA recommended that eligibility for a new home- and community-based benefits program be income-related and that private insurance be encouraged for those who can afford such coverage. They favor this encouragement to take the form of minimum federal standards, relieving the burden of state regulation, and tax clarification, increasing the affordability and legitimacy of this type of coverage.

The topic of insurance standards is beyond the scope of this chapter, but it is worth noting that the language of the Clinton plan has been viewed alternately as a barrier and a support for private insurance development. Resolving this conflict is necessary if private insurance is to be an effective complement to public financing efforts. However, the Clinton plan fell short of embracing private long-term care insurance precisely because of opposition to means testing reforms, and the desire by those favoring a comprehensive solution that private insurance not become a barrier to a larger public program at some later time.

For a private market to be an effective partner, the boundaries on the role of the public sector should be clearly defined and understood by everyone concerned. More precisely, the distinction between what the public sector can do versus what it will do needs to be made clear. Then the partitioning of the risks and responsibilities between the public and private sectors must be established. It remains to be seen if and how such a compromise might be struck.

State-Private Insurance Partnership

One strategy for supporting private insurance market development considered by the Clinton team was to link the purchase of private long-term care insurance to Medicaid eligibility as a form of Medicaid buy-in for middle- and upper-income persons. The idea is based on the Partnership for Long-Term Care, a state-based program undertaken with the support of the Robert Wood Johnson Foundation to promote the development of high quality and affordable long-term care insurance options through public-private cooperation (Meiners, 1993). It is intended to be at least budget neutral for governments, with some potential to reduce the pressure on Medicaid budgets from long-term care.

The key feature of the partnership program is that it offers to make long-term care more affordable and appealing to consumers. Under special arrangements with the state, insurance companies specializing in long-term care can assure their policyholders that they no longer have to go broke to qualify for Medicaid. The assets protected under the partnership can mean the difference between autonomy and dependence if policyholders exhaust their insurance and still need assistance.

This poverty protection incentive is designed to make partnership insurance more attractive than the private insurance alone. The policies carry a stamp of approval from the state, indicating that they meet special state certification requirements. As part of the program, educational campaigns are conducted to increase awareness among elders and their families about the lack of protection and about their financial options. All participating insurers are required to provide the state with data for program monitoring and special studies.

The intent is to significantly broaden the role of private insurance in paying for long-term care by bringing into the market many who might not consider this option because they have limited resources to protect and cannot comfortably spend enough on insurance to get meaningful lifetime protection from impoverishment. Without the partnership, only inflation-protected lifetime coverage can give complete assurance that a person will not be impoverished by long-term care expenses. With the partnership, this same assurance can be obtained from more limited, less expensive coverage. Recent analysis of this approach suggests that the partnership benefit might increase the potential market for long-term care insurance by as much as 100 percent (Goss and Meiners, 1994). If it can serve as an alternative to the growing trend toward "gaming the system" and transferring assets, it will save Medicaid expenditures.

Four states — California, Connecticut, Indiana, and New York — are participating in the program. The poverty protection incentive being used in California, Connecticut, and Indiana features a dollar-for-dollar model. It provides a dollar of asset protection for each dollar paid out by a state-certified private long-term care insurance policy. It allows for a wide variety of product designs, with benefits ranging from one year of coverage on up. This allows persons of different means the option of choosing the amount of protection they can best afford (Mahoney and Wetle, 1992).

The model of choice in New York is designed to protect all assets (Holubinka, 1992; Nussbaum, 1992). It is structured on the basis of time rather than the amount of coverage purchased. Certified policies must cover three years in a nursing home or six years of home health care. The minimum daily amount of coverage for 1994 is $110. Once the benefits of a certified policy are exhausted, the Medicaid eligibility process will not consider assets at all. Protection will be granted for all assets, but an individual's income must be devoted to the cost of care.

The prime motivation behind the New York approach differs from that of the other states. New York's approach is primarily intended to offer a viable alternative to transfers of assets to become eligible for Medicaid.

Transfer of assets is thought to be quite common in New York and to be such a growing phenomenon that any strategy that encourages individuals to take responsibility for their own care could yield savings to the state.

The partnership strategy did not ultimately become part of the Clinton proposal for health care reform, for many of the same reasons noted above regarding the opposition to means testing and private insurance. Still, it seems to fit well with the key aspects of the plan — support for state-based initiatives to improve public programs for long-term care and support for a complementary role for private insurance. In fact, the system improvements sought by the Clinton plan will be needed if the partnership insurance strategy is to become more generally applicable. Many state Medicaid programs do not offer comprehensive home and community benefits or a system of needs assessment and care management which supports the continuity of care desired in such a partnership.

If a comprehensive long-term care program is neither fiscally or politically feasible, as is indicated by the fate of the Clinton plan, then incremental improvements to current efforts must be accepted as the direction of the future. However, improvements to long-term care programs cannot be sustained unless affordable and appealing private market financing options are available.

The partnership strategy is in the early stages of implementation, with few lessons as yet discernible about its market appeal. Connecticut and Indiana have reported early success with their effort to broaden the market to those who feel they can afford to cover only one or two years worth of benefits (Kyzivat, 1994; Leich, 1994). The partnership effort in New York is reported to have given a boost to the credibility and sales of the entire New York long-term care insurance market (Holubinka, 1994).

The partnership strategy is only a piece of the long-term care puzzle and not a panacea for reforming our current financing maze. However, the basic strategy seems flexible enough to accommodate potential advances in benefit designs, including those that seek to better integrate acute and long-term care.

Integrating Acute and Long-Term Care

There is general recognition of the need to improve the health care delivery system for those with chronic care needs. A commonly accepted premise is that to make progress we must improve the integration and coordination of acute and long-term care (see Chapters 3, 6, and 7). To do this, providers must experiment with new systems of care and financing. Perhaps, then, one of the most significant elements of the Clinton plan was the proposed development and study of integrated systems of care for chronically ill and disabled persons in as many as 25 demonstration sites. The proposal called for $50 million for new service costs over and above those in any publicly or privately financed program, along with $7 million in 1996, to cover the cost of technical assistance, research, and evaluation, and $4.5 million in each of the six succeeding years.

This proposal is noteworthy because support for experimentation has declined over the past decade and a half. Demonstrations as a way to foster new ideas have been subject to complaints from both extremes in the debate on long-term care. Those who want much more progress on this front had grown tired of demonstrations and viewed them as poor substitutes for action. Those who fear the increased cost of new benefits see demonstrations as a foot in the door to just such an outcome. As a result, demonstration programs have faced difficult times since the early 1980s. Achieving the necessary waivers to try new approaches has been at best difficult and consumes so much time and effort that financing and delivery system innovations have been severely limited.

But the fact is that Medicare policy and Medicaid policy have contributed to the fragmentation of our system of care. Unnecessary hospitalizations of those in nursing homes are encouraged by low Medicaid reimbursements, bed-hold day payments, and case-mix payment incentives for short-stay hospital admissions. Physician payments are biased toward hospital care instead of care in the office, home, or nursing home. More emergency room visits, medical transportation, and readmissions result.

These examples suggest the need for new incentives, along with payment methods that encourage providers to work together to overcome those problems. Pooled capitation payments combined with managed care and greater flexibility are the mechanisms often suggested to encourage providers to work together in creating cost-effective care packages (Bringewatt, 1994).

Further development is likely to build on the efforts of the social health maintenance organizations and the On Lok/PACE community-based care projects; two of the best-known long-term care demonstration efforts that have survived, these programs are now being replicated. Though few in number, these models provide evidence that will help further developments.

The social HMO model emphasizes home and community care within a limited managed long-term care benefit package and is designed to appeal as a supplement to Medicare HMO benefits for chronic care (Leutz, et al., 1985). It is marketed mostly to healthy private payers but is not limited to that segment of the population. As this model has evolved, it has been criticized for being simply a benefit add-on without the system integration needed to improve chronic care delivery. In 1990 Congress authorized a second generation of the social HMO model, to refine its population targeting, financing methods, and benefits design.

The Health Care Financing Administration has chosen to put more emphasis on a geriatric care model in the social HMOs (Health Care Financing Administration, 1994). Four new sites will be supported to accomplish the following improvements:

— drug monitoring to avoid misuse and adverse effects of pharmaceutical agents
— improved decisionmaking regarding acute medical and surgical problems to avoid unnecessary hospitalizations
— greater use of alternative facilities in place of hospital care
— greater use of alternatives to nursing home care
— more attention to making critical decisions about care choices
— more attention to end-of-life decisions
— protocols for better evaluating and managing common geriatric conditions
— standardized assessment protocols to screen persons at risk of medical complications, or at risk of inadequate social supports
— leadership by geriatricians and geriatric nurse practitioners

In contrast to the social HMO, the On Lok model and its ten-site replication demonstration, PACE (Program for All-Inclusive Care for the Elderly), focuses on the other end of the continuum of need (Ansak, 1990; see also Chapter 3). It is targeted to community-based frail elderly persons who are "nursing home certifiable" and likely near the end of life. The key service component is adult day care, which serves much like a geriatric care clinic, offering daily activities designed to allow for a stimulating environment and close observation and supervision that would otherwise be available only by institutionalizing the patient.

The PACE model is probably the best available example of successful integration of acute and long-term care under managed care arrangements. It has much more of the geriatric care orientation being sought in the second generation social HMOs, but the model is primarily targeted to those eligible for both Medicare and Medicaid. Nonetheless, there is growing interest in making this model of care more appealing to private pay populations who need similar care. The trick will be to get people to accept the need for this care earlier (to pay the premiums) while making a commitment to the prescribed delivery system. One approach that might work is to offer this care system as a preferred provider arrangement under long-term care insurance contracts.

A new more comprehensive approach to long-term care financing and organization is represented by the Minnesota Long-Term Care Options Project (LTCOP), a program in the early planning stages that builds on the accomplishments of the above demonstrations (Minnesota Department of Human Services, 1993). The LTCOP is seeking to demonstrate that integration of acute and long-term care financing can stimulate delivery system changes that will reduce cost shifting between Medicare and Medicaid and improve care outcomes. Its focus is those "dually eligible" for both Medicare and Medicaid. This population provides a good starting point for learning what it means to integrate acute and long-term care. Those who are Medicaid eligible tend to be relatively high cost users of care, and there is interest in gaining insight about their patterns of care.

The project is a direct response to the desire to eliminate the financing barriers to more cost-effective care for elderly persons. Currently, states have little incentive to address chronic care needs, because the savings are more likely to accrue on the Medicare side, for which the states have no fiscal responsibility, while potentially increasing utilization of state-financed Medicaid services. Incentives are strong for states to have as much care pushed to the acute care side as possible because there is no state cost sharing of Medicare expenditures.

The LTCOP project differs from the On Lok model in that its targeted population is broader than community residents who are nursing home certifiable. The intent is to include, in addition, those in nursing homes who are dually eligible and the well elderly in the community. It differs from the social HMO because it will concentrate on serving the Medicaid eligible, and the benefit package is not limited to home and community care services.

The LTCOP has the advantage of building on the prepaid medical assistance program (PMAP) in several Minnesota counties that require Medicaid eligible persons to enroll in one of several participating managed health care plans. While all Medicaid services except long-term care are covered under PMAP, these services are limited and do not address the coordination of acute and long-term care. PMAP does, however, provide an administrative base that could be used to integrate the benefits offered by Medicare, PMAP, and the new long-term care program. The idea is to give enrollees a choice between an LTCOP plan or the PMAP plan. To reduce consumer resistance to the new and unknown program, enrollees will be allowed to withdraw from it to the regular PMAP program.

It remains to be seen how HCFA will react to the details, but it seems likely that successful integration of acute and long-term care will need to allow for the pooling of Medicare and Medicaid dollars if progress is to be made. Once systems of care are redesigned to deal with chronic illness for those eligible for both Medicare and Medicaid, it may be possible for chronic care benefits to be accepted in the private insurance market.

State Initiatives in Long-Term Care

It is not surprising that states have been the focal point in the reform of long-term care. Much of long-term care is related to daily living needs rather than health care needs. This tends to make the approach to care more the concern of individuals and their communities. Perhaps even more important, the financing and administration of long-term care under the Medicaid program has been an increasing burden for states. Their desire to find alternatives to nursing home care has provided most of the program innovation.

There are arguments for and against state-based reform of long-term care (Friedman, 1994). State governments can act more quickly. States are more likely to implement a program of their own making. State initiatives are more likely to be better enforced. States represent multiple and smaller laboratories, allowing more learning and limiting the size of possible failures. If the federal effort does not work, at least states will have reforms in place.

But states may be reluctant to implement reforms because they are not confident in how to proceed or do not have the resources. Those states that do take action could be victimized by neighboring states seeking to shift their fiscal burden. State legislatures are typically not stable entities in terms of personnel, thus limiting knowledge and available expertise. They also have extensive contact with local lobbyists, which can make consensus difficult.

States are hungry for workable models to help deal with their long-term care responsibilities. One example of this is the response to the implementation of the Partnership for Long-Term Care program. By the summer of 1993, as many as twenty-one states had passed enabling legislation of one type or another so as to implement some version of that program and encourage greater private insurance financing. Hawaii carefully considered that approach but concluded that a better model for them was universal social insurance, which would be funded by new income taxes (Hawaii, Executive Office on Aging, 1991). The research and development from the Hawaiian effort became the basis for a similar plan in Vermont (State of Vermont Health Care Authority, 1993). Neither of these plans has yet been adopted, but along with the partnership programs they illustrate the role that state-based initiatives can have in designing strategies for financing long-term care.

Encouraged by these state-based efforts at long-term care reform, the Robert Wood Johnson Foundation launched a program for innovative states seeking to revamp their systems of financing and delivering long-term care. Under this program, long-term care includes chronic care services ranging from home and community care to institutional care for people of all ages. This broad focus is meant to encourage states to consider a wide range of alternative delivery systems and financing arrangements.

By the end of the planning phase of this initiative, participating states will be expected to have identified the reform(s) they wish to pursue, analyzed the implications for long-term care access and costs, and outlined specific steps necessary for implementation. This initiative is seeking to give state and national policymakers additional examples of how to build the political support and technical capacity to move forward with long-term care reform.

Conclusion

Several things about the future of long-term care financing and organization seem clear. States will have a major role in reforming the current system. Whether as the innovators of state-based strategies or as the implementers of a national plan, states will be challenged to build the political support and technical capacity to move forward. Neither the public nor the private sector alone is capable of providing an adequate solution. The basic message of the Clinton Health Plan was that long-term care is important but expensive.

The key public policy question is how to engineer an effective partnership of resources. For progress to be made, the Clinton team concluded, we must proceed incrementally, encouraging innovation by states in the area of home and community care, improvements in means-tested public programs, and support for private sector responsibility. Acceptance of these goals is a step in the right direction as we proceed with long-term care reform.

Significant progress will require a public-private financing partnership by design, not default. The private market will need governmental support to experiment with new systems of care and financing. Government already is heavily involved in long-term care, and private markets need incentives to innovate. Public and private sectors must give special attention to the needs of the rapidly aging population for chronic care services. To get on the fast track, government must take the lead in supporting innovation through the Medicaid program, because it is the principal payer for long-term care.

The dilemma we face in moving forward with long-term care reform is that different approaches, for example universal social insurance versus means testing, make compromise difficult. But, there is a need to commit to a vision for the future, because providing long-term care incurs a financial risk that will require prefunding if it is to be affordable, either privately or publicly. Incremental solutions would seem to make sense in terms of both the cost and the experience necessary for solid progress.

Incremental improvements invariably will depend, in one way or another, on means testing. The improvements could take the form of revisions to Medicaid, such as giving more financial support and flexibility to states for developing innovative approaches; replacement of Medicaid's role in long-term care with a new means tested program specifically for long-term care; or reforms to Medicare, such as better chronic care benefits to facilitate subacute needs. The reality is that there will need to be a program that is for poor people only. For the gaps that remain, individuals will have to pay out of pocket until they qualify for the public means-tested program or they will have to buy private insurance to fill the gaps.

Effective private financing options require a clear delineation of where the public role ends and personal responsibility begins. This is especially the case if people are expected to plan for their risk of chronic disability. If planning does not occur, more people will be dependent on public support. This places even more pressure on limited public budgets.

The Clinton plan, on the one hand, supported private action and preparation through tax clarification and national insurance regulations. On the other hand, it proposed a home and community care benefit that left the impression that governmental programs would be sufficient to meet individual needs, even though the details really suggested a capped entitlement to states — in practice, a much more limited intervention. There was considerable nervousness on the part of states about how to implement the proposal, because they already saw themselves in fiscal crisis and were worried about how to afford such a system if not allowed to means test for eligibility.

Means testing is the approach states are more familiar with because they have experience with it through Medicaid, but means testing is unacceptable to some policy analysts and interest groups. It is viewed as leading to poorly funded, inadequate programs because the political constituency is not broad enough to keep this from happening. Strategies need to be considered to minimize this risk, so that this opposition can be overcome.

Concerns about a "two-tiered" health care system are inevitable when there is only enough in the budget to provide a base of support for the most needy. Those who can afford more will want to use their resources as they see fit, including to purchase more care if that is what they prefer. A way to eliminate the concern that a program for the poor becomes a poor program, because it lacks the political constituency to keep it adequately funded, is to structure a linkage of the means-tested program with long-term care insurance, as is being done in the Robert Wood Johnson Foundation's Partnership for Long-Term Care Program. This strategy is intended to help secure middle- and upper-class support for a viable and decent means-tested program, by making it part of what they may need to depend on in the face of otherwise catastrophic long-term care expenses.

The partnership long-term care insurance model and an improved means tested long-term care program in the states would be mutually complementary. Currently the applicability of the model to other states is limited by the variability in Medicaid programs. Many state Medicaid programs do not offer the comprehensive home and community benefits or the system of care management which support the continuity of care desired in such a partnership. Furthermore, states that have not developed strong programs for the poor will have trouble justifying efforts at preventing poverty. On the other side, improvements to the Medicaid program cannot be sustained unless affordable and appealing private-market financing options can serve to keep people from using those benefits unless it is as a legitimate last resort. By linking the partnership incentive to Medicaid (or a new means-tested long-term care program), the constituency for the means-tested program should be enhanced rather than eroded.

Consumers need affordable and appealing options that encourage them to save for long-term care expenses. Incremental strategies that encourage as much personal responsibility as possible are necessary for progress to be made. The existence of a government program as a backup, like Medicaid, makes the financing structure of long-term care relatively unique. Building on Medicaid, a state-centered approach allows for the development of financing reforms that are consistent with the reality of economic and political considerations. It seems that the logical way to proceed from the structure laid out in the Clinton plan is to support a new means-tested program for long-term care that is designed to complement private market options.

It is important to recognize that when we talk about the role of the private sector we are talking about more than just private enterprise. Most long-term care is either provided by family and friends directly or purchased by them out of pocket. The interrelationship between these two forms of support can be complicated, but the simple fact is that any realistic intervention must support, not replace, our willingness to accept personal responsibility for our long-term care needs.

Where private enterprise enters into the equation is that it needs to help this happen to the greatest extent possible. This means that good-quality, affordable products that meet the need as perceived by consumers and their families must be developed and marketed. We are just beginning to see this happen. Examples that have recently emerged include the growing number of home and community care options, assisted living communities, and long-term care insurance. These developments should be encouraged.

To make the system work, it is necessary now and for the future to spell out the structure of public and private responsibilities clearly. Long-term care, by its very nature, requires prefunding or shifting of resources from now to the future. Whether this happens through new taxes or through a private premium, it is best to get started now, before the problem only gets more difficult.

References

Adams, K. E., Meiners, M. R., and Burwell, B. O. (1993). Asset spend-down in nursing homes: Methods and insights. *Medical Care* 31 (1): 1–23.

Ansak, M.-L. (1990). The On Lok model: Consolidating care and financing. *Generations* 14 (spring): 73–74.

Bringewatt, R. (1994). Reforming managed care financing to support service integration. *NCCC Update* 4 (5): 1–2.

Burwell, B. (1991). *Middle-Class Welfare: Medicaid Estate Planning for Long-Term Care Coverage.* Lexington, Mass.: Systemetrics/McGraw Hill.

Clinton administration (1993). Description of President's "Health Security Act of 1993." Bureau of National Affairs, Washington D.C., September 7.

Congressional Research Service (1993). *Medicaid Source Book: Background Data and Analysis.* Report to the Subcommittee on Health and the Environment, Committee on Energy and Commerce, U.S. House of Representatives. Washington D.C.: U.S. Government Printing Office.

Coronel, S. (1994). Long-term care insurance in 1992. Health Insurance Association of America, policy and research findings brief, February.

Etheredge, L. (1988). Financing and management of home and community based services. In *State Long Term Care Reform: Development of Community Care Systems in Six States* (pp. 115–45). Washington, D.C.: National Governors' Association.

Friedman, E. (1994). Getting a head start: The states and health care reform. *Journal of the American Medical Association* 271 (11): 875–78.

Garner, R. (1993). Statement of HIAA on Health Security Act implications for long term care before the Ways and Means Committee, Subcommittee on Health, U.S. House of Representatives, Washington D.C. November 2.

Goss, S. C., and Meiners, M. R. (1994). Increasing the market for long-term care insurance by reducing the risk of impoverishment: The effect of the 'dollar-for-dollar' partnership model. Paper presented at the 1994 annual meetings of the American Economics Association, Boston, Mass.

Hawaii, State of, Executive Office on Aging (1991). *Financing Long-term Care: A Report to the Hawaii State Legislature.*

Health Care Financing Administration (1994). Social health maintenance organization demonstration, phase II: Request for proposals. Washington, D.C.: U.S. Department of Health and Human Services.

Holubinka, G. (1992). New York partnership for LTC insurance. *LTC News and Comment* 3 (2): 9–10.

Holubinka, G. (1994). Personal communication with project director, New York Partnership for Long-Term Care.

Kennedy, E. M., and Wofford, H. (1994). Senate Bill 1833, 103rd Congress, 2nd session, February 7.

Kyzivat, L. (1994). Data collection and evaluation: The key to LTC partnerships. *LTC News and Comment* 4 (6): 10–12.

Leich, J. (1994). Indiana partnership: One year later. *LTC News and Comment* 4 (12): 8.

Leutz, J., Greenberg, N., Abrahams, R., Prottas, J., Diamond, L. M., and Gruenberg, L. (1985). *Changing Health Care for an Aging Society: Planning for the Social/Health Maintenance Organization.* Lexington, Mass.: Lexington Books.

Liu, K., Perozek, M., and Manton, K. (1993). Catastrophic acute and long-term care costs: Risks faced by disabled elderly persons. *Gerontologist* 33:299–307.

Mahoney, K. J., and Wetle, T. (1992). Public private partnerships: The Connecticut model for financing long-term care. *Journal of the American Geriatrics Society* 40:1026–30.

Meiners, M. R. (1993). Paying for long term care without breaking the bank. *Journal of American Health Policy* 3 (2): 44–48.

Minnesota Department of Human Services (1993). Health care reform: Acute and long term care integration for Medicare/Medicaid dual eligibles. Concept paper.

Neuschler, E. (1987). *Medicaid Eligibility for the Elderly in Need of Long Term Care*. Washington D.C.: National Governors' Association.

Nussbaum, S. (1992). The New York State partnership for long-term care. *The Bulletin: Official Publication of the New York City Association of Life Underwriters 72* (3): 27–36.

State of Vermont Health Care Authority (1993). Universal access plans. Report to the General Assembly (pp. 93–116). November 1.

White House Task Force on Health Reform, Long-Term Care Work Group (1993a). Long-term care. Draft. September 7.

White House Task Force on Health Reform, Long-Term Care Work Group (1993b). Toll gate: Five talking points. April 15.

Wiener, J. M. (1994). Financing long term care: The current system. Presentation at the Agency for Health Care Policy and Research user liaison program, workshop on long term care. Miami, Fla., December 6.

10

The Politics of Enacting
Long-Term Care Insurance

Robert H. Binstock, Ph.D.

Analyses throughout this volume provide a rich and detailed picture of how the organization and financing of long-term care is evolving in the United States. This chapter deals with but one of these elements. It focuses on the broad political factors that are likely to determine whether a new federal program of long-term care insurance will be enacted in the foreseeable future.

The general principle that a new public long-term care program should be established seemed to have been accepted in the early 1990s by national Democratic leaders and some Republicans (although, as Meiners indicates in Chapter 9, there were divergent views on details). Indeed, proponents of long-term care insurance were optimistic about its passage during the 103rd Congress of 1993–94, until the broader effort at health care reform, in which it was embedded, collapsed.

Now, in the mid-1990s, the old-age advocacy groups and other constituencies interested in the establishment of public long-term care insurance have shifted their political focus from offense to defense. The Republican-dominated 104th Congress has ushered in what appears to be a new era in the politics of domestic public policy. Proposed changes in federal policies are part of a sweeping agenda for limiting the role of government, redistributing responsibilities of the federal government to state governments, and bringing the annual federal budget into balance. Congress is contemplating substantial overall expenditure cutbacks in Medicaid, currently the principal government program paying for long-term care, as well as structural changes that will likely reduce the resources specifically available for long-term care. Unless the balance of power in Washington changes substantially and quickly, the enactment of public insurance for long-term care is very unlikely by the end of the century.

The chapter begins with an overview of the current political context, which has become problematic for the enactment of major policies to expand benefits to older people, and distinguishes it from earlier eras in the politics of aging. Second, it discusses the saga of the Medicare Catastrophic Coverage Act, passed in 1988 and largely repealed in 1989, to draw a lesson about what may be required politically if any future policy initiative for public funding of long-term care is to succeed. Third, the chapter examines why younger and older disabled persons seem to have difficulty in forming a strong coalition in support of new long-term care legislation. Fourth, it provides an analysis of why the broader constituency of older Americans has yet to coalesce as a potent grassroots force supporting long-term care insurance. And finally, it explores some factors that may change and thereby increase the political feasibility of enacting such a policy.

The New Political Context of Policies on Aging

The Earlier Eras

From the establishment of Social Security in 1935 through the mid-1970s, stereotypes of older Americans in popular culture were largely compassionate, and the role of government in responding to their needs grew continually. The media tended to portray older people as poor, frail, dependent, and, above all, deserving (see Binstock, 1983). The American polity responded to this compassionate construct through the New Deal's Social Security program, the Great Society's Medicare and the Older Americans Act, special tax exemptions and credits for being age 65 or older, and many other measures enacted during President Nixon's New Federalism, creating what has been termed an old age welfare state (Myles, 1989). Most programs that provided benefits and protection to older persons were structured primarily on the basis of old-age criteria, without much reference to substantial variations in economic and health status, and social conditions within the older population.

Starting in 1978 and continuing into the mid-1990s, new stereotypes emerged in popular culture, depicting older people as prosperous, hedonistic, selfish, and politically powerful "greedy geezers." The most important factor contributing to this reversal of stereotypes was that academicians (e.g., Hudson, 1978) and journalists (e.g., Samuelson, 1978) began to recognize a tremendous growth trend in the proportion of government dollars expended on benefits to older Americans, which by 1995 exceeded one-third of the annual federal budget (U.S. Congress, 1995).

Various public figures, academicians, and policy analysts focused on programs for the elderly as an important tradeoff element in any attempt to deal with American economic and social problems, in the present and future. Comparisons between expenditures on older people and on other social and economic causes were thematically unified and publicized as issues of so-called intergenerational equity by organizations such as Americans for Generational Equity (see Quadagno, 1989) and the Concord Coalition (1993). The theme of intergenerational equity and conflict was adopted by the media and a number of academics and policymakers, as a routine perspective for describing many social policy issues (Cook et al., 1994). The essence of the generational equity paradigm was expressed succinctly by the president of the prestigious American Association of Universities when he asserted, "The shape of the domestic federal budget inescapably pits programs for the retired against every other social purpose dependent on federal funds, in the present and the future" (Rosenzweig, 1990, p. 6).

Within this political climate of the 1980s and early 1990s the age-categorical principle for distributing benefits and burdens among older people through programs on aging eroded substantially. Starting in 1983, Congress made a number of incremental changes—in Social Security, Medicare, the Older Americans Act, and other programs and policies—that reflected the diverse economic situations of older persons (Binstock, 1994a). Some of these reduced benefits to comparatively wealthy older persons; others targeted benefits to relatively poor older persons.

President Clinton's 1993 proposal for health care reform (White House Domestic Policy Council, 1993) attempted to maintain this trend of differentiating among older people with respect to their economic status. Under the plan, high-income Medicare participants, individuals earning $100,000 and couples earning $125,000, would have paid Medicare Part B premiums at a higher rate than others. Co-insurance payments for long-term care were proposed as sliding scale payments for those persons above 150 percent of the federal poverty line. Subsequent proposals for amending Medicare and Social Security have also discriminated among older persons with respect to their economic status. And a 1994 report on how to reduce entitlement program spending, issued by the Congressional Budget Office (U.S. Congress, 1994) focused exclusively on means testing and progressive individual taxation of entitlement benefits as measures for achieving that goal.

The New Era

The new era in the politics of aging, which emerged in 1995, is distinct from the previous eras in two fundamental respects. First, it is shaped predominantly by a larger political agenda than the status of older persons or issues of intergenerational equity. Second, the reforms being proposed for programs affecting older Americans may have substantial and grave consequences for large segments of the present and future elderly populations, especially those who are not well-off economically, as opposed to the effects of the minor incremental policy changes enacted in the 1980s and early 1990s.

The larger political agenda of the 104th Congress, expressed in the so-called Contract with America, is structured by the following basic principles that have long been staples of conservative Republican ideology: Government should play a less intrusive role than it does in American society and in the lives of individuals. Citizens and businesses can make more effective use of their money if it remains in their hands, as opposed to being confiscated through taxes to support governmental activities. Intricate social programs funded by federal grants-in-aid should be administered with substantial discretionary authority by state governments. In addition, Republicans, and some Democrats, now adhere to the principle that the annual budget of the federal government should be brought into balance by sharply reducing expenditures.

This last concern, to balance the budget, has weighed heavily in the proposals for large reductions in Medicare and Medicaid expenditures that have been championed by the Republican leadership. Congress enacted a budget resolution in the summer of 1995 calling for a $270 billion reduction in projected Medicare spending by 2002. It also resolved to cap the rate of growth in Medicaid, to achieve savings of $182 billion in the same time period, and to turn over administration of the program to state governments by delivering allocations in block grants (Eaton and Diemer, 1995). How these goals would be achieved remained to be worked out as Congress attempted to pass for fiscal 1996 an Omnibus Budget Reconciliation Act that President Clinton would not veto.

Although large cuts in Social Security could also help achieve a balanced budget, the Republican leadership did not propose any in 1995. On the contrary, early in the year the House of Representatives passed a bill designed to raise the ceiling on earnings allowed to retirees before reductions are made in their Social Security benefits and to reduce the percentage of benefits subject to taxation for higher-income recipients.

There are several possible explanations for this choice to focus expenditure-reduction on Medicare and Medicaid rather than on Social Security, and they are not mutually exclusive. From a policy analysis perspective, it makes more sense to tackle Medicare and Medicaid expenditures in balancing the budget. Spending projections for these programs indicate that they will contribute substantially to increases in federal spending by the end of the century unless they are significantly changed (U.S. Congress, 1994). In contrast, large increases in Social Security outlays are not expected until several decades from now, when much of the baby boom cohort will join the ranks of old age.

It also makes more sense from a political perspective to deal with the growth of Medicare and Medicaid rather than tackle Social Security in attempts to balance the budget. Cuts in the health care programs are in keeping with the philosophy of the Contract with America, but cuts in retirement benefits would be contrary to it. Medicare and Medicaid do not put money in the hands of beneficiaries but in the hands of health care providers and suppliers. Accordingly, the programs are largely perceived as vast governmental bureaucracies. (Medicare is still portrayed by some political commentators as "socialized medicine.") Social Security, on the other hand, does put money directly into the hands of individuals; to take much of it away would be counter to the Republican principles and would have a direct impact on voters. The Republican leadership may also have made a calculated decision to enact Social Security changes that would leave more money in the hands of comparatively well-off older persons as a tradeoff tactic to moderate political opposition by mass-membership old-age interest groups to the proposed cuts in Medicare and Medicaid.

Regardless of explanations for the choice to concentrate deficit-reduction efforts on Medicare and Medicaid, the possible effects of the proposed measures are likely to be unfortunate for relatively poor older persons. This is especially the case with respect to Medicaid, which pays for the care, at least in part, of about three-fifths of nursing home patients (Wiener and Illston, in press) and for 28 percent of home- and community-based services (American Association of Retired Persons, 1994).

Some analysts predict that substantial reductions in current state Medicaid spending will almost certainly occur unless states are required to increase their funding for the program (U.S. General Accounting Office, 1995). According to one analysis (Kassner, 1995), the 1995 congressional proposals for limiting Medicaid's growth would trim long-term care funding by as much as 11.4 percent by 2000 and mean that 1.74 million Medicaid beneficiaries and potential beneficiaries would lose or be unable to secure coverage. This analysis also assumed that states would make their initial reductions in home- and community-based care services (because nursing home residents have nowhere else to go) and concluded that such services would be substantially reduced. Five states were projected to completely eliminate home- and community-based services by the end of the century, and another 19 to cut services by more than half. Whether or not these predictions come true, capping and block-granting Medicaid is almost certain to engender conflict within states regarding the distribution of limited resources for long-term care and other forms of health care that are reimbursed by the program.

A Lesson from Medicare Catastrophic Coverage Act

The new political context established by the 104th Congress makes it highly unlikely that public funding for long-term care insurance will be on the policy agenda in the mid-1990s. Perhaps by the turn of the century or shortly thereafter a new political order will be established in Washington in which long-term care policy initiatives may reemerge. Even if that happens, however, chances are that any proposal for a new long-term care program will be structured (as was the Clinton proposal for long-term care) on the premise that it is to be financed in substantial measure by program beneficiaries themselves. This was the case with the Medicare Catastrophic Coverage Act (MCCA) of 1988, which was swiftly repealed in 1989. Therefore, it is worth reviewing briefly the chronicle of the MCCA for the perspective it can provide on the politics of future attempts to establish a new public long-term care program.

The MCCA included the first major expansion of benefits to older persons in sixteen years. It provided insurance coverage for economically catastrophic hospital and physician bills, outpatient prescription drugs, and for some elements of long-term care. About one-third of these new benefits were to be financed through increased premiums paid by all Medicare Part B enrollees, and two-thirds through a progressive, sharply escalating surtax levied on middle- and higher-income Medicare enrollees — about 40 percent of program participants. This approach was a substantial departure, of course, from the traditional model of social insurance programs under the Social Security Act, such as Old Age and Survivors Insurance and Medicare Hospital Insurance, which are financed through the Federal Insurance Contributions Act payroll tax on employees and their employers.

The MCCA was developed through the initiatives of public officials in the White House, Congress, and the bureaucracy who were focused on their own agendas for social and economic policy (see Iglehart, 1989). During a period of nearly two years between the introduction of the bill and its enactment as law, neither Congress nor the old-age advocacy groups floated "trial balloons" to enable older Americans to understand what sorts of benefits they would receive through the new MCCA, and who would pay for them. Consequently, when the proposal finally did become a law, there was no popular constituency supporting it. But there was distinct opposition to it from those older persons who had to pay the most new taxes and who perceived that they already had private insurance coverage for the benefits provided through the new law (Crystal, 1990; Day 1993; Holstein and Minkler, 1991). They were a small numerical minority, yet they were dispersed through every congressional district. When they protested vociferously against the act, Congress received no evidence of countervailing popular support for the MCCA. If there had been such support, it is likely that Congress would have withstood the protests of the minority of older persons who expressed their dissatisfaction with the legislation. Indeed, following the repeal of the law, several congressional leaders publicly lamented that they had not had the courage to stand up to a small number of comparatively wealthy older constituents (Tolchin, 1989).

The experience of the MCCA provides a lesson for assessing the politics of any major initiative for expanding public long-term care insurance that calls for significant financing by program participants. Such a program will probably require broad political support from a grassroots constituency that articulates its desires and demands actively within congressional districts throughout the nation.

The Politics of Public Long-Term Care Insurance

The Emergence of Earlier Proposals

Although disabled persons of all ages have long-term care needs, the major initial impetus for public long-term care insurance was successful advocacy efforts on behalf of older people. Particularly noteworthy in this regard were the efforts undertaken by a political coalition concerned about Alzheimer disease which began to form in the mid-1970s (Fox, 1989). By the mid-1980s, advocates for older and younger disabled people began meeting to explore their common policy interests (see Brody and Ruff, 1986; Mahoney, Estes, and Heumann, 1986). And in 1989 a broad coalition named the Long-Term Care Campaign was formed. A Washington-based interest group claiming to represent 140 national organizations with more than 60 million members, it had as one of its key legislative goals that "long term care services should be available to all who need them, regardless of age" (Long-Term Care Campaign, 1990).

A specific policy link was forged between younger and older disabled people in 1989 when Representative Claude Pepper introduced a bill to provide comprehensive long-term home care insurance coverage for persons of any age who were dependent in at least two activities of daily living (ADLs). Since then, a number of such long-term care bills have been introduced, with projected expenditures ranging from $10 billion to $60 billion, depending on provisions regarding the specific populations to be eligible and on details regarding the timing, nature, and extent of insurance coverage.

The long-term care component in President Clinton's 1993 health reform package carried forward the principle of age irrelevance in determining eligibility for benefits. It posited that to be eligible for publicly financed services, an individual must meet one of the following conditions: (1) require personal assistance, stand-by assistance, supervision, or cues to perform three or more of five ADLs — eating, dressing, bathing, toileting, and transferring into and out of bed; (2) present evidence of severe cognitive or mental impairment as indicated by a specified score on a standard mental status protocol; (3) have severe or profound mental retardation; or (4) be a child under the age of six who is dependent on high technology or otherwise requires hospital or institutional care (White House Domestic Policy Council, 1993, pp. 171–72).

Neither the Clinton proposal nor the earlier proposals, of course, came close to being enacted by Congress. Nonetheless, these proposals did firmly establish the principle that any federal long-term care policy should rely on criteria involving need for services rather than on an age-categorical approach.

Disparate Perspectives of Younger and Older Disabled People

Although some congressional and administrative policy leaders have been committed to this principle of age irrelevancy, it remains to be seen whether it will prove to be politically viable. Even if the fiscal costs of such a program come to be perceived as manageable, it is far from certain that older and younger disabled people — the latter including persons with spinal cord injury, cerebral palsy, mental retardation, AIDS, and other disabling conditions — will emerge as a powerful unified constituent coalition to back such legislation. Unity would require substantial resolution of divergent outlooks and needs among the constituencies to be served.

Traditionally, advocates for the aged and for younger disabled populations have not been united in supporting long-term care initiatives, and they have sometimes engaged in sharp conflict (see Torres-Gil and Pynoos, 1986). From the perspective of older persons long-term care has been seen as a problem besetting elderly people, categorically, to be dealt with through a "medical model" of health and social services. And a major, though not exclusive, element of their interest in public insurance has been generated by an economic concern. That concern is the possibility of becoming poor through "spending down," that is, depleting one's assets to pay for long-term care and then becoming dependent on a welfare program, Medicaid, to pay subsequent long-term care bills. There is a distinct middle-class fear — both economic and psychological — of using savings and selling a home to finance one's own health care. This anxiety reflects a desire to preserve estates for inheritance, as well as the psychological intertwining of personal self-esteem with one's lifetime accumulation of material worth and sense of financial independence. This kind of concern has little political appeal beyond segments of the old-age constituency, of course, in the contemporary political environment.

In contrast to older persons, younger disabled persons and their advocates do not perceive long-term care insurance as mostly an issue of whether the government or the individual client and/or family pays for the care. At least as important to them is the issue of basic access to services, technologies, and environments that will make it feasible to carry forward an active life. They argue that they should have assistance to do much of what they would be able to do if they were not disabled.

The Americans with Disabilities Act of 1990 will help to eliminate discriminatory as well as physical barriers to the participation of people with disabilities in employment, public services, public accommodations and transportation, and telecommunications. But it will not provide the elements of long-term care desired by disabled younger adults, such as paid assistance in the home and for getting in and out of the home, peer counseling, semi-independent modes of transportation, and client control or management of services.

Although younger disabled people have advocated for long-term care services, they have rejected a medical model that emphasizes long-term care as an essential component of health services. This is understandable, given their strong desires for autonomy, independence, and as much normalization of daily life as possible. By the same token, disabled younger people have tended to eschew symbolic and political identification with elderly people, because of traditional stereotypes of older people as frail, chronically ill, declining, and "marginal" to society.

Beyond issues of disparate philosophy lie specific divergences in service needs. For example, as A. E. Benjamin points out in Chapter 4 of this volume, persons disabled through spinal cord injuries tend to remain in stable medical and functional condition for many years, and persons with AIDS have a trajectory of decline, punctuated by intermittent and continual episodes of acute illness. Although the trajectory for many elderly persons in long-term care is gradual decline, on average their need for acute care is not as frequent as that of persons with AIDS.

Even among older persons in long-term care there are divergent needs. For instance, the cognitive impairments of people with dementia often require that the nature of a service be altered. A dementia patient often fails to understand and cooperate with service providers; at the same time, many service providers are not especially knowledgeable about or skilled at working with patients who have dementia (see U.S. Congress, 1990).

Despite their traditional differences, advocates for the aged and for the disabled did work together temporarily in the planning process for President Clinton's 1993 initiative on long-term care. This was reflected in the fact that the president's proposal incorporated many specific concerns that have been put forward by advocates for the younger disabled population over the years, for example, the principle that clients should be able at their own discretion to hire and fire service providers. But this unity eroded shortly thereafter in the context of considerable reservations that the respective constituencies had regarding the overall Clinton plan for health care reform (see Binstock, 1994b).

The Political Power of the Aged

The prospects for the development of a substantial political coalition among the younger and older constituencies of the disabled seem dim, despite occasional optimistic exhortations to the contrary (e.g., Rubenfeld, 1986). But some 33 million Americans ages 65 and older (as well as their families) have much at stake in the enactment of national long-term care insurance. Is it likely that grassroots political support of older people will be mobilized in a fashion powerful enough to bring about the passage of such legislation?

Media stereotypes frequently portray older persons as a monolithic bloc of voters who promote and defend their self-interests successfully. And old-age-based organizations are conventionally depicted as one of the most powerful constituencies in American politics. In 1990, for example, when President Bush and congressional leaders agreed on a budget proposal that included changes in Social Security benefits and taxes, a

New York Times reporter predicted a political explosion: "America's older citizens are among the nation's most potent constituencies. They vote at higher rates than most other Americans. . . . In addition their organizations, lead [sic] by the American Association of Retired Persons, swing great weight on Capitol Hill" (Oreskes, 1990, p. 12). A brief examination of the role of older people in American politics will indicate, however, that these nuggets of conventional wisdom are very oversimplified. To date, older people have not been a cohesive political constituency.

Political Attitudes

The political attitudes of older people are diverse. A study by Day (1990), for instance, analyzed polls conducted from 1972 to 1986 by three different national opinion surveys to test for attitudinal differences among older, middle-aged, and younger adults with respect to policy areas that affect older persons most directly (e.g., Social Security and Medicare). Her analysis suggests that the attribute of old age is not an important factor in shaping political attitudes and that there is no evidence of so-called intergenerational conflict to be found in comparing age group attitudes toward policy issues. She found that "older people are nearly indistinguishable from younger adults [both middle-aged and younger] on most issues including aging policy issues" (p. 47).

When Day examined the responses of older persons in subgroups defined by various combinations of socioeconomic characteristics and partisan attachments, she confirmed the findings of numerous studies that show clear relationships between such combinations and political attitudes among adults of all ages. For example, "pluralities of people who were low-income, nonwhite, less educated, working-class, Democratic, or liberal favored increases in Social Security and Medicare, while pluralities of higher income, white, well educated, middle-class, Republican, or conservative people expressed satisfaction with current spending levels" (p. 53). This theme is echoed in National Opinion Research Center (1986–91) surveys of views of spending for Social Security. Among black older persons, a group that experiences a very high rate of poverty, 68.1 percent felt that we were spending "too little on Social Security." In contrast, only 43.8 percent of white older persons shared this view.

Voting Behavior

Older Americans vote in large numbers, composing between 16 and 21 percent of people who voted in national elections from 1980 through

Table 10.1

Distribution of Votes, by Age Group and Gender, in Presidential Elections, 1980, 1984, 1988, 1992 (percentages)

	1980			1984		1988		1992		
	Reagan	Carter	Anderson	Reagan	Mondale	Bush	Dukakis	Clinton	Bush	Perot
All Voters										
all ages	51	41	7	59	40	53	45	43	38	19
18–29 years old	43	44	11	59	40	52	47	44	34	22
30–44 years old	55	36	8	57	42	54	45	42	38	20
45–59 years old	55	39	5	60	40	57	42	41	40	19
60 years and older	54	41	4	60	40	50	49	50	38	12
Men										
all ages	55	36	7	62	37	57	41	41	38	21
18–29 years old	47	39	11	63	36	55	43	38	36	26
30–44 years old	59	31	4	61	38	58	40	39	38	22
45–59 years old	60	34	5	62	36	62	36	40	40	20
60 years and older	56	40	3	62	37	53	46	49	37	14
Women										
all ages	47	45	7	56	44	50	49	46	37	17
18–29 years old	39	49	10	55	45	49	50	48	33	19
30–44 years old	50	41	8	54	45	50	49	44	38	18
45–59 years old	50	44	5	57	42	52	48	43	40	17
60 years and older	52	43	4	58	42	48	52	51	39	10

Source: Adapted from *New York Times*/CBS News Poll, "Portrait of the Electorate," *New York Times*, November 5, 1992, p. B9.

1992 (*New York Times*/CBS News Poll (1992). They also vote at much higher rates than most other Americans. The overall voting participation rate in the 1988 presidential election was 65.9 percent (National Opinion Research Center, 1986–91). The youngest age group, 18–29, had the lowest rate of participation, just 44.8 percent; with each successive older age group the rate increased, until it peaked in the age ranges of 60–69 years (79.5% voting) and 70–79 years (81.7% voting).

Even though older people vote at a high rate, they are as diverse in their voting patterns as any other age group; their votes divide along the same partisan, economic, social, and other lines as those of the electorate at large. Older and middle-aged voters were rarely more than a few percentage points apart in presidential elections from 1952 through 1980 (Campbell and Strate, 1981). And, as can been seen in Table 10.1, presidential elections from 1980 through 1992 exhibited the same pattern — sharp divisions within each age group and very small differences between age groups.

In the 1992 U.S. presidential election, older voters departed somewhat from their usual pattern. Although they voted for Republican George Bush in the same proportions as did other age groups, they voted for Democrat Bill Clinton at a higher rate and for Independent Ross Perot at a lower rate than did younger voters. A possible explanation for this distinctive distribution of votes by older persons may lie in their comparative reluctance to accept Perot as a serious candidate. Older persons tend to have a greater attachment to traditional political institutions. Accordingly, they have been consistently less supportive of independent candidates than have younger age groups (Binstock and Day, 1996).

These data should not be surprising. There is no sound reason to expect that an age cohort — constituted of all races, religions, ethnic groups, economic and social statuses, political attitudes, and every other characteristic in American society would suddenly become homogenized in its political behavior when it reaches the "old age" category (Hudson and Strate 1985; cf. Cutler 1977). As Heclo (1988) observed, "'the elderly' is really a category created by policy analysts, pension officials, and mechanical models of interest group politics" (p. 393).

Moreover, the very assumption that mass groupings of the American citizenry, such as elderly people, vote primarily on the basis of self-interested responses to single issues is, in itself, problematic (Simon, 1985). To the extent that issues have an impact within a heterogeneous group, such as older persons, self-interested responses to any single issue are likely to vary substantially. Even in the context of a state or local referendum that presents a specific issue for balloting, such as propositions to cap local property taxes or to finance public schools, the best available studies show that old age is not a statistically significant predictor of the distribution of votes (Button and Rosenbaum 1989; Chomitz 1987). Overall, the weight of the evidence indicates that older people's electoral choices are rarely, if ever, based on age-group interests.

Old-Age Interest Groups

The last three decades have witnessed a tremendous expansion in the number, the memberships, the visibility, and the political activity of old-age interest groups (see Pratt, 1993). Although there are literally hundreds of contemporary organizations that engage on an ad hoc basis in the politics of policies and programs affecting older persons, dozens of them — often referred to as the "gray lobby" (Pratt, 1976) — are more or less exclusively preoccupied with national issues related to aging. As indicated in Table 10.2, some of them are mass membership organizations, and others have been organized to advocate for selected constituencies of older persons or for professional and trade interests associated with old age. About 40 of these have constituted themselves as the Leadership Council on Aging, which attempts to speak with one voice.

By far the largest of these aging-based organizations is the American Association of Retired Persons (AARP), which claims some 35 million members and has 4,000 local chapters, 1,700 employees (*New York Times,* 1995), and revenues that totaled $469 million in 1994 (Pear, 1995). Whatever AARP chooses to do (or not do) tends to define the political position of the old-age lobby, overall. By the same token, the strategies of the rest of the old-age-based organizations tend to be politically insignificant if AARP does not take the lead on them. Although AARP lobbies actively in national politics, its political activities appear to be less important as membership incentives than the material and associational incentives (see Clark and Wilson, 1961) provided through its investment funds, insurance programs, pharmaceutical discounts, credit cards, publications, travel packages, local chapter educational and cultural programs, and a variety of other activities.

Only limited political power is available to AARP and the other aging-based interest groups. As implied by the evidence from voting behavior, there is no indication that such organizations have been able to shift even marginally the votes of older persons, let alone produce a cohesive old-age vote.

Organized demands of older persons have had little to do with the enactment and amendment of the major old-age policies such as Social Secu-

Table 10.2
National Old-Age Interest Groups (Selected)

Mass Membership Organizations
    American Association of Retired Persons (35 million members)
    Gray Panthers (70,000 members)
    National Alliance of Senior Citizens (2 million members)
    National Association for Older Persons
    National Association of Retired Federal Employees (490,000 members)
    National Committee to Preserve Social Security and Medicare (5 million members)
    National Council of Senior Citizens (5 million members)
Advocacy Organizations for Special Older Constituencies
    Alzheimer's Association
    Asociacion Nacionale Pro Personas Mayores
    Families U.S.A. Foundation (poor older persons)
    National Caucus and Center on Black Aged
    National Citizens Coalition for Nursing Home Reform
    National Foundation for Long-Term Care
    National Hispanic Council on Aging
    National Indian Council on Aging
    National Pacific/Asian Resource Center on Aging
    Older Women's League
Professional and Trade Organizations
    Alliance for Aging Research
    American Association of Homes and Services for the Aging
    American Association for International Aging
    American Federation for Aging Research
    American Geriatrics Society
    American Society on Aging
    Association for Gerontology in Higher Education
    Gerontological Society of America
    National Academy of Social Insurance
    National Association for Home Care
    National Association of Area Agencies on Aging
    National Association of Foster Grandparents
    National Association of Meals Programs
    National Association of Nutrition and Aging Services Programs
    National Association of RSVP[a] Directors
    National Association of Senior Living Industries
    National Association of State Units on Aging
    National Council on the Aging
    National Senior Citizens Law Center

Source: Adapted from Van Tassel and Wilkinson Meyer (1992).
  [a]Retired Senior Volunteer Program

rity and Medicare. Rather, such actions have been largely attributable to the initiatives of public officials in the White House, Congress, and the bureaucracy who have focused on their own agendas for social and economic policy (on Social Security, see Derthick, 1979; Light, 1985; on Medicare, see Cohen, 1985; Iglehart, 1989). The impact of old-age-based interest groups has been largely confined to relatively minor policies that have distributed benefits to professionals and practitioners in the field of aging rather than directly to older persons themselves (Binstock, 1972; Binstock, Levin, and Weatherly, 1985; Estes, 1979; Fox, 1989; and Lockett, 1983).

Some forms of power, however, are available to old-age interest groups. In the classic pattern of American interest group politics (Lowi, 1969), public officials find it both useful and incumbent on them to invite such organizations to participate in policy activities. In this way, public officials are provided with a ready means of being "in touch" symbolically with millions of older persons, thereby legitimizing subsequent policy actions and inactions. A brief meeting with the leaders of AARP and other old-age organizations can enable an official to claim that he or she has duly obtained representative views of a mass constituency.

The symbolic legitimacy that old-age organizations have for participating in interest group politics gives them several forms of power. First, they have easy informal access to public officials: members of Congress and their staffs, career bureaucrats, appointed officials, and occasionally the White House. They can put forth their own proposals — regarding long-term care, Social Security, Medicare, and a variety of other matters — and work to block the proposals of others. To be sure, their audiences or targets may be unresponsive in subsequent policy decisions, but access provides some measure of opportunity.

Second, their legitimacy enables them to obtain public platforms in the national media, congressional hearings, and in national conferences and commissions dealing with old age, health, and a variety of subjects relevant to policies affecting aging. From these platforms the old-age organizations can initiate and frame issues for public debate, and respond to issues raised by others.

A third form of power available to the old-age interest groups might be termed "the electoral bluff." Although these organizations have not demonstrated a capacity to swing a decisive bloc of older voters, incumbent members of Congress are hardly inclined to risk upsetting the existing distribution of votes that puts them and keeps them in office. Few politicians, of course, want to call the bluff of the aged or any other latent mass constituency if it is possible to avoid doing so. In fact, the image of "senior power" is frequently invoked by politicians when — for one reason or another — they desire an excuse for doing nothing or for not differentiating themselves from their colleagues and electoral opponents.

Nonetheless, these forms of power are limited in their impact. Most of the legislative changes enacted since 1983 which have introduced economic criteria in old-age programs, discussed above, were unsuccessfully opposed by AARP and other old-age organizations. The 1989 repeal of the MCCA was a substantial defeat for AARP, which had heartily endorsed the bill developed by Congress and futilely lobbied in opposition to the repeal legislation. Moreover, vociferous opposition to the MCCA by many AARP members — and reported subsequent cancellations of several million memberships — has led the organization to be more cautious in taking unequivocal positions on legislation.

When the Clinton administration began to develop its 1993 plan for health care reform, it involved AARP in the process, early and deeply. The organization's chief lobbyist became a White House "insider" in health care reform and worked for many months to promote the Clinton plan with a wide range of constituencies. Yet AARP was never willing to officially endorse the Clinton proposal, even though it included a program of long-term care insurance and an expansion of Medicare to cover prescription drugs. In the waning weeks of the 103rd Congress the organization finally endorsed watered-down health care reform bills favored by the Senate and House majority leaders (Pear, 1994), but even then, many AARP members immediately expressed their outrage at this endorsement (*New York Times*, 1994a, 1994b). A few months later, for the first time, a president of AARP publicly acknowledged that the organization could not speak for all its members in such matters (Lehrman, 1995).

Today, the organization's staff and volunteer leaders are very cautious in their lobbying activities. Its tactical approach is relatively moderate, forgoing massive investments of financial and staff resources in conventional lobbying approaches and eschewing efforts at militant activities that would involve mobilizing millions of older people to express their needs or protests through their immediate physical presence. AARP now seems inclined to establish a record of "fighting a good fight," win or lose, but not in a fashion that threatens to jeopardize the stability of the organization's membership and financial resources.

What Lies in the Future?

The present political context makes a new initiative in funding public long-term care insurance very unlikely in the years immediately ahead.

Perhaps by the end of the decade or early in the twenty-first century — if the political climate changes — an important new long-term care proposal may be put forth by national political leaders. Even if it is, however, substantial grassroots support from the constituencies that would most likely benefit from such a program may not be forthcoming. The tenet of providing benefits on the basis of need for services, without regard to age, has been established. Yet, younger and older disabled persons have so far failed to find a common ground that is solid enough to develop a powerful political coalition. Although elements of the old-age constituency, such as victims of Alzheimer disease and their families and the Alzheimer's Association, are committed to achieving public long-term care insurance, the broader constituency of older persons does not appear to be very committed as yet. To be sure, many old-age interest groups support this goal, but the political heterogeneity of older persons, even with respect to aging-related policy issues, makes it difficult for these organizations to develop broad, effective constituent support.

Yet, extrapolation from the past and present is not always a good mode of prediction. Changing factors, especially in the lives of older persons and their families, could engender much broader and deeper popular support for long-term care legislation in the future than has been observed to date. Some analysts have argued for years that an "age consciousness" will develop among older persons and, in turn, transform them into a cohesive political force (Bengtson and Cutler, 1976; Cutler, 1981; Cutler, Pierce, and Steckenrider, 1984). Although such predictions have not been accurate in general, the development of age consciousness may be possible with respect to the issue of long-term care.

As earlier chapters in this volume make clear, projections are that disabling conditions will affect ever-increasing numbers of older persons and their families. As they do, the frustrations of financing and obtaining adequate supportive services may become even more pervasive within the American population than they are now. Such frustrations might engender broader and deeper public support than there is today for government financing of long-term care.

It is also possible that new long-term care bills, if eventually introduced in Congress, will be more appealing to both the younger and older disabled constituencies than was the 1993 Clinton proposal. For one thing, they may be more carefully crafted, to assure the disparate groups that none of them will be shortchanged in either their share of program resources or the appropriateness of services for different types of clients and the suitability of arrangements through which they are available.

Perhaps more important, if such new initiatives are introduced without being part of an overall plan for reforming the nation's health care system, the various constituencies may embrace them far more readily than they did the Clinton long-term care plan. The latter, of course, was part of a broader proposal that engendered significant reservations among advocates for younger and older disabled persons regarding provisions affecting the acute care arena.

On the one hand, advocates for the younger disabled were concerned that persons with what they term "special needs" would receive short shrift in the acute care range of needs if their health care were provided in the context of the limited budgets of health maintenance organizations, preferred provider organizations, and the other health care provider groups that would have been assembled for the purchasing alliances. On the other hand, old-age interest groups, particularly AARP and the National Committee to Preserve Social Security and Medicare (see McSteen, 1993), were concerned with what they regarded as inequities between the insurance provided to Medicare enrollees as compared with the coverage that the president's plan proposed for most other Americans. Moreover, a provision that would have allowed states to integrate Medicare into purchasing alliances raised the specter of unofficial rationing of health care on the basis of old age, a fear paralleling that expressed by advocates for younger disabled persons (see Binstock, 1994c).

In the last analysis, even if substantial grassroots support for public long-term care insurance does develop, enactment of such legislation will also require strong national leadership. As indicated above, none of the major policies that have composed the welfare state for the elderly — such as Social Security, Medicare, and the Employee Retirement Income Security Act — came about because of pressure from old-age interest groups or in response to broad popular demands for their enactment. Public long-term care insurance will need to be perceived by a president and congressional leaders as an essential response to a social issue of national importance.

References

American Association of Retired Persons, Public Policy Institute (1994). *The Costs of Long-Term Care*. Washington, D.C.: American Association of Retired Persons.

Bengtson, V. L., and Cutler, N. E. (1976). Generations and intergenerational relations: Perspectives on age groups and social change. In R. H. Binstock and E. Shanas, eds., *Handbook of Aging and the Social Sciences* (pp. 130–59). New York: Van Nostrand Reinhold.

Binstock, R. H. (1972). Interest-group liberalism and the politics of aging. *Gerontologist* 12:265–80.

Binstock, R. H. (1983). The aged as scapegoat. *Gerontologist* 23:136–43.

Binstock, R. H. (1993). Healthcare costs around the world: Is aging a fiscal "black hole"? *Generations* 17 (4): 37–42.

Binstock, R. H. (1994a). Changing criteria in old-age programs: The introduction of economic status and need for services. *Gerontologist* 34:726–30.

Binstock, R. H. (1994b). Older Americans and health care reform in the 1990s. In P. V. Rosenau, ed., *Health Care Reform in the Nineties* (pp. 213–35). Thousand Oaks, Calif.: Sage Publications.

Binstock, R. H. (1994c). The Clinton plan, Medicare integration, and old-age-based rationing—the need for public debate. *Gerontologist* 34:612–13.

Binstock, R. H., and Day, C. L. (1996). Aging and politics. In R. H. Binstock and L. K. George, eds., *Handbook of Aging and the Social Sciences,* 4th ed. (pp. 362–87). San Diego: Academic Press.

Binstock, R. H., Levin, M. A., and Weatherley, R. H. (1985). Political dilemmas of social intervention. In R. H. Binstock and E. Shanas, eds., *Handbook of Aging and the Social Sciences,* 2nd ed. (pp. 589–618). New York: Van Nostrand Reinhold.

Brody, S. J., and Ruff, G. E., eds. (1986). *Aging and Rehabilitation: Advances in the State of the Art.* New York: Springer Publishing.

Button, J. W., and Rosenbaum, W. A. (1989). Seeing gray: School bond issues and the aging in Florida. *Research on Aging* 11:158–73.

Campbell, J. C., and Strate, J. (1981). Are older people conservative? *Gerontologist* 21:580–91.

Chomitz, K. M. (1987). Demographic influences on local public education expenditures: A review of econometric evidence. In Committee on Population, Commission on Behavioral and Social Sciences and Education, National Research Council, ed., *Demographic Change and the Well-being of Children and the Elderly.* Washington, D.C.: National Academy Press.

Clark, P. B., and Wilson, J. Q. (1961). Incentive systems: A theory of organizations. *Administrative Science Quarterly* 6:219–66.

Cohen, W. J. (1985). Reflections on the enactment of Medicare and Medicaid. *Health Care Financing Review* (ann. suppl.): 3–11.

Concord Coalition (1993). *The Zero Deficit Plan: A Plan for Eliminating the Federal Budget Deficit by the Year 2000.* Washington, D.C.: Concord Coalition.

Cook, F. L., Marshall, V. W.., Marshall, J. G., and Kaufman, J. E. (1994). The salience of intergenerational equity in Canada and the United States. In T. R. Marmor, T. M. Smeeding, and V. L. Greene, eds., *Economic Security and Intergenerational Justice: A Look at North America* (pp. 91–129). Washington, D.C.: Urban Institute Press.

Crystal, S. (1990). Health economics, old-age politics, and the catastrophic Medicare debate. *Journal of Gerontological Social Work* 15 (3/4): 21–31.

Cutler, N. E. (1977). Demographic, social-psychological, and political factors in the politics of aging: A foundation for research in "political gerontology." *American Political Science Review* 71:1011–25.

Cutler, N. W. (1981). Political characteristics of elderly cohorts in the twenty-first century. In S. Kiesler, J. N. Morgan, and V. K. Oppenheimer, eds., *Aging: Social Change* (pp. 127–57). New York: Academic Press.

Cutler, N. E., Pierce, R., and Steckenrider, J. (1984). How golden is the future? *Generations* 9 (1): 38–43. ,

Day, C. L. (1990). *What Older Americans Think: Interest Groups and Aging Policy.* Princeton: Princeton University Press.

Day, C. L. (1993). Older Americans' attitudes toward the Medicare Catastrophic Coverage Act of 1988. *Journal of Politics* 55:167–77.

Derthick, M. (1979). *Policymaking for Social Security.* Washington, D.C.: Brookings Institution.

Eaton, S., and Diemer, T. (1995). Congress approves balanced budget plan. *Cleveland Plain Dealer,* June 30:1.

Estes, C. L. (1979). *The Aging Enterprise.* San Francisco: Jossey-Bass.

Fox, P. (1989). From senility to Alzheimer's disease: The rise of the Alzheimer's disease movement. *Milbank Quarterly* 67:58–102.

Heclo, H. (1988). Generational politics. In J. L. Palmer, T. Smeeding, and B. Boyle Torrey, eds. *The Vulnerable* (pp. 381–411). Washington, D.C.: Urban Institute Press.

Holstein, M., and Minkler, M. (1991). The short life and painful death of the Medicare Catastrophic Coverage Act. In M. Minkler and C. L. Estes, eds., *Critical Perspectives on Aging: The Political and Moral Economy of Growing Old* (pp. 189–208). Amityville, N.Y.: Baywood.

Hudson, R. B. (1978). The "graying" of the federal budget and its consequences for old age policy. *Gerontologist* 18:428–40.

Hudson, R. B., and Strate, J. (1985). Aging and political systems. In R. H. Binstock and E. Shanas, eds., *Handbook of Aging and the Social Sciences,* 2nd ed. (pp. 554–85). New York: Van Nostrand Reinhold.

Iglehart, J. K. (1989). Medicare's new benefits: Catastrophic health insurance. *New England Journal of Medicine* 320:329–36.

Kassner, E. (1995). *Long-Term Care: Measuring the Impact of a Medicaid Cap.* Washington, D.C.: Public Policy Institute, American Association of Retired Persons.

Lehrman, E. L. (1995). Health-care reform at the crossroads. *Modern Maturity* (January–February): 12.

Light, P. (1985). *Artful Work: The Politics of Social Security Reform.* New York: Random House.

Lockett, A. (1983). *Aging, Politics, and Research: Setting the Federal Agenda for Research on Aging.* New York: Springer Publishing.

Long-Term Care Campaign (1990). Pepper Commission recommendations released March 2nd. *Insiders' Update* (January–February): 1.

Lowi, T. H. (1969). *The End of Liberalism.* New York: W. W. Norton.

Mahoney, C. W., Estes, C. L., and Heumann, J. E., eds. (1986). *Toward a Unified Agenda: Proceedings of a National Conference on Disability and Aging.* San Francisco: Institute for Health and Aging, University of California, San Francisco.

McSteen, M. (1993). Testimony before the Subcommittee on Health, Committee on Ways and Means, U.S. House of Representatives. Washington, D.C.: October 21.

Myles, J. (1989). *Old Age in the Welfare State: The Political Economy of Pensions.* Lawrence: University Press of Kansas.

National Opinion Research Center, University of Chicago (1986–91). Data provided by the Roper Center, University of Connecticut, Storrs.

New York Times (1994a). Endorsement riles members of retiree group. August 12, p. A10.

New York Times (1994b). Not all in A.A.R.P are behind health plan. August 13, p. 7.

New York Times (1995). G.O.P. senator investigates finances of retirees' group. April 9, p. Y13.

New York Times/CBS News Poll (1992). Portrait of the electorate. *New York Times,* November 5, p. B9.

Oreskes, M. (1990). Social Security: A tinderbox both parties handle gingerly. *New York Times,* September 28, p. 12.

Pear, R. (1994). Two bills in Congress backed by association of retirees. *New York Times,* August 11, p. A10.

Pear, R. (1995). Senator challenges the practices of a retirees association. *New York Times,* June 14, p. A14.

Pratt, H. J. (1976). *The Gray Lobby.* Chicago: University of Chicago Press.

Pratt, H. J. (1993). *Gray Agendas: Interest Groups and Public Pensions in Canada, Britain, and the United States.* Ann Arbor: University of Michigan Press.

Quadagno, J. (1989). Generational equity and the politics of the welfare state. *Politics and Society* 17:353–76.

Rosenzweig, R. M. (1990). Address to the president's opening session, 43rd annual scientific meeting, the Gerontological Society of America. Boston, November 16.

Rubenfeld, P. (1986). Ageism and disabilityism: Double jeopardy. In S. J. Brody and G. E. Ruff, eds., *Aging and Rehabilitation: Advances in the State of the Art* (pp. 323–28). New York: Springer Publishing.

Samuelson, R. J. (1978). Aging America: Who will shoulder the growing burden? *National Journal* 10:1712–17.

Simon, H. A. (1985). Human nature in politics: The dialogue of psychology with political science. *American Political Science Review* 79:293–304.

Tolchin, M. (1989). House acts to kill '88 Medicare plan of extra benefits. *New York Times,* November 5, p. A1.

Torres-Gil, F. M., and Pynoos, J. (1986). Long-term care policy and interest group struggles. *Gerontologist* 26:488–95.

U.S. Congress (1990). Office of Technology Assessment. *Confused Minds, Burdened Families: Finding Help for People with Alzheimer's Disease and Other Dementias.* Washington, D.C.: U.S. Government Printing Office.

U.S. Congress (1994). Congressional Budget Office. *Reducing Entitlement Spending.* Washington, D.C.: U.S. Government Printing Office.

U.S. Congress (1995). Congressional Budget Office. *The Economic and Budget Outlook: Fiscal Years 1996–2000.* Washington, D.C.: U.S. Government Printing Office.

U.S. General Accounting Office (1995). *Medicaid: Restructuring Approaches Leave Many Questions.* GAO/HEHS-95-103. Washington, D.C.: U.S. Government Printing Office.

Van Tassel, D. D., and Wilkinson Meyer, J. E. (1992). *U.S. Aging Policy Interest Groups: Institutional Profiles.* New York: Greenwood.

White House Domestic Policy Council (1993). *The President's Health Security Plan.* New York: Random House.

Wiener, J. M., and Illston, L. H. (1996). Health care financing and organization for the elderly. In R. H. Binstock and L. K. George, eds., *Handbook of Aging and the Social Sciences,* 4th ed. (pp. 427–45). San Diego: Academic Press.

11

Reflections on Some Ethical Issues in Long-Term Care

Nancy Neveloff Dubler, LL.B.

The ethical issues in any care system reflect the nature of the care provided, the setting in which the care takes place, the capabilities of the care recipients, the commitments of the care providers, and the social and financial arrangements that society has created to structure and reimburse the activities of caring. At this point in American society, all of the these features of the long-term care system are changing.

Moreover, the needs of society are changing. The population is "graying" and in so doing is coming to need more care, especially as the "oldest old" emerge as a significant cohort. There has been a resurgence of AIDS among younger gay men, and the disease has gathered new force among women of color, children, and adolescents (Centers for Disease Control and Prevention, 1994). The orphans of the AIDS epidemic are just now emerging as a distinct population (Dane and Levine, 1994; Levine, 1993; Levine and Stein, 1994; Michaels and Levine, 1992) that may already have swamped and outgrown the ability of the foster care system to provide them adequate care. The future contours of long-term care will be set by the needs of these various populations.

How the multiple settings in which long-term care is provided will evolve will determine which ethical questions emerge as the most compelling. All we can make now is an educated prediction, with the caveat that such intellectual projections are likely to be broad of the mark.

For my purposes, I will take the following definition of long term care:

> services for the health and well-being of chronically disabled persons, many of whom are elderly. Services include nursing home care; congregate living arrangements with supportive personal care and home-

making assistance; community-based services such as home health care, congregate and home-delivered meals, transportation, and shopping assistance; and other services to help maintain quality of life and to assist family care providers, such as visiting companions and professional treatment for chronic illnesses. Services may be delivered formally, by an agency or other licensed health care provider, or informally, by family, friends, and neighbors. (Barnes, 1992, p. 635)

This is an expansive and inclusive definition. What I shall do, as much in the spirit of reform as of reflection, is examine some of the most pressing issues of our day and explore how health providers, citizens, and legislators might change the present configurations of long-term care to strengthen those aspects of the system that most support the kinds of moral values Americans cherish, and redesign those parts that are ethically problematic or distasteful.

I would suggest that the dialogues and debates on ethics and values in the practice of medicine over recent decades have first identified and then reaffirmed a set of moral principles commonly shared and agreed applicable to acute and long-term care. Those shared ethical precepts include the value of individual autonomy, the central place of liberty, and the importance of beneficence and nonmaleficence (Beauchamp and Childress, 1994) for care providers and for care-providing institutions.

The recent aborted excursion into health care reform and the decade-long and successful efforts to reform state guardianship statutes have served to highlight unresolved ethical issues. Are we in fact morally responsible for the health and well-being of our neighbors? Do we have the right under the law (Tronto, 1993), and should we under an ethic of caring, intervene in the life of a person existing on the fringe of conventional behavior but committed to independent existence? Should we reassert the validity of the *parens patriae* stance of government? Are we willing to act only as long as these commitments stay within the preordained limitations of the fisc or are we ready to commit new funds to the support of persons judged to be in danger or in pain? We have explored these issues over recent years with, I would suggest, no clear community response.

The Rise of Patient Autonomy

In medicine the past decades have seen the struggle between the paternalism and clinical expertise of professionals and the strongly held positions of individual patients resolved largely in favor of patient choice. In judicial opinions and scholarly exegesis the rights of patients to choose have been supported and vindicated. Patients in acute care and residents in long-term care have the right, protected by the doctrine of informed choice, to select which of the possible diagnostic and treatment interventions they will accept or refuse. In the process of winning this most basic of patients' rights, however, patients may have lost the support of some care providers who were offended by the adversarial nature of the conversations and disillusioned by being relegated to the role of purveyors of information rather than wise advisors.

The years since the passage of the 1987 Omnibus Budget Reconciliation Act have seen a new era in "residents' rights" in long-term care. New emphases on individual liberty and choice have reinforced the ability of residents to make decisions about their lives within confined settings. Perhaps most noticeable in this movement has been the change of practice in the use of physical and chemical restraints. In 1992, the American Health Care Association adopted practice guidelines to lessen the use of restraints, to ensure they are used only to treat medical symptoms and not to punish patients or restrain them for the convenience of health care providers.

Discussing autonomy in long-term care is particularly complex, given the debates about the meaning of the term. Lidz and Arnold (1993, p. 606), in a comprehensive and well-structured article, reviewed the meanings ascribed to autonomy in prior scholarly work. They highlighted various definitions, including: "an individual's exercise of the capacity to form, revise and pursue personal plans for life" (the President's Commission); "being one's own person, without constraint either by another's action or by psychological or physical limitations" (Beauchamp and Childress); "the ability to identify with the decisions that one makes" (citing Gerald Dworkin and George Agich); and not "a unitary concept but . . . a group of related notions" (citing Collopy and Thomasma). They grouped the discussions about autonomy into three types of related theories: autonomy as total independence, indicating a radical self-sufficiency; autonomy as free action, reflecting a process that is intentional and voluntary; and autonomy as effective deliberation, indicating understanding, consideration, and judgment.

To this maelstrom of definitions the authors add their own. In concentrating on autonomy in long-term care, Lidz and Arnold chose to focus on patterns of living rather than discrete decisions. In the context of long-term care they argue for a conception of autonomy as consistency, emphasizing that "the autonomous activity be consistent with an individual's commitments, values and life plans — that the person's activities are roughly consistent with the individual's self. It is an individual's involvement with, or acceptance of, an activity or series of activities that makes them autonomous" (p. 619).

A major value of this definition is its insistence on the importance of the setting. If the facility or program is one that encourages and permits consistent decisions, then autonomy will be well served even if the setting is one of a total institution, in the Goffman sense, that, by its very nature, limits the a priori conception, as well as the implementation, of choices.

As Kane and Caplan (1991) discovered in an innovative project they conducted in the early 1990s, what nursing home residents prize most highly is their ability to decide independently such things as when and under what conditions to use the telephone. Given this perspective, complex, nuanced definitions that focus on the appropriate path of medical care remain interesting but merely tangential to the core human needs that animate long-term care residents themselves.

Brian Hofland, of the Retirement Research Foundation, directed a foundation initiative in the mid-1980s that focused exclusively on autonomy in long-term care. The findings of that initiative were summarized by Hofland and David (1990) in a special issue of *Generations*. Their conclusions are particularly striking as an indictment of the conventions of dealing with individual difference in systems that value sameness. The authors concluded that personal autonomy, whatever its definition, is severely constricted in any long-term care setting. Particularly germane to this endeavor, they also note that "it is quite likely that future cohorts of clients will demand greater direct involvement in the formulation and execution of care plans. As the baby boom generation ages and enters the long-term care system, it is likely that their autonomy goals will be higher than those expressed by current cohorts" (p. 92).

This educated hunch of two scholars familiar with the literature and with long-term care practice is a bridge to speculation. What will we, aging professionals in an aging society, now engaged in the hurly-burly of life, demand when we need the supports that only long-term care can provide?

The growth of life-care communities suggests that many of us who can afford and manage doing so will seek out communities that have a continuum of services, including housing, catering support, and the existence of long-term care residential and medical facilities should we lose the ability to provide for ourselves. These communities have allowed many retired professionals to continue their intellectual and social lives in retirement settings without contemporary restrictions but with clear and supported future expectations. These communities, which replace the extended families and stable villages of prior societies, provide the sort of security for the future that permits individuals to maximize their activities in early old age without worries about later unmet needs. From my present vantage point they look too homogeneous and sheltered for my taste. But even I, committed New Yorker that I am, can envision coming to fear the anomie, crime, and logistical barriers to easy movement in the large American city. Suburban and rural settings, less expensive than urban real estate, provide the protection and comfort that increasingly dependent elders demand.

But what if a nursing home is the destination of some of the baby boomers? How those facilities will look and function in the future will depend, for the most part, on how they are funded and regulated, a set of issues that I will address shortly. But, if the residents are not demented and can conceive of individual choice, they might demand such as the following: single rooms that can be furnished with their own possessions, double rooms for married couples or life partners, more flexible meal and facility schedules, unlimited access to telephones (made increasingly possible by new developments in communications technology) and to e-mail and the Internet. We increasingly relate to expanded modes of communication as if they were forever a part of our emotive capabilities. That feeling will not and should not disappear when we are part of long-term care.

Ethical Issues and Health Care Reform

Whether we have single rooms or double, as now decreed by regulation and reimbursement, will depend, in large measure, on what happens to health care reform and how long-term care is conceived of in that package. It was my pleasure to co-chair, with Marian Gray Secundy, professor of bioethics at Howard University, the Ethical Foundations of the New Health Care System Working Group in the National Health Care Reform Task Force in 1993. In that process, the place of long-term care assumed a special status.

The notion of universal access and large-scale health reform has largely disappeared. Because of that political demise, the work of the American College of Physicians and the American Geriatric Society, jointly published in the *Journal of the American Medical Association*, stands as a coda to the debate rather than a contribution. In the article, the groups present suggestions and commentaries on long-term care that highlight some of the ethical issues of financing (Weiner, 1994). They argue that "long-term care differs from acute care in that it involves 'life choices,' such as where and how to live" (p. 1526), and that the subject thus straddles the health and social service systems, which should be responsible jointly for the expense. The article estimates that "in the cohort of all people turning 65 in 1990, the average lifetime cost of nursing home care is $27,600, and total required is $60 billion" (p. 1525). Will we as a society be willing to shoulder some proportion of these costs, or will individuals be granted or denied access based on the extent of their personal funds? Furthermore, will we continue to let the savvy shelter their assets and qualify for public funding while the less knowledgeable and less sophisticated "spend down" and see their nest eggs eaten by the predatory bird of Medicaid eligibility? These are some of the central questions we face as we contemplate the future.

In the ethics working group there was uniform agreement that health care services are a continuum and that primary and preventive care form the basis for acute care services, which in turn form the foundation for long-term care. The major barrier to creative thinking on the task force was the inability or unwillingness of the long-term care working group to opt for one of two routes for reform. There was never a clear choosing between a social insurance system for paying for long-term care or a private indemnity plan. Needless to say, there are serious ethical consequences that flow from either of these choices. There are also useful lessons to be learned from other countries in evaluating the relative merits of the two financing systems.

Using social insurance to fund long-term care would require substantial new demands on the Social Security system or on some new system designed exclusively to fund chronic and long-term care. These demands could be met only by an increase in general tax revenues, by increasing the Social Security tax, or by establishing a new tax to meet future needs. The first seems politically impossible, the second highly unlikely, and the third probably unthinkable. As any new program would require an identified funding stream, the likelihood of a long-term care system funded by social insurance is low. It is interesting to note that even the American Association of Homes for the Aging, which testified before the Senate Finance Committee's Subcommittee on Medicare and Long-term Care, could not present a single funding strategy. Sheldon Goldberg, testifying for the association, urged a private insurance system for those who can afford it and public resources for the "truly needy" (Congress urged, 1992).

Consigning long-term care to the individual indemnity system, however, will continue an inequitable and unfair system under which access is governed by ability to pay. It seems ironic, as we grapple with the inequities of primary and acute care systems funded by indemnity plans, to create a new system plagued by similar moral design defects.

In considering the moral foundations of any health care reform effort, the ethics working group identified three categories of principles that were relevant to the moral analysis of any plan: caring for all, making the system work, and choice and responsibility (Brock and Daniels, 1994).

The first category, caring for all, contains such concepts as universal access, comprehensive and equal benefits, intergenerational solidarity, and the communal sharing of risks by people who pay according to their ability. This package of concepts goes to the equity and fairness of the system, which in any new formulation, it was argued, had to meet the needs of all of the citizens who need or might in the future need care. The same ethical considerations are relevant to evaluating the characteristics of a to-be-created long-term care system.

The second bundle of ethical perceptions and arguments were collected under the heading "making the system work." Some might argue that good business practice and efficient management technique demand efficiency and quality. The ethics working group argued, however, that such concepts as wise allocation, quality assurance, and efficient management were all justified by an ethical analysis. Were health care inefficient and poorly managed it could, and probably does, take up more of the nation's economic resources than is wise. There are other national priorities; bridges need to be fixed, schools run creatively, and art museums supported. If money is squandered in an inefficient and poorly managed system, these other "goods" will not be readily available. So too with quality. Only good-quality health care should survive the scrutiny of evaluators, and only high-quality care should be an option for health care consumers. All other options are a kind of fraud, in which, past indicators show, the poor fare the least well.

Finally, the working group identified a set of concerns including individual choice, personal responsibility, professional integrity, and fair procedures. These issues speak to the relationship between the individual and the system. These concerns argue for an accessibility of data that will permit individuals to choose the right sort of care to meet special, or even idiosyncratic, needs. In a parallel vein, the systems must respect the wisdom, skill, and judgment of relevant professionals and offer to both professionals and patients a fair process to resolve misunderstandings, disagreements, and disputes.

The above analysis is as applicable to long-term care as it is to primary and acute care. Whether chronic and long-term care will be included in any gradual health care reform (clearly the only possible option remaining at this time) will determine to the very greatest extent how equitable the systems will be. If the same inequities that pervade the provision of long-term care at present survive into the future, then that will be, at least in my judgment, the central ethical dilemma. As long as access to long-term care depends on ability to pay and as long as some elderly, disabled, and AIDS patients — dependent on ever-diminishing public funding — receive substandard care and thereby experience suffering, that will remain the central ethical issue.

Conflict Management in Long-Term Care

Consider how long-term care might function if access were assured and only fair and due process were used to resolve disputes. In such a system, discussions would be informative and supportive; and misunderstandings, disagreements, and disputes would be identified quickly and addressed fairly. This notion of a dispute resolution system was also pondered by members of the health care reform task force.

In any system of long-term care some conflict is inevitable; human beings disagree about what their primary goals are and how best to reach them. An understanding that conflict is a part of life and of the delivery of health care, not a negative comment on the abilities and commitment of care providers, is central to thinking about the generation and resolution of disagreements in long-term care.

Conflict is part of the human condition. For those of you who have children, or know families with more than one child, consider how often children, or for that matter children and their parents, can be in the same setting for more than a brief time without developing a misunderstanding, disagreement, or dispute. The difference between the hearth and the hospital, however, is often the difference between life and death. The issue is not whether conflict exists but rather how it is dealt with and how a system must be structured to manage conflict in the most expeditious and helpful way.

The nature of conflict in medicine is changing, and one can posit that the same changes will emerge soon out of long-term care relationships and arrangements. In medicine the tradition has been to settle conflicts through the malpractice system, although most experts agree that the system reaches only a scant percentage of the patients harmed by medical interventions, does little to improve the quality of care, and provides money largely to the trial lawyers bar. Nonetheless, petitions charging negligence have increasingly plagued medicine over the past four decades and have had measurable effects on the practice of some subspecialties, such as obstetrics and gynecology. In the past few years there has been an increase in the number of suits challenging the decision of an insurance company or managed care network on the issue of coverage and reimbursement and of suits challenging whether a particular intervention is experimental or part of standard care. These suits are not the result of the alleged "bad acting" of a provider but of endemic conflict and the lack of a standing institutional ability to identify conflict and provide a route for resolution.

The ethics working group made this series of assumptions in regard to conflicts in health care provision:

— Misunderstandings, disagreements, and disputes will always exist as a natural part of delivering health care, especially if interpretations of the benefit package are required.
— Training in effective communication and dispute resolution can reduce the number of disagreements that will otherwise escalate into full-blown disputes.
— Health plans should be strongly encouraged or required to design dispute mediation systems in which issues, whenever possible, are resolved by the parties themselves.
— Conflict resolution at the site of care avoids determinations by higher authorities that accentuate rights (rather than interests), encourage power tactics, and tend to disempower marginalized persons who have little access to legal services.
— Conflict resolution strategies should be speedy, open, user-friendly, and flexible. (Dubler and Marcus, 1994, p. 6)

I would argue that a long-term care system, even more than an acute care system, needs to have a regular conflict-response plan. Conflicts in long-term care tend to grow and fester unless identified and addressed. One response to this sort of conflict is the appointment of an individual or the creation of a team that can be consulted on ethical issues. An increasingly common solution in long-term care institutions is the creation of an ethics committee (Wilson Ross et al., 1993). Either an individual consultant or a committee can be helpful, depending on the character of the organization or facility. Home care agencies are also experimenting with ethics committees in meeting the needs of their clients.

What links ethics directly to conflict management is the fact that ethical dilemmas are really conflicts. There are two ways of thinking about an ethical problem. One way emphasizes the clash between opposing principles of ethical or legal analysis. For example, providing sufficient morphine to ease a certain patient's suffering, as the patient requests, would support patient autonomy. But, others could argue that providing sufficient morphine might hasten his death and thus show a disrespect for life. Forests have been felled in search of the perfect analytic framework for resolving these problems.

In contrast, consider the origins and dynamics of this conflict. It turns out that the patient is an older man who has had a difficult relationship with his providers. At one point his clinic advised him that he would no longer be welcome, because he was disruptive and was the source of constant complaints to a regulatory agency. He was referred to a new clinic, which was equally troubled by his behavior but managed to identify one provider to whom the patient could relate and who assumed the task of primary provider. That person admitted the patient to the hospital for what appeared to be a final episode of chronic obstructive pulmonary disease. The bioethics consultant and mediator arranged a meeting, attended by the patient, primary physician, nurses, and pulmonary specialists. The discussion explored the perspective and wishes of the patient, the reluctance of the pulmonologist, the hesitancy of the primary provider, and the squeamishness of the nurses. A discussion of the prognosis, the patient's suffering, and the lack of alternatives led to a note in the chart documenting the process, the issues, and the decision to accommodate the patient's request for pain control. A short time after the morphine drip was started the patient died comfortably.

This same sort of disagreement can take place in home care or in a nursing home. We think of these settings as less high-tech and stressful than an acute care hospital, but recent data indicate that the hospital is moving into the home and that the sorts of disagreements once limited to acute care are invading long-term care (Arras and Dubler, 1994). Long-term care must have the power to resolve all sorts of disagreements, from those over access to telephones or whether a resident's roommate has to take a bath to those that involve starting or stopping total parenteral nutrition for a home-care patient with end-stage AIDS.

The dilemmas in home care can be even more intractable than those in acute or residential care, because there are greater numbers of parties with real and weighty interests in the outcome of the decision process. It is relatively easy to see that the patient has the most at stake in consenting to or refusing an amputation for a gangrenous foot, even though ethics analysis has moved beyond a totally patient-centered analysis of decisions (Blustein, 1991). Autonomy and liberty do not consign the patient to isolation, even if they protect her from the imposition of a care plan by others.

In home care, the real and weighty concerns and interests of others must be put, directly, into the calculation of risks, benefits, and possible alternative plans. Let us assume that Mr. X, a patient in acute care who has recently undergone hip surgery to repair a fracture, wants to go to the home of his daughter after discharge from the hospital. Let us further assume that the only place to put the hospital bed that her father would need would be on the first floor of the house in the living room. Let us further assume that this particular daughter is not overly fond of her father who, she feels, much preferred her younger sister. It is clear that the decision where to go affects the interests of the daughter as much as the interests of the patient and that she is, therefore, a part of, and not peripheral to, the decision (Dubler, 1992). The decision of a patient to go home cannot be governed exclusively by the principle of autonomy; it is more properly considered under the rubric of accommodation.

What is important about the above example, however, is not only the variation in principle that it requires to reach a just solution but also the process by which the decision is reached. Have the father and daughter been permitted to lock horns in combat, or has someone intervened to help manage the conflict and leave the underlying relationship as strong as possible given the present tensions and prior grievances (Dubler, 1994)?

Other sorts of conflicts cry out for management in long-term case situations. At present many nursing homes feel caught between respecting the wishes of the patient and family and complying with the letter of regulatory oversight. The ongoing debate about the place of artificial nutrition and hydration for a dying patient provides one example. Many state departments of health classify fluid and artificial food as comfort care and consider the nonprovision as abuse. Medical authorities, and the courts, are more likely to classify artificial nutrition and hydration as treatments, which should be dealt with under the rules for withdrawing or withholding treatments that have been refused by or are not indicated for the patient. Recent data even indicate that patients may be more comfortable in the terminal stage of illness if they are not regularly provided with unrequested food and fluid (McCann, Hall, and Groth-Juncker, 1994). The fact remains that patients or families who are permitted to refuse food or fluid may cause the nursing home to be cited by the supervising authority (Kaufman, 1988). This situation calls for a process by which the apparent conflict among the regulators, providers, resident, and family can be resolved fairly and in a timely manner.

Until now I have talked largely about the chronically ill disabled and the elderly, but there are other populations in long-term care, such as persons with AIDS and the orphans of the AIDS epidemic. Just imagine how our long-term care system will be changed if some fraction of the orphans of the AIDS epidemic need to be accommodated within the system. Michaels and Levine (1992) predict that 100,000 children will be orphaned in the 1990s. This explosion of orphans has not been equalled since the flu epidemic of 1918, and it can probably not be accommodated by the foster care systems in the major cities. New York City has seen its foster care population almost triple in the past decade; currently there are nearly 46,000 children in the New York City foster care system (Perez-Pena, 1994). Orphanages are back in discussion. Will we recreate congregate institutions for these new orphans and will we count these facilities as part of long-term care? If we do, it will certainly change the nature and character of the enterprise and the ethical dilemmas encountered.

Focusing on the Future

Which ethical dilemmas will be central in the future of long-term care? Answering this question must wait for American society to resolve a series of policy debates: Who will be receiving long-term care? Will communities and institutions be restricted to the rich and the qualifying poor, as the case is now, or will some notion of a sliding scale of payment and universal access govern? Who will be providing care? Will it be the same mix of paid workers and family members as now exists, or will some equitable method of payment and tax credits reimburse family and friends for their efforts and devotion? Will we continue to provide funding for long-term care through Medicaid, thus limiting the funding to the poor and the "arranged to be poor," or will we come to see provision of long-term care as part of the continuum of services that a caring and just society must provide?

Years ago I made a prediction to my medical school class about a question facing the U.S. Supreme Court regarding whether or not poor women had a constitutionally protected right to government financial support for abortion. I gave what I considered to be an eloquent and persuasive argument supporting access. I was wrong. The Supreme Court held that the existence of a right does not require government to assure equal access. With that in mind I am reluctant to make predictions about the coming ethical issues. Let us say that who we become as a nation will determine the urgent ethical issues we will face in long-term care and how they will be resolved.

References

Arras, J. D., and Dubler, N. N. (1994). The technological tether: An introduction to ethical and social issues in high-tech home care. *Hastings Center Report.* Suppl. (September–October).

Barnes, A. P. (1992). Elder law: Beyond guardianship reform: A reevaluation of autonomy and beneficence for a system of principled decisionmaking in long-term care. *Emory Law Journal* 41:633.

Beauchamp, T. L., and Childress, J. F. (1994). *Principles of Biomedical Ethics*, 4th ed. New York: Oxford University Press.

Blustein, J. (1991). *Care and Commitment: Taking the Personal Point of View.* New York: Oxford University Press.

Brock, D. W., and Daniels, N. (1994). Ethical foundations of the Clinton administration's proposed health care system. *Journal of the American Medical Association* 271:1189–96.

Centers for Disease Control and Prevention (1994). Update: Impact of the expanded AIDS surveillance case definition for adolescents and adults on case reporting—United States, 1994. *Morbidity and Mortality Weekly Report* 43: 160–61, 167–70.

Congress urged to give long-term care higher priority. (1992). (Recent Health Care Developments, News Briefs) *Health Care Financing Review* (summer): 203.

Dane, B. O., and Levine, C., eds. (1994). *AIDS and the New Orphans: Coping with Death.* Westport, Conn.: Auburn House.

Dubler, N. N. (1992). Accommodating the home care client: A look at rights and interests. In C. Zuckerman, N. N. Dubler, and B. Collopy, B., eds., *Home Health Care Options: A Guide for Older Persons and Concerned Families* (pp. 141–66). New York: Plenum Press.

Dubler, N. N., and Marcus, L. J. (1994). *Mediating Bioethical Disputes: A Practical Guide.* New York: United Hospital Fund.

Hofland, B. F., and David, D. (1990). Autonomy and long-term care practice: Conclusions and next steps. *Generations* 14:91–95.

Kane, R. A., and Caplan, A. L. (1991). *Everyday Ethics: Resolving Dilemmas in Nursing Home Life.* New York: Springer Publishing.

Kaufman, A. (1988). Bioethical issues and the long-term care facility. *Nursing Homes* 37 (2): 32.

Levine, C., ed. (1993). *A Death in the Family: Orphans of the HIV Epidemic.* New York: United Hospital Fund.

Levine, C., and Stein, G. L. (1994). *Orphans of the HIV Epidemic: Unmet Needs in Six U.S. Cities.* New York: Orphan Project.

Lidz, C. W., and Arnold, R. M. (1993). Rethinking autonomy in long-term care. *University of Miami Law Review* 47:603.

McCann, R. M., Hall, W. J., and Groth-Juncker, A. M. (1994). Comfort care for terminally ill patients: The appropriate use of nutrition and hydration. *Journal of the American Medical Association* 272: 1263–66.

Michaels, D., and Levine, C. (1992). Estimates of the number of motherless youth orphaned by AIDS in the United States. *Journal of the American Medical Association* 268 (4): 3456–61.

Perez-Pena, R. (1994). Report finds the limbo of foster care is growing longer. *New York Times,* December 22, p. B1.

Tronto, J. C. (1993). *Moral Boundaries: A Political Argument for an Ethic of Care.* New York: Routledge, Chapman and Hall.

Weiner, J. (1994). Financing long-term care: A proposal by the American College of Physicians and the American Geriatrics Society. *Journal of the American Medical Association* 271:1525–29.

Wilson Ross, J., Glaser, J. W., Rasinski-Gregory, D., McIver Gibson, J., Bayley, C. (1993). *Health Care Ethics Committees: The Next Generation.* Chicago: American Hospital Publishing.

12

American Culture and Long-Term Care

Otto von Mering, Ph.D.

This chapter examines important cultural traditions, or rather cultural markers, that have shaped and continue to define the distinctive story of long-term care in the United States. It is a discourse on the deep structure of shared presuppositions about age and age grading in everyday life, and of special understandings about correct individual behavior in ordinary circumstances and under altered conditions of living, such as chronic illness and disability.

An Age-Graded Culture

In the era of prolonged life expectancy, the American ways of age grading the life course, of *defining* who is young or old, who is of working age or on welfare, retirable and eligible for a level of economic security benefits, and of *specifying* who receives acute treatment or care for chronic disease or disability, affects how long-term care is practiced today and will look tomorrow. If we did not live in our particular kind of age-graded society we would not have our particular definitions of *old* or *old age*, or *retirement* nor our special forms of social legislation. If we did not have our distinctive views about individual life, work-dependent health care, and postretirement economic benefits, we would not have our special patterns of short- and long-term caregiving for the frail young or for the elderly afflicted with an acute or chronic condition. Moreover, given these patterns, we have evolved our characteristic ways of dealing with those who are physically disabled and with those who are mentally ill or "demented" at any given point in their life, or are so afflicted throughout their life.

What then can we say about our age-graded culture? It has been well studied in the book *How Old Are You? Age Consciousness in American Culture* (Chudacoff, 1989). Age distinctions were blurred in the agrarian society of America before 1850. With average life expectancy around the mid-forties, there was a general lack of age and stage-of-life consciousness, and no special differentiation of teenager from mid-lifer, nor of either of these from elder.

In subsequent decades, the age grading of people became a more official part of life, especially for the young, with the rise of the primary and secondary education system and its uniform curricula, textbooks, and discipline. By 1890, the sequencing of elementary, secondary, and college education was set. In addition to this age grading, medical experts had begun to differentiate a special branch of medicine devoted to children. During the 1890s, an age-graded schedule of growth and development was articulated for youth (Chudacoff, 1989). Medical experts also indicated that the loss of memory and intelligence would normally occur in old age, that debility was natural and inevitable. In general, age requirements and norms became a common feature of the educational system. Indeed age and educational achievement were becoming characteristics fraught with expectations and fears about occupational success as an adult.

Between 1900 and 1920 an intensification of age norms took hold. Starting in 1900, U.S. census takers recorded people in age categories. The new "science" of mental testing standardized expectations of intellect and further solidified age grading, categorization, and peer grouping. Juvenile justice courts had started to separate "wayward youths" from "juveniles." Compulsory attendance at school, where physical education further grouped people into different age categories with different expectations, became a normative way of keeping the young out of the labor force (Chudacoff, 1989). All this was coeval with the ever more rapid industrialization of America, a process which also enshrined the division of labor between men and women — in the work place and at home as a caregiver, respectively.

After World War I there was a "discovery" of middle age as a distinct life stage, and advanced age began to be viewed as a time of dependency. The cult of youth spread rapidly, so that by 1930 and from then on popular music, like other aspects of America culture, became clearly age and peer oriented (Chudacoff, 1989). After World War II, the graying of America became gradually more evident to everyone. A concomitant change was increased public interest in the cosmetic and exercise-based rejuvenation of face and body during midlife and preretirement years.

In particular, increased public awareness that more people were living into advanced years of life and experiencing difficulty in coping with its economic and social consequences contributed to the passage of Medicare, in 1965. This social mechanism reinforced age-grading as a means of rationalizing what we do to people and with people of different ages and in different circumstances of living and ill-being. Quite apart from the fact that Medicare is seen as one of the milestones in American social legislation since the Great Depression, it is akin to many pieces of federal legislation which epitomize the use of age categories as an organizing principle of social policy. These other laws, in turn, became the criteria for the competitive coexistence and targeted distribution of specified economic resources and of defined health services for special classes and age cohorts of patients (von Mering and Earley, 1965).

Moreover, in an industrialized society like the United States, the customary approach to how we age in what we do and who we are consists of counting years and fixing dates. "Our interests and curiosity, our energies and talent count for less. Our capacity to learn and to change with the human and physical environment as we grow old is devalued. Indeed, age-bound thinking has increased its stranglehold on our behavior with one another. Age has become deeply embedded in custom and law, in our ideas of attainment, in our so-called 'plunge' into the adult world, and our descent into senescence" (von Mering, 1992, p. 124), and in our continued existence in a context of long-term care.

It is important to acknowledge that our dominant cultural penchant for using chronological age markers to identify the social performances and caregiving ways of young and old has gotten out of step with today's rising biosocial fact of extended personal longevity (p. 125). In the European Community, as in the United States, "the number of people over 75 is growing faster than any other age group. It has become less and less true that work-enders are near to being life-enders" (Young, 1990, p. 14).

When we consider the demographic facts, we recognize the absurdity of using "age altogether as *the* governing criterion for marking the transition from one phase of life to another" (p. 14), from a time of youthful vitality to an end period of infirmity. And yet, we persist in our habit of chunking up our life time into a procrustean bed of time-controlled experiences of independence and dependence, of living through special "nonproductive" rather than productive periods during the teen years and the old years. This runs counter to our best judgment of human potential and performance in all seasons of life (von Mering, 1992, p. 126).

The Culture of Caregiving and Retirement

Above all, our age-graded society has had a distinct effect on what we may call the culture of caregiving. As such, caregiving is a fundamental trans-cultural behavioral category of curative and preventive support, succor, and nurturing between people of any age across the life course. It is advocated and practiced in all cultures and in all manner of domestic units, be they a biological family or other small or large groups of related or unrelated persons in a given society. Every society evolves and abides by a different shared template of rules and standards for the performance of particular caregiving tasks that are appropriate to the needs of the individual requiring or deriving care. A single set of cultural guidelines forms a kind of mental map for everyone within a given cultural group, indicating when and what kind of care is needed to promote a basic quality of everyday living and to advance survival among the ill or disabled.

In this connection it is important to note that the ways in which people care for each other in sickness and in health is a fundamental activity of cultural survival. It is apparent that the pervasive age grading of life in the United States has contributed significantly to the professional segmentation of lifelong caregiving practices into infant care, child care, youth care, adult care, and senior care. Moreover, this age-based thinking and acting about the giving of care has made it simple to segregate professionally acceptable forms of caregiving according to location in the larger community. These special places are, of course, the hospital or health center, the nursery school, the kindergarten, community centers for teens, adults, and elders, the clinic, and the nursing home (von Mering and Earley, 1965). As a consequence, it is only recently that the natural occurrence of long-term care, or shall we say informal "seamless care" patterns across and between generations in the community has become a significant issue for formal health care providers. Such life-giving care, though not uncommon within large three-generation extended kin groups, within informal networks of unrelated fictive kin, or in domestic units headed by a single adult, has been difficult for the formal health care sector to incorporate.

The American way of age grading has shaped what we have come to see as a "natural" path of caregiving, especially long-term care for people of different ages. This becomes even clearer when we examine the evolution of our thinking about and our practice of retirement since the days when the United States was a predominantly agrarian society. "Historically, retirement was defined in personal terms before it became a major institution in this century. . . . Noah Webster defined retirement as 'private abode; habitation secluded from much society, or from public life.' Yet none of Webster's definitions applied exclusively to the aged" (Achenbaum, 1994, pp. 12–13). During the latter half of the nineteenth century, retiring had also come to be a transitive rather than intransitive verb: it signified that under defined circumstances and at a given age someone else than yourself decided that your time to retire had come.

At the time of the Great Depression and thereafter, however, disabling ill-being continued to be the primary reason why people stopped working and retired. A survey in the 1920s of retirees in eleven eastern cities revealed that "28.1 percent gave 'old age' as their reason for quitting; another 30 percent mentioned either chronic illness or rheumatism. Miners, factory workers, and men in steel mills were said to 'become prematurely aged.' Nevertheless, the boundary between disability and old age remained unclear" (pp. 19–21). Indeed, "prior to 1952, the availability of old age insurance (Title II) benefits seldom prompted voluntary retirement, . . . [and] prior to the 1980s poor health still accounted for more than half of all retirements, particularly among those in low-paying jobs" (p. 22).

The formal cultural linkage between ill health and retirement and old age actually began with the Social Security Act of 1935. "By 1974, 93 percent of all people over 65 were eligible for benefits. In the process, age 65, the system's eligibility baseline, became the benchmark for determining who was 'old' in America" (p. 20). The public linkage between receiving retirement benefits and becoming a likely subject to more illness episodes became more culturally fixed with the passage of Medicare and Medicaid in 1965. Moreover, it reinforced the fundamental philosophical premise that benefits from such programs are principally earned after having reached "a certain level of past work-related contributions, . . . financed entirely through payroll taxes" (Monk, 1994, p. 6).

Clearly, "the actual event of retirement, coupled with the [official] transition to old age, triggers a unique set of circumstances and creates conditions that bear no resemblance to those of other stages of life" (p. 8). With "life expectancy in the year 2000 anticipated to be 75.3 for males and 80.4 for women . . . people may well spend a quarter of their entire lives, in some cases a third, in retirement" (p. 4). Moreover, much of the time, some may find themselves coping with more than one chronic health condition largely on their own. Others will require intermittent or prolonged formal professional long-term care services. But most people who will live into their eighties or nineties anticipate or hope to receive some care and support informally from biological or conjugal relatives and significant others.

This overview of silent cultural historical markers in the American experience with the life course in health and illness bears directly on today's public understanding of what action is feasible and desirable in the short- and long-term care of people at any age, but particularly of those who have stopped working or are retired and too sick to take care of themselves. Indeed, the current national discussion over the eventual design of a scheme of "health security" for all is connected intimately with the traditional underlying American assumption of the primacy of individual responsibility in all matters of life, work, and well-being. This assumption has even made it legitimate for some members of Congress to consider social legislation that is largely indifferent to a national guarantee of help for the most vulnerable citizen, regardless of age. These cultural markers individually and interactively bespeak the absolute importance of the self-reliant avoidance of public subsidy in matters of personal economic and physical well-being.

Individual and Collective Responsibility

Woven into this individualistic view of a personal security is the idea that society cannot cushion indefinitely all people from serious unemployment, prolonged disability, or unremitting poor health. Spending a life time of medicated survival, or living out a duration of abject retirement at public expense is not supposed to be the "American Way." In the main, the American Way rejects the idea that in good or bad times every citizen must be his brother's helper or sister's keeper, or for that matter, regard health care as a basic social good or inalienable right.

Historically speaking, the expectation of relying on a commons of caring for everyone is no more American than living off a commons of grazing land. Only the individual, or rather private, pursuit of well-being is truly American, as if choosing good health were like trading in an old car for a new model. Though chronic ill-being is becoming an unwelcome part of life for more aging Americans every day, and is not readily dealt with by individual effort alone, health care in general and long-term care in particular are not supposed to be like welfare schemes. Rather, they are viewed as marketable commodities. By this definition, health care is a manageable item of consumption which can best be distributed according to exacting criteria of utility, need, and insurance "risk pools," much like toothpaste or computers (Angell, 1993).

Today, most Americans are inclined to view health security much like life insurance, and hence as an essentially private act of providence which is at least partly backed by the employer through a standard fringe benefit program. Having a prepaid or partially paid personal health benefit is predominantly seen as a part of the normal compensation for being or having been a *working* American. It is expected to facilitate the early return to work status after a bout with an acute health condition. It is only beginning to be thought of as a way to also plan for some preventive protection from the long-term care costs of dealing with a chronic condition, especially after retirement from work.

Short- and long-term health care security has become economically personalized. It is viewed as an entitlement for working Americans who so-to-speak have paid their dues. Hence, it is thought that personal health care is not a benefit that can readily be generalized for everyone and that attempting to do so is imprudent, especially when the costs must be paid out of general revenues, rather than be derived from something like the Social Security trust funds. It seems reasonable to suggest that these pronounced individualistic and work-force-dependent criteria for enjoying a well-cared-for old age are keys to the general American problem of how to make more people healthier, however that may be defined. Designing disease preventive initiatives and undertaking public health-promotion programs to help everyone to 'choose' more health, as well as the particular problem of how to shape new forms of long-term care for chronic conditions, become highly chancy political and economic issues for everyone.

Not surprisingly, a chorus of lamentations has been heard about the land concerning the lack of coverage for pre-existing conditions, the stigma enveloping inadequate mental health care, the spending down of life savings on prescriptions drugs, and the use of an ever-increasing amount of wages, salaries, or retirement checks on insurance premiums, minimum payments, and co-payments for hospitalization, convalescent care, and long-term care. As the 1993 Robert Wood Johnson Foundation report on Chronic Health Conditions stated: "Clearly, until now, the incentives of the marketplace have been perverse. On the one hand, they reward insurance carriers and health plans that avoid people with chronic illnesses. On the other hand, for those already in the medical care system, such as Medicare patients receiving fee-for-service care, providers are rewarded for providing expensive, high technology care and penalized for spending resources on integrating care in the community" (Robert Wood Johnson Foundation, 1993, p. 21). However, it is not marketplace forces alone, as we have seen, which have created an individual and societal problem out of the provision of long-term care for chronic conditions.

The Continuing Care Retirement Community

It seems best now to draw attention to the distinct kinds of experiences Americans do have with current private initiative-based and insurance-driven long-term care living arrangements on the one hand, and with public purse-dependent and regulation-laden long-term care programs on the other. Our discussion starts with a generic definition of long-term care. A culture-syntonic and timely definition appears in the 1994 *Columbia Retirement Handbook*: "Long-term care generally refers to the medical and social support services needed by people whose capacity for independently performing the activities of daily living (ADL) is impaired, according to recognized or approved standards, for a prolonged period of time by a chronic illness or deteriorating condition. Long-term care may be provided at home, in the community, or in a nursing home (at the level of custodial, intermediate or skilled care)" (Chen, 1994, p. 561).

This definition suggests the possibility of a great range of places of habitation within which long-term care may take place in America today. The most complete model of combined formal paid-for and informal voluntary long-term care for older Americans is a life-care community or continuing care retirement community (CCRC). A more common, spontaneous, and informal kind of long-term care takes place within social networks of different kinds of domestic units (i.e., places of continuous shared residence, composed of related and unrelated adults, children, and grandchildren). There, long-term care patterns function with a minimum of input from professional community resources.

In 1990 it was estimated that some 800 CCRCs in the United States, housed approximately 230,000 elderly inhabitants. As many as 1,500 such community living places are expected to be the primary domicile for 450,000 persons by the year 2000 (von Mering and Neff, 1993, p. 5). A formal definition is useful. The American Association of Homes and Services for the Aging defines a continuing care retirement community as a habitat "that offers a full range of housing, residential services and health care to serve its older residents as their needs change over time. This continuum consists of housing where residents live independently and receive certain residential services such as meals, activities, housekeeping and maintenance; support services for disabled residents who require assistance with activities of daily living (ADLs); and health care service of those who become temporarily ill or who require long-term care" (von Mering and Gordon, 1993, p. 167).

Regardless of their size, great differences in the quality of extended assisted living and health services exist among CCRCs. However, the majority, in addition to offering 24-hour nursing home care, try to provide at least two general types of residential support services, one for physically "frailing" but mentally alert individuals and the other for mentally "fraying" persons who are physically able. The former group of residents experience increasingly debilitating conditions like arthritis, hypertension, and diabetes, as well as problems with ADLs, requiring some assistance with bathing, toileting, grooming, ambulation, eating, or medication. The latter group includes people who have exhibited demented behavior, including rising difficultly in comprehending the environment, becoming more easily confused or lost in a familiar setting, and eventually showing persistent restlessness, irritability, and problematic conduct (von Mering and Neff, 1993, p. 6).

The most sophisticated of these villages of long-term caring function as "total communities," which have succeeded in creating many formal and informal layers of residential treatment environments, to the extent that their nursing facilities have come to be viewed as subacute hospitals, where only the most impaired residents need be domiciled. "This layering and mixing of different individual case-indicated treatments is made possible by an on-site, comprehensive home care program. It ranges from homemaker and instrumental activities of daily living services (e.g. cleaning and personal assistance in going to the doctor or grocery shopping) to post-hospital recuperative health care, as well as continuous or intermittent on-site clinical service visits by skilled physical therapists, occupational therapists, respiratory therapists and nurse practitioners" (von Mering and Gordon, 1993, p. 168).

It is granted, the great majority of older Americans do not enjoy this high quality of long-term care. CCRCs are representative of the successful fully-funded individualistic solution to prolonged assisted living with chronic disease conditions. Only a few of these communities have existed for a century or more, and those have been sponsored by religious and fraternal organizations. The vast majority are of recent vintage. Overall, these elder communities require individually planned financial support or prepayment of one's assets in return for later high-intensity personal services and care, in combination with Social Security and Medicare benefits, as well as the voluntary contribution of in-kind or other financial resources by residents (von Mering and Neff, 1993, p. 6).

It is important to note that this long-term care model, which offers opportunity for positive aging despite declining vitality and health, represents "a renewed expression of the long history of social movements in the U.S. where people are creating special small communities to rediscover their own worth, survivability, and maybe even their soul" (von Mering and Neff, 1993, p. 4). Specifically, older people discover a strong affinity with their and their age cohort's needs, and they turn this realization into the creation of a small community of personal attachments and long-term caring which fits their middle-class means and the fact of extended longevity. It is as if they have found a post-work-a-day kind of lifestyle of "ordered and balanced adjustment of interests, in which each individual shall have a place and part and privilege, *but* at the same time hold sacred the part, the place, the privilege, of every other" (von Mering and Neff, 1993, p. 5).

The CCRC long-term care model, while culturally syntonic with the American Way, must seem like the "Abode of the Blest" to most long-living persons in the United States. The persuasive power of this world-wide folkloric legend, however, accounts in part for the intermittent push in American society to do better than increase the scattered warehousing in board and care homes or nursing facilities of the majority of frail and old persons who are economically less fortunate.

To capture this prototypical image of better health for all regardless of age, but especially for the old, it is worth recalling the classic description of the Abode of the Blest. It is a place, where "their hair is crowned with golden bay leaves and they hold glad revelry, and neither sickness nor baneful 'old' mingles among that chosen people; but aloof from toil and conflict, they dwell afar" (Pindar, as quoted by Gruman, 1966, p. 22). The urge to prolong the good life in the pattern to which one has become accustomed, or to find a lifestyle to which one would like to become accustomed, dwells in everyone, regardless of station and worldly means. At the very least, the mirage of endless well-being enables most everyone to gloss over the inner negative meaning of receiving chronic disease care: meekly experiencing a personal future that features an intractable health condition.

The Forgotten Elderly

Given our particular American cultural presuppositions about aging and ways of assuring personal well-being and physical and mental health, it should not come as surprise that a very large number of older persons live out their lives as the "forgotten elderly," beyond the reach of long-term care from formal health and rehabilitation agencies. They may actually be living within a sheltering network of informal support, and, as we shall see, they may be busy inventing their own special versions of small communities of mutual caring and support. However, as a rule, they are only referred to as "special populations" with "special needs." They tend to be tucked away in rural poverty pockets, or they live isolated in crime-ridden urban enclaves where there are few or no readily accessible formal health and human services. Moreover, they have come to be viewed as "the most difficult group" of older persons to reach by formal community services.

Some descriptive statistics are in order. The life situation of "special" older U.S. populations has not changed substantially since 1989, even though newer statistics have been made available via the U.S. census (Cohen, Van Nostrand, and Furner, 1993; Older Women's League, 1993; Sotomayor and Garcia, 1993; U.S. Senate, Special Committee on Aging, 1991). Overall, U.S. elderly constituted about 15 percent of the non-metropolitan population, but only 12 percent of the metropolitan population (Cohen, Van Nostrand, and Furner, 1993). While the elderly are about as likely as younger people to be poor, in 1989 a greater proportion of the elderly (27.2%) lived near the poverty level than did younger people (21.2% of those under 65). The poorest elderly are minorities, women, the "oldest old" (85 years or older), and persons who live alone (Cohen, Van Nostrand, and Furner, 1993).

In 1988, the poverty rate among black elderly (33.2%) was more than triple that of white elderly (10%), and among Hispanic elderly (22.4%) it was more than double that of whites. Retired Hispanics are more likely than non-Hispanic whites to live with Social Security as their only source of income (Sotomayor and Garcia, 1993). In 1992, 39 percent of black women and 24 percent of Hispanic women aged 65 or over were listed as living below the poverty level. This increases to 40 percent for Hispanic women and 50 percent for black women if the "near poor" are included (Older Women's League, 1993). Elderly black persons in nonmetropolitan areas are more likely to be poor than those in metropolitan areas (Cohen, Van Nostrand, and Furner, 1993).

In 1989, the median annual income of elderly women was $7,655, or 58 percent of the income of elderly men ($13,107). The oldest women were found to be the poorest: more than one in five women 85 years or older lived in poverty in 1989. This trend is growing. More elderly women live alone. Older men tend to remain married while women become widows or divorced. In 1992, "39 percent of all women alone and 64 percent of Black women alone live in the South. Fifty percent of Hispanic women alone live in the West." In 1992, 23.3 percent of older women living alone were below the poverty level. "Widows age 65 and over are the largest group of poor elderly in all areas of the United States, whether rural or urban" (Older Women's League, 1993, p. 3).

The nonmetropolitan elderly are twice as likely as metropolitan elderly to have to travel for more than 30 minutes to reach their usual source of health care (Cohen, Van Nostrand, and Furner, 1993). In terms of health, more than four out of five people aged 65 or older have at least one chronic condition, and multiple conditions are commonplace, especially among older women. Eighty percent of those caring for frail older persons, either as family members, friends, or neighbors, are women.

Of critical importance here is the adequacy of housing occupied by the majority of women. As they grow older, their housing choices become more restricted. Housing adequacy in the later years centers around affordability and adaptability to changes at different life stages and depends on the availability of social- and health-related assisted living services. Each is needed for assuring independent living at home for as long as possible. Without providing for these three critical quality-of-life areas, women become vulnerable to persistent housing problems and restricted choices as to where and how they live (Older Women's League, 1993, p. 3), and to what kind of long-term care is possible.

Overall, the principal long-term health care issues in the United States revolve around the accessibility and appropriateness of services for the old and very old, no matter where they live. However, it is well to note here that "about four times as many frail elders requiring some long-term care services reside in the community as live in nursing homes" (Tilson, 1990, p. xix). Moreover, "informal caregivers are not only the most common providers of care, but they also provide far and away the greatest amounts of care" (Kemper, 1992, p. 447).

These statistics paint a striking socioeconomic picture of being alive but not well, of what it is like to live longer as an old, poor, and benignly neglected resident of the United States. Most significant of all is the "feminization" of old age and the fact that "four out of every ten older women are poor or near poor." In particular, "women aged 65 or older are more likely to rely on Social Security as their sole source of support than are men of the same age, . . . and only 22 percent of older women receive a pension, either public or private, based on their work record or that of their spouse" (Kuriansky, 1992).

Given the American presuppositions about the strictly personal pursuit of individual health and secure well-being, as well as the above enumerative picture of living poorly into the later years, we can reach certain conclusions. Becoming a financially and health-disadvantaged female and/or ethnic senior is not the result of U.S. health care policies, although they have had a selective impact on these special populations. This state of affairs is an unintended side-effect of the American cultural mind-set of separating general social and economic welfare from enlightened individual economics and health care initiatives.

Becoming an old disadvantaged female is readily linked to the common judgmental tendency to dwell on how "some people" cause their own health hazards or contribute to their disease or obesity. Being disadvantaged is also connected to the popular inclination to gloss over the actual negative impact on health of occupational and economic inequities, at the group or special population levels. These are matters, of course, over which an individual often has no control. Certainly, the cultural habit of linking Social Security and medical benefits to monetary contributions made while still in the workforce has significantly influenced the shape of the problem of available and accessible high-quality long-term care for older women. The majority of them were not in the formal workplace as were their male age mates, and thus have become merely secondary beneficiaries of Social Security legislation.

Coping and Caring, Informally

"The prevailing U.S. distrust of socialized solutions and big government combined with an insistence on self reliance" (Filinson, 1992, p. 274), as well as a palpable shift from patient-centered to device-centered care by formal care providers, has complicated the task of targeting services for older adults, especially women, in a balanced manner (Nahmiah, 1994). In light of this, it is perhaps not surprising that there has been a notable rise in popular reliance on "hands on" care through informal unpaid voluntary effort and a resort to services by alternative health care providers. This is especially notable among elderly women and minorities, who have a life-long experience of unequal access to formal health care and monetary support because of their traditionally unequal participation in the labor market.

There is growing albeit still incomplete evidence that a goodly number of the "invisible" poor elderly have discovered ways to blunt the daily sting of social and economic disadvantage. Clearly, the manner in which someone in the company of others experiences the structural limits of his or her existence is the key to what action the person takes. The individual and the cultural traditions and social changes which everyone is subject to across the life course shape what kinds of health demands a person is likely to make and how "well" he or she lives. How a person copes with the daily rising limitations of function that can come with advancing years depends on how much the person lives in isolation from others in a world of limited good.

Longitudinal behavioral studies in the United States and the United Kingdom confirm that informal social networks in the community, particularly in low-income neighborhoods, are a key element in the experience of long-term care and support among old persons (Henderson, 1990; Henderson et al., 1993; Wenger, 1992). It remains highly problematic, however, how many disadvantaged persons can locate and use successfully unexpected opportunities for help within the severe socioeconomic constraints of their habitat. The very awareness among many of the "forgotten" elderly of being able to cope better when in the company of people in similar predicaments is a powerful motivating force for fashioning self-enhancing changes in their well-being. For them, the problem is not a matter of "locating support," "service delivery," and "case management" but a practical question of care and sharing.

On the one hand, the elderly of all walks of life in our society know that they face a later and perhaps darker date with death than did their forebears (von Mering, 1992). Their elongated life course has become as ordinary as early death in previous historical eras. On the other hand, many older women and some men, through extensive voluntary informal support networks, contradict the public's and policymakers' uninformed as well as gloomy impression of the plight of the single and lonely, low-income and frail old person. Although living in small quarters with insufficient government support, they struggle bravely with the infirmities of long life, going forward with cane, umbrella, and shopping bag for their own and others' necessities of daily living. While doing so they also provide long-term care for those who are more frail or vulnerable than themselves, regardless of whether they be older or their great-grandchildren.

A few statistics document this social reality. "In the United States today, approximately 75 percent of all nonmedical care for the 'frail elderly' is provided by informal caregivers, . . . a substantial percentage of them are also elderly and often in need of support themselves, . . . [and overall], 70 percent of caregivers are women" (von Mering, 1992). "In 1992, three million grandchildren, 5 percent of all children under age 18, lived in homes maintained by their grandparents. Of that group, 45 percent lived with a grandmother alone" (Older Women's League, 1993, p. 12). Though often poor, the people in the fourth age of life continue to demonstrate their ability and willingness to do long-term care for others, and not just care about their personal well-being.

Quite outside of government policy, more and more elderly women are developing their collective potential as a human resource for long-term health management. Creating new domestic units of interdependent care and resource utilization among kin and nonkin, they rely on Aid to Families with Dependent Children and Supplemental Security Income, food stamps and Medicaid, and they generate "income" via the fruits of barter to contribute to the survival of individual members of the household (von Mering, 1992). In a real sense, with their long-term care intergenerational efforts, they have rediscovered "the small community," or rather, reinvented a naturally occurring supportive habitat in the midst of disjunctive social, economic, and formal health care circumstances. Their small-scale caring human environments are a far cry from the CCRC, but they may well spring from the same cultural tradition that has made the United States the host to more millenarian communities than any other country.

The complex interactions of this so-called informal support and care sector of U.S. health and human resources are not yet well understood as a key variable in the differential impact of available formal long-term care services in the community. Most often, formal caregivers prescribe case management long before reaching a proper understanding of the many varieties of nearly-cashless-but-cared-for survival with some dignity. Without an identifiable benefit of formal long-term care services, there exists a great range of supportive, long-lasting activity that engages informal caregiving partnerships between two or more persons in a domestic unit. A formal professional agency caregiver who works on behalf of individual members of special populations may well discover that trying to provide equivalent long-term care for equivalent needs in highly unequivalent social habitats is a troublesome undertaking.

It is becoming more evident that there exist slowly expanding groups of informal carers who in many so-called blighted neighborhoods develop a high degree of personal and behavioral affinity with each other. They become informal long-term carers, perhaps even "health managers," as they age in special small, shared housing settings or in neighborhood housing for the elderly provided by county or city agencies. Over time, they devise informal, private cooperative solutions for handling most of the IADLs and also some of the less burdensome ADLs within their informal support networks. This is seen as "private knowledge," not readily communicated to representatives of state and local agencies charged with serving the public at large.

In sum, a growing number of the frail and not yet frail elderly poor, banding together in supportive affinity-bonded groups while aging in place, have turned themselves into a practical, informal long-term care alternative. They have done this despite their well-documented partial exclusion from ready access to formal health and long-term well-being care (von Mering, 1992). Like all of us, they are not able to stave off their ultimate state of confinement to one small earthly space. But together, many have prevented and do prevent themselves from slipping into a prolonged existence that is drastically curtailed by external economic forces. Together, they are also demonstrating their capacity to deny premature social death and precipitous consignment to a Medicaid-defined nursing home status.

Looking to the Future

Although the above-described approach of informal long-term care by the poor may pose little resemblance to the CCRC solution of the middle classes, it is testimony to the inventiveness of individuals in harnessing forgotten and publicly invisible resources to achieve a basic level of long-term care, even in the most unlikely circumstances. Even in environments where the air may not be decent to breathe, where children and old people find it often unsafe to play or sit, where regular paid-for work is scarce or unavailable, and where few find confidence to look forward to the future, the individualistic American culture of caregiving can find promising expression. It seems important that we learn how to link up with these hidden renewable human resources when planning and doing formal long-term care services.

We have shown that giving care and receiving benefits is an interactive process, over time and across generations. The contrasting examples of CCRCs and the informal small networks of long-term care, whether in the inner city or the countryside, illustrate this. In a manner of speaking, the contribution of in-kind resources and of individual support, so often given at great personal sacrifice by one generation or affinity-bonded network of older persons, can alleviate many of the "deficits" in life quality experienced by another generation or group.

A question about the future of long-term care in the United States has therefore less to do with the reported disappearance of the family as the primary informal source of long-range caregiving than with the timely prevention of informal caregivers' overextension and gradual exhaustion during a prolonged period of providing support. Designing more sensitive ways of allocating formal publicly funded grants and respite services to those social networks that give signs of having difficulty in sustaining the level of care needed for its aging members may be a future option. The current gradual rise of more sophisticated and comprehensive voluntary adult day care centers in small and large towns as well as cities holds some promise for better long-term care outreach in the future.

Much may also be achievable through planning new communities or "retrofitting" old neighborhoods in such a way that public facilities and gathering places (Kercher, 1993) like stores, branch libraries, and day care centers are closer to a functioning community network of support. Individual income maintenance and pension schemes for the poor are insufficient protection by themselves for an era of prolonged life expectancy. The public sector of health care has to relate creatively to the inner workings of informal small support networks, where barter and other nonmonetary forms of exchange of value make long-term care possible for the old, the alone, and the poor, and make health management feasible for the parentless young as well.

As the Older Women's League has observed, there is much room for improvement along many fronts of social and health security for older Americans, but especially for older women. Most important of all, perhaps, it is time for everyone to embrace the idea that aging is more a matter of human resource and enterprise development than a prolonged, burdensome, terminal process accompanied by the medicated postponement of the final fatal infirmity. To accomplish this conceptual shift, we must first make a cultural shift away from the current "episodic sickness" model of health care toward a long-term partnership among provider, consumer, payer, *and* informal caregiver "shadow worker" on behalf of chronic care. It is a step that clearly "focuses on achieving the maximum wellness possible for every individual" (Smith et al., 1993, p. 9). Once this cultural paradigmatic shift becomes accepted, it will also be feasible not to go on regarding long-term care as a private health insurance issue primarily of concern to, if not wholly dependent on, the formal health care system (Morris and Morris, 1993; Tilson, 1990).

The open public airing of competing predictions and perspectives on health and well-being care for aging Americans will, it is hoped, remove the shackles of yesterday's traditions and presuppositions and help us embrace the best caregiving directions for tomorrow. Today, health care insurers, employers, and the public are wrestling with the insufficiences of the relatively new "managed care system." They are beginning to recognize that this system of health care delivery has been designed one-sidedly, to handle both acute care and long-term chronic care via traditional, facility-dependent "supply-side" initiatives (e.g., the local hospital, clinic, day surgery, and regional health center). That is to say, it relies on limiting access to care through "gate-keeping" practices mandated by insurance companies and carried out by primary care physicians.

Fortunately, as a countervailing force for community well-being and health management, a focus on the demand side of care services and self-care is developing in corporate America. New, demand-side initiatives are being tried to intercept the individual precipitants of inappropriate (i.e., too late or too soon) emergency room visits and to provide those in need of health maintenance and urgent care with suitable knowledge and the support necessary to navigate successfully the complicated health care delivery system.

A current corporate initiative delivering health benefit management to seniors and the general population of corporate employees and their dependents may serve as an example. It represents a significant conceptual shift from the supply side to the demand side of providing effective health care, and it thereby achieves a much-improved corporate "bottom line" as well. It provides its "Senior Choice" members in California with toll-free access to nurses specially trained in the art of nondirective care counseling. Callers are provided with information and direct support advice for medical and well-being decisionmaking. For the aging adult and caregiver, this type of service modality, integrated with concurrent clinical care benefits, signifies a natural opportunity to promote the capacity to manage the personal demand for care and support (von Mering, 1995).

It is not just simple remedies for the signs and symptoms of our changing bodies and minds that we need to address; it is the social, economic, and personal discomforts and the hidden human resources associated with our passage into the country of the old that we must study more wisely. The design of the best long-term care choices for aging well lie in that pioneer territory.

We need a new language about persistent poverty and ill-being in old age, a language that knows of the beneficent reality of informal self-health care and support. We must become more knowledgeable about the shape and drift of cultural presuppositions about caregiving if we wish to move beyond conventional treatment decisions when we care for the robust, the dying, the frail, the demented, and all the other unique younger and older persons who require long-term care. Becoming a "shape shifter" of ideas is a clear and present need for everyone who accepts long-term care as an integral part of a future health security for all.

References

Achenbaum, W. A. (1994). U.S. retirement in historical context. In A. Monk, ed., *The Columbia Retirement Handbook* (pp. 12–28). New York: Columbia University Press.

Angell, M. (1993). How much will health care reform cost? *New England Journal of Medicine* 328 (29): 1778–79.

Chen, Y. (1994). Financing Social Security, Medicare, Medicaid and long term care. In A. Monk, ed., *The Columbia Retirement Handbook* (pp. 551–69). New York: Columbia University Press.

Chudacoff, H. P. (1989). *How Old Are You? Age Consciousness in American Culture*. Princeton: Princeton University Press.

Cohen, R. A., Van Nostrand, J. F., and Furner, S. E. (1993). Chartbook on health data on older Americans: United States, 1992. *U.S. PHS Report Series 3-29*, (PHS) 93-1413. Washington, D.C.: National Center for Health Statistics.

Filinson, R. (1992). Ethnic aging in Canada and the United States: A comparison of social policy. *Journal of Aging Studies* 6 (3): 273–87.

Gruman, G. J. (1966). A history of ideas about the prolongation of life. *Transactions of the American Philosophical Society,* n.s., vol. 56, part 9 (December), pp. 1–102. Philadelphia.

Henderson, J. N. (1990). Anthropology, Health and Aging. In *Anthropology and Aging: Comprehensive Reviews,* edited by R. D. Rubinstein, pp. 34–68. Boston: Kluwer.

Henderson, J. N., Gutierrez-Mayka, M., Garcia, J., and Boyd, S. (1993). A model for Alzheimer's Disease support group development in African-American and Hispanic populations. *Gerontologist* 33 (3): 409–14.

Kemper, P. (1992). The use of formal and informal home care by the disabled elderly. *Health Services Research* 27 (4): 421–51.

Kercher, W. C. (1993). Co-location of public buildings and facilities: Build communities while we build facilities. *Florida Planning* 5 (8): 5.

Kuriansky, J. (1992). *Old, Poor, and Forgotten: Elderly Americans Living in Poverty*. Washington, D.C.: Older Women's League. Quoted in testimony before the House Select Committee on Aging, June 24.

Monk, A. (1994). An introduction. In A. Monk, ed., *The Columbia Retirement Handbook* (pp. 3–11). New York: Columbia University Press.

Morris, J. N., and Morris, S. A. (1993). Aging in place: The role of formal human services. In J. J. Callahan, ed., *Aging in Place* (pp. 73–88). Amityville, N.Y.: Baywood.

Nahmiah, D. (1994). Targeting services to older adults at risk: A balancing net. *Canadian Journal on Aging* 13 (1): 1–4.

Older Women's League (1993). *Mother's Day Report — Room for Improvement: The Lack of Affordable, Adaptable, and Accessible Housing for Midlife and Older Women*. Washington, D.C.: Older Women's League.

Robert Wood Johnson Foundation (1993). *Annual Report: Chronic Health Conditions*. Princeton, N.J.: Robert Wood Johnson Foundation.

Smith, Q., Smith, L., King, K., Frieden, L., and Richards, L. (1993). *Health Care Reform, Independent Living and People with Disabilities, and Issues in Independent Living Report*. Houston: Institute for Rehabilitation and Research, Independent Living Research Utilization Program.

Sotomayor, M., and Garcia, A. (1993). *Elderly Latinos: Issues and Solutions for the Twenty-first Century*. Washington, D.C.: National Hispanic Council on Aging.

Tilson, D. (1990). *Aging in Place: Supporting the Frail Elderly in Residential Environments*. Glenview, Ill.: Scott, Foresman.

U.S. Senate, Special Committee on Aging (1991). *Aging America: Trends and Projections*. Washington, D.C.: Government Printing Office.

von Mering, G. (1995). Contemporary health plan designs: Focusing on demand. Aetna Lecture before Fibre Box Association, Health Care Benefits Workshop, November 9. Hartford, Conn.: Aetna Life Insurance.

von Mering, O. (1992). Societies in transition: The impact of longevity on generations. *Educational Gerontology* 18:123–34.

von Mering, O., and Earley, L. W. (1965). Major changes in the western medical environment. *Archives of General Psychiatry* 13:195–201.

von Mering, O., and Gordon, S. (1993). Elder villages: Ghettos or godsends? In K. Tout, ed. *Elderly Care: A World Perspective* (pp. 166–72). London: Chapman and Hall.

von Mering, O., and Neff, L. (1993). Joining a life care community: An alternative to 'frailing' into a nursing home in the U.S.A. *Generations Review* 3 (4): 4–8, 26.

Wenger, C. (1992). *Help in Old Age — Facing up to Change: A Longitudinal Network Study*. Institute of Human Aging, Occasional Paper 5. Liverpool: Liverpool University Press.

Young, M. (1990). Down with age. *London Review of Books*, October, pp. 13–14.

EPILOGUE

13

Foreseeing the Future of Long-Term Care: The Highlights and Implications of a Delphi Study

Dennis L. Kodner, Ph.D.

The current system of long-term care presents consumers, providers, payers, and policymakers alike with a number of urgent shortcomings and dilemmas. Financial critics are concerned that Americans are not adequately protected against the catastrophic costs of long-term care and that the level and growth rate of public costs for such care are unacceptably high — especially in the absence of universal coverage. Performance critics of long-term care, on the other hand, consider that the system is too heavily slanted to institutional care, overly medicalized, poorly coordinated, inefficient, and that the care it delivers is lacking in adequate quality.

If long-term care is not overhauled before we enter the twenty-first century, most observers now agree, these problems will worsen and ultimately overwhelm a seriously imperfect system. Despite the fact that the first cohort of baby boomers will begin to swell the ranks of the elderly population by the year 2010, surprisingly little systematic thought has been given to identifying and realistically assessing the most probable forces and trends that will shape the long-term care system between now and then.

In long-term care as in other fields, forecasting is a difficult task that often carries a high likelihood of error. Nonetheless, making predictions can be a useful exercise — one that should perhaps be tried more often. Obtaining insights into the future can broaden and enrich the context in which good policymaking and planning should be done. With reasonable forecasts in hand, stakeholders can more effectively steer the course of long-term care and creatively respond to tomorrow's developments.

What will long-term care look like by the year 2010, and how will this picture challenge major actors? Answering these questions was the goal of Project 2010, a study conducted between the years 1991 and 1992 at the Institute for Applied Gerontology of Metropolitan Jewish Health Care System. The purpose of this research was not to present an idealized version of how long-term care should develop, but rather to generate a broad and empirically based forecast and to explore its consequences. This chapter summarizes that study (Kodner, 1993). Because Project 2010 produced literally hundreds of forecasts, particular attention is given here to identifying the major drivers of change in long-term care as well as the most significant developments that are anticipated in this complex field. It also explores the impacts on stakeholders, as well as important issues that they and society-at-large must face as the long-term care system undergoes change.

Using the Delphi Method to Foresee the Future

The subject being examined — the future of long-term care — does not lend itself neatly to precise quantitative techniques. Because tomorrow's long-term care will ultimately reflect the complex interplay between facts and values, Project 2010 began with an a priori assumption that the knowledge, insights, and opinions of experts in the field could be used to make predictions. This was the premise for our choice of the Delphi method.

The Delphi method is a systematic, iterative forecasting technique that pools the individual judgments of a geographically dispersed panel of experts to generate consensus about a particular question or problem (Linstone and Turoff, 1975). Utilizing a structured group process, this qualitative method combines anonymous panel interaction, multiple questionnaires, and controlled feedback to produce results (Rowe, Wright, and Bolger, 1991).

Like other group research techniques, the Delphi method is based on the notion that two heads are better than one (Cornish, 1977; Helmer, 1983; Millet and Honton, 1991). According to Helmer, when group opinion is dominated by individual personalities, this often produces skewed results. However, in contrast to face-to-face decisionmaking, the Delphi method guarantees a process that is free of the "bandwagon effect." Therefore, the Delphi method is capable of producing a strong and valid picture of long-term care by the year 2010.

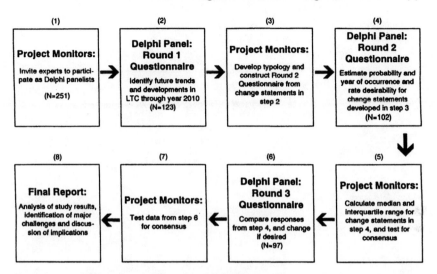

Figure 13.1.   The sequence of steps in Project 2010

Figure 13.1 depicts the sequence of the eight steps in our study. Researchers determined that three rounds of questionnaires would be satisfactory to generate consensus.

Expert Panel

A reputational approach was used to compile the names of 251 experts in the long-term care field, as broadly defined. Potential subjects came from 19 different backgrounds and disciplines. Nearly half of the invited experts on this list initially agreed to participate as panelists. As shown in Table 13.1, 123 panelists were involved in Round 1, 102 in Round 2, and 97 in Round 3. This represents a 95 percent completion rate, which is considered exceptionally high for a Delphi study.

Data Collection and Analysis

Round 1. Asked to make ten short, simple statements about the future of long-term care, panelists generated a total of 1088 statements. Researchers independently categorized these unedited statements and then agreed on the construction of a final typology consisting of 22 categories (Table 13.2).

Round 2. Panelists were provided with a structured, close-ended questionnaire listing 200 "change statements" — each representing a future

Table 13.1
Invitees and Respondents in Delphi Study, by Category or Discipline

Category/Discipline	Invitees	Respondents		
		Round One	Round Two	Round Three
Health policy and research	31	15	15	15
Gerontology	30	14	11	10
Geriatrics or biomedical research	19	9	9	8
Federal or state government	18	9	6	6
Long-term care facilities	15	9	5	5
Consulting	14	7	7	7
Home and community care	13	6	4	4
Long-term care insurance	11	6	6	5
Consumer or family caregiver	9	5	4	4
Corporations	10	5	3	3
Ethics and legal	11	5	4	4
Aging network	12	4	4	4
Demography or epidemiology	8	3	2	2
Social work	10	3	2	1
Hospitals	8	3	3	3
Foundations	6	3	2	2
Nursing	6	2	2	2
Housing	5	2	2	2
Miscellaneous	15	13	11	10
Total	251	123	102	97

trend or development in one of the issue categories listed in Table 13.2. This list was constructed from the content analysis of the unedited statements derived in Round 1. For each change statement, participants were asked to:

1. make a 50 percent probability estimate and a 90 percent probability estimate of whether these changes would happen;
2. forecast the anticipated year of occurrence for each of these estimates; and
3. rate the desirability of each of these changes, whether or not considered likely to occur, on a five-point Likert scale, with 1 meaning very undesirable and 5 meaning very desirable.

For the purposes of this study, the median and interquartile ranges were used to statistically represent consensus and the spread of opinion, respectively. Consensus was considered reached when 75 percent or more of the responses to any item were found between the first and third quartiles. Calculations were performed for each of the 600 responses in the Round 2

Table 13.2
Categories of Long-Term Care Issues and Concerns
Developed in Delphi Study

1. Social, political, and economic developments
2. Demographics and health status
3. Biomedical and clinical breakthroughs
4. Medical care delivery and financing
5. Lifestyles and values
6. Health promotion, prevention, and self-care
7. Informal caregiving
8. Long-term care supply and demand
9. Long-term care system
10. Nursing homes and other long-term care facilities
11. Home and community long-term care services
12. Hospitals and long-term care
13. Housing-related long-term care options
14. Technological and design innovations
15. Regulation, quality, and planning
16. Geriatric medicine
17. Personnel issues
18. Ethical concerns and intergenerational issues
19. Research
20. Long-term care financing and reimbursement
21. Corporate America and long-term care
22. Miscellaneous

questionnaire and then tested for consensus according to this stopping criteria. The results of Round 2 consensus were as follows: 42 percent of the 50 percent probability items achieved consensus, as did 73 percent of the 90 percent probability items and 70 percent of the desirability items.

Round 3. Panelists were requested to revise their own probability estimates (if they wished) for each of the items failing to reach consensus in the previous round, based on feedback of the median and interquartile ranges. If the panelist chose to remain outside the boundary of consensus, a brief written justification was also required. One hundred percent of the items achieved consensus in Round 3.

Highlights of Results

Project 2010 generated 600 separate forecasts on 22 major topics in long-term care. This chapter can present only highlights from these results. The highlights presented here in narrative form are based on the 90 percent probability estimates and represent the best and most confident projection of the future by the expert panel. Although the study included point-in-time forecasts, only trends and developments are summarized here. To assist the reader, these highlights are broadly divided into two parts, progenitors of change and the future long-term care landscape.

Progenitors of Change

To begin, we consider the six major progenitors of change that will affect the direction and shape of long-term care by the next century.

Aging Baby Boomers. When aging baby boomers start retiring in the year 2010, the resulting surge in the number of long-lived citizens will contribute to a substantial rise in the need for long-term care throughout the first several decades of the twenty-first century.

Changing Burden of Illness. The burden of chronic illness among the elderly will continue to engulf the long-term care system. While elderly people will remain the predominant users of long-term care as we enter the next century, more younger persons with chronic and medically complex conditions — AIDS patients, for example (see Chapter 4) — will use nursing homes and other long-term care services.

Biomedical and Clinical Breakthroughs. There will be important breakthroughs in the prevention, diagnosis, and treatment of at least three disabling conditions associated with the risk of long-term care: Alzheimer disease, osteoporosis, and osteoarthritis. In the case of Alzheimer disease, however, none of these advances will lead to prevention or cure of the disease by the year 2010.

New Generation of Elderly. The next century will find a cohort of elderly people quite different from its predecessors. While pockets of poverty will persist among the elderly, tomorrow's 65-plussers will be wealthier. They will also be better educated, work longer before retirement, and be more assertive about their needs and wants. However, not all of the anticipated changes will be positive. Because many Americans will be single, divorced, or separated, growing old will translate into less family support when the need for long-term care arises; this trend will be exacerbated by future work and household demands.

Restrained Governmental Role. Antigovernment and antitax senti-ments will prevent Washington and the states from shouldering total re-sponsibility for major new social programs, especially those benefiting the elderly. Medicare and Medicaid, in particular, will continue to be tempt-ing targets for budget-cutters as they wrestle with a perpetual deficit.

Growing Concern about Long-Term Care. Understanding of long-term care and the need for catastrophic protection will grow, especially among older Americans. Baby boomers will add their voices to the long-term care debate, and advocates for the elderly and disabled will work together to promote new policies and programs. This will make long-term care reform an important national priority. The next generation of better-educated and more insistent elderly people will also transform themselves from today's "invisible" long-term care consumers to tomorrow's de-manding long-term care customers. They will be more sensitive to quality and value concerns and play a stronger role in deciding which services should be delivered and from what site. Providers, therefore, will have to pay more attention to the needs and preferences of elderly clients and patients if they want their business.

Future Long-Term Care Landscape

The preceding drivers of change will result in an almost entirely trans-formed long-term care landscape. Ten major developments are antici-pated by the year 2010.

Public-Private Financing. The idea of a universal, publicly financed comprehensive long-term care program will never gain widespread po-litical acceptance. However, Congress will ultimately enact a combined public-private long-term care financing system covering citizens of all ages. The federal government will pay for a package of home- and community-based services plus limited "front-end" or "back-end" coverage of nurs-ing home stays. Private insurers will then be encouraged to offer gap-filling policies that will be based on uniform standards. The states, in turn, will use Medicaid to buy these policies on behalf of eligible persons who cannot afford the cost of premiums, co-pays, and uncovered long-term care services.

Capitation and Case-Mix Reimbursement. With a new public-private long-term care system in place, fee-for-service payment for nursing homes and home care providers will rapidly give way to capitation, case mix, and other innovative forms of reimbursement designed to control costs. Reimbursement will also be linked to the quality of care provided.

Coordinated Access to Services. Public utility — like agencies will become the local command centers for the future long-term care system. Regardless of the source of payment, these local access agencies will evaluate client needs, determine eligibility, make referrals to community providers, and coordinate care. They will also use standardized assessment tools and case management protocols, and payment will be based on their authorizations.

Managed Long-Term Care. Future emphasis on cost control and coordination will give rise to managed long-term care plans. Like today's On Lok/PACE and social health maintenance organization programs, these integrated provider networks will afford convenient, one-stop access to a continuum of acute and long-term care services for disabled persons of all ages. Prepaid funding would come from public and private premiums. These plans will gain widespread popularity among consumers and payers and ultimately dominate the long-term care system.

Focus on Home and Community Services. Long-term care will continue its shift toward home- and community-based services. These noninstitutional services will be at the core of the future system. However, the drive for efficiency and quality, along with changing consumer preferences, will alter the way traditional in-home and community care will look and operate; new services and modalities of care will emerge by the year 2010.

Different Kind of Nursing Home. The nursing home of the future may end up being several different types of facilities. A growing pool of patients with acute illnesses being treated outside of the hospital will require short-term stays for subacute care and intensive rehabilitation. On the other hand, the heavy emphasis on noninstitutional services will fill nursing homes with patients whose complicated needs can no longer be met in lower levels of care; these are today's hard-to-place patients. Finally, there are the patients in between — Alzheimer disease victims, for example — who will need a less costly, but more homelike environment. Because of its flexibility, today's assisted living facility model will play an increasingly important role as a provider of residential care in the future, for reasons of both cost and quality.

The future nursing home will also be more diversified. Survival in the twenty-first century will demand major adjustments to changing patient needs as well as a restructured long-term care system. Therefore, many more facilities will establish adult day care centers, supportive housing, and even home care agencies.

Finally, the freestanding nursing home will begin to disappear. In the future, local nursing homes will find it in their best interest to join national or regional for-profit chains and nonprofit alliances. These multiple-facility networks will assist providers in improving management capabilities, enhancing competitiveness, forging links with managed long-term care plans, and increasing access to needed capital.

Patient-centered Care. The next two decades will see a shift to better quality care, with the needs of the patient being placed at the center of the long-term care system. Long-term care providers will inevitably view quality as a consequence of carefully managed resources. Outcomes will be adjusted to reflect the effects of case mix, and standards will apply to clients and patients with equivalent needs rather than common services or settings. With the active involvement of providers in quality management activities, the states will assume more of an oversight role. External review agencies will make periodic quality checks with the involvement of local consumer groups, and these ratings will be figured into the reimbursement rate. In this quality-conscious environment, superior providers will receive bonus payments and poor performers will find it increasingly difficult to survive.

Housing as a Long-Term Care Resource. Housing will receive more attention, as the site of long-term care. By the year 2010, more flexible housing arrangements with on-site supportive services will allow elderly and other long-term care users to remain in the community except for the most serious changes in health status or personal situation. More elderly people will live in congregate rental housing and continuing care retirement communities. In addition to these upscale housing alternatives, there will be more options for low- and moderate-income persons. Many housing programs in the future will be sponsored by nursing homes and hospitals and will benefit from links with long-term care financing.

Preventive Gerontology. As research begins to yield clues about how to treat, manage, and even prevent some of the major disabling conditions, the emerging discipline of preventive gerontology will capitalize on the growing wellness wave and ultimately become an accepted part of the future long-term care system.

Persistent Staffing Problems. Personnel problems in long-term care will persist in the future. While training and salaries will improve somewhat and increasing use will be made of labor-saving "gerotechnology," it will still be difficult for providers to attract and retain caring and motivated workers, especially paraprofessionals.

Implications of Results

A paradigm shift in long-term care is likely to occur. If the trends and developments forecasted by Project 2010 ensue, they will fundamentally remake long-term care as we know it today. These potentially significant changes can best be understood through the following cross-cutting discussion of the challenges posed to key stakeholders both now and in the future.

Prevent Disability

Chronic illness and disability are the dark side of aging. They also drive need and economics in long-term care. Biomedical advances in disorders that cause the greatest disability in elderly people can significantly influence the future size of the long-term care population and the ultimate costs of care. Changes in education, income, lifestyle, and other factors may also make important contributions. Therefore, prevention in the broadest sense holds the promise of greater vigor and independence in later years, enriched quality of life for the next generation of elderly people, and big savings of increasingly limited health care dollars.

Although preliminary findings by Manton, Corder and Stallard (1993) suggest that disability rates among elderly people may already be on the decline, common sense dictates that we should expand efforts in the arena of prevention. With the hope that disability can be managed, reduced, and even prevented, funding must be found in today's and tomorrow's difficult economic climates to support both basic and applied research in this crucial area. Additionally, the fruits of this research must be quickly mainstreamed into acute and long-term care so that "preventive gerontology" can indeed play a major role in cushioning the effects of increased survival and chronic illness.

Strengthen Informal Care

The family is the front line of long-term care, providing some 80 percent of the day-to-day personal assistance received by community-dwelling elderly persons (U.S. General Accounting Office, 1982). Various studies have shown, however, that these informal services are most commonly used in conjunction with formal or paid help (Soldo, Agree, and Wolf, 1989). That families play a major role in caring for their older relatives, and in deciding when and if institutionalization is necessary, is a well-established fact (Brody, Poulshock, and Masciocchi, 1978; Horowitz, 1985; Stone, Cafferata, and Sangl, 1987). In the future, the home will become an even more important long-term care setting. However, according to our panel, this will be counterbalanced by the decline in the availability of family support.

There are compelling reasons to strengthen informal care. Family members and other unpaid helpers enhance the quality of life of elderly persons, and they have a major impact on the utilization and costs of formal services. Despite the accumulated knowledge about the importance of informal care, there has been little response to the needs of families in the current long-term care system.

The challenge is to develop a viable partnership between both types of care. The formal system is capable of supplementing the work of families and other unpaid caregivers and should take over from these efforts when the burden is too great or family is lacking. This is a complex problem whose ultimate solution will require the involvement of both the public and the private sectors. Of necessity, future answers must cut across policies and programs related to long-term care financing, service delivery, taxation, and employment. The potential use of other gap-filling community resources — churches, synagogues, volunteer programs, and elder care cooperatives, for example — should not be overlooked. Finally, additional research should be encouraged to complete our knowledge base on the informal needs of special populations (e.g., minority and low-income elderly persons and elderly persons living alone), the effectiveness of various caregiver interventions, and better methods of targeting support services.

Improve Management and Service Delivery

Long-term care is becoming increasingly complex. By the next century, services will be more diversified and move away from their traditional settings. Providers will be expected to continuously improve and streamline the care they offer. Organizations will begin to vertically and horizontally integrate the delivery of services. The focus will shift from isolated providers and fee-for-service reimbursement to multiple-provider long-term care networks and capitation or other new forms of payment. In this future, long-term care providers will have to adapt not only to these new organizational, reimbursement, and service delivery realities but also to a different and more demanding clientele. The net effect of all these changes will be that providers will need to become more sophisticated about how they manage and deliver services.

This presents four main challenges. First, the long-term care industry must professionalize itself and develop a new generation of managers — both administrative and clinical — with an essential orientation to systems, quality outcomes, and markets. Second, a high level of leadership and investment will be needed to design, develop, and perfect managed long-term care plans. Third, in order to work, these future comprehensive long-term care programs will require new or enhanced technologies, from assessment to service coordination to quality management to information systems. And fourth, providers of various kinds will have to join forces and integrate services to operate successfully in the future long-term care system.

Increase and Enhance Personnel

Long-term care is a people-intensive endeavor. Quality in this field cannot be high without an adequate supply of caring, motivated, and properly trained personnel. Unfortunately, there is a lack of able-bodied workers today, and our study expects this shortage to continue into the next century at least until the year 2010.

The personnel problem in long-term care stems from a complex combination of factors: licensing and other regulatory requirements, reimbursement caps, more competitive salaries in and out of the health care industry, relatively poor benefits and working conditions, limited advancement opportunities, restrictive labor contracts, and inherent biases in society-at-large and the workforce against elderly people and long-term care in general.

Clearly, this problem must be attacked on several fronts. The recruitment and retention of a competent workforce should receive first priority; such issues as salary and benefits, job security, scheduling flexibility, and career advancement must be addressed. Next, creative approaches must be found to use personnel more efficiently and effectively, including by redefining jobs in both the home and nursing home settings. Finally, attention should be given to the education and training of personnel on all levels, so they can meet the new challenges of long-term care.

Promote Technology

Technology offers a tremendous potential that should not be overlooked in the redesign of long-term care. Technology can shape the home and community environments to enhance independence, assist individuals to overcome physical deficits, facilitate the monitoring of services, and even supplement or substitute for some hands-on personal care.

More research and development attention is needed to achieve technological breakthroughs that are relevant to long-term care. The various human dimension and ethical factors must also be explored. Last, realistic consideration must be given by the policy, planning, and reimbursement sectors to the proper diffusion and management of these new long-term care technologies.

Rethink Residential Care

There is general agreement that the focus of long-term care should be on the home, an idea that is especially appealing to elderly people and their families. The government has of late come to that same belief, primarily for cost-containment reasons. As a result, home- and community-based services have been growing rapidly, and states have kept a tight lid on the supply of nursing home beds. The future long-term care system is likely to maintain this posture. Nonetheless, many of tomorrow's long-term care clients will be older, sicker, and more disabled and will require heavier care. Many in this group will probably need to be admitted to some type of long-term care facility before they die.

Most people fear the prospect of living in a nursing home. Moreover, the quality of care in these facilities is far from excellent, and the costs of care are high. Now is the time to rethink what residential care should look like in the future.

Long-term care is essentially a problem of housing, inasmuch as nursing homes are actually residential facilities with an intensive array of services. Smaller and more flexible assisted-living facilities already cater to disabled elderly persons who fit the nursing home profile — except for the most vegetative or medically unstable patients. These mostly privately funded facilities offer one prototype for residential care in the next century, according to Project 2010. This raises some important questions: What is the best assisted-living model? What steps should be taken now to expand the supply of these facilities? How can we get existing nursing homes to operate more like these programs?

Developing affordable supportive housing is the other critical challenge. It is believed that such housing can promote independent community living and take some of the pressure off nursing homes. The increasing number of elderly people will make housing-based approaches to long-term care much more important in the future. However, a major obstacle that must be overcome is the lack of an existing relationship between long-term care and housing policies on the federal level. To solve this problem, the government must embrace an "aging in place" policy that recognizes that the best place to provide long-term care is where elderly people currently live. We must also understand the best and most cost-effective strategies for delivering supportive services in housing environments. Finally, there will be a need for more funding and other incentives to modify existing housing and construct new special-purpose housing units to meet anticipated needs.

Emphasize Quality

Quality has always been one of the weakest aspects of long-term care, especially in nursing homes. While the quality of service has steadily improved over the last several years, this critical dimension of care is still less than optimal.

Good-quality care will be even more important in the next century. Consumers will be smarter about the quality issue and more insistent on receiving good care. The continued shift to home- and community-based services will raise concern about whether quality can be effectively monitored and maintained in noninstitutional settings. And the emergence of capitation financing will generate important questions about whether clients can be shortchanged in the new world of managed long-term care.

Providing high-quality long-term care to meet the broad spectrum of physical, medical, and psychosocial needs is a complicated undertaking. It takes competent management, a well-trained, caring staff, and the right resources and facilities. Moreover, there are other challenges in achieving good care.

First, the quality of long-term care must be clearly delineated in terms of outcomes, and uniformly accepted criteria and standards must be developed. Second, regulatory systems on the federal and state levels must be totally overhauled to monitor the performance of the next generation of long-term care providers. Third, the future long-term care financing system must consider the relationship between reimbursement and quality. There is obviously a minimal reimbursement level below which it becomes impossible to provide adequate care; this must be carefully defined.

Fourth, individual client preferences, and concerns about client autonomy, must take center stage in long-term care decisionmaking.

Create an Affordable Financing System

Few reforms can be successfully implemented without changing the current method of paying for long-term care. Indeed, one of the findings of our study is that there is a strong probability that some kind of public-private program for long-term care will be in place by the year 2010 — this despite the advantages of universal, totally publicly financed long-term care insurance.

In 1994, the Clinton administration proposed a long-term care program as part of its American Health Security Act, which was not passed by Congress. This block grant program, which was to be phased in between the years 2000 and 2003, would have been administered by the states and would have covered expanded home- and community-based services for citizens of all ages who were severely disabled, cognitively impaired, mentally retarded, or (in the case of children under age six) technology dependent. It would also have liberalized Medicaid nursing home coverage and encouraged the development of gap-filling private insurance through national standards, consumer education and protection, and more favorable tax treatment.

The Clinton long-term care proposal was a harbinger of things to come. While the program did not fully address all of the important concerns — it did not include non-Medicaid nursing home coverage and stopped short of encouraging managed long-term care, for example — the bill strongly suggested that our study's vision of the future might be realistic.

Despite the possibilities, any long-term care program faces a potentially big stumbling block in the form of cost. The first question will be: How will the new program be paid for? In a period of budgetary constraint and antipathy to major new governmental initiatives, finding a satisfactory answer to this question will determine the probability that any long-term care proposal will find broad acceptance with the president, the Congress, and the American people.

The other major obstacle that must be addressed is deciding where long-term care should stand on the health policy queue. In effect, which should come first: general health care reform or a new long-term care program? Or an overall plan that could be phased in to allow both problems to be resolved, without substantially increasing the deficit or incurring new taxes?

For long-term care to move ahead on the domestic agenda, three conditions must be met: (1) the public and key interest groups must recognize the importance of long-term care and the need for fundamental change in the financing system; (2) they must agree on a path for change; and (3) there must be strong political leadership to translate this consensus into reality. If these conditions are ultimately satisfied, a public-private program of long-term care is achievable by the beginning of the twenty-first century.

A Concluding Note

Project 2010 generated a multidimensional picture of how long-term care will look by the first decade of the next century. The forecasts produced by the study, however, should not be misunderstood. They are not prophecies or predictions, exact indications of the future; the future cannot be foretold. Rather, the results are estimates of future probabilities made by a particular group of experts at a particular point of time. Therefore, it is conceivable that other views of the future exist. Nonetheless, if this limitation is clearly recognized, data from the study can be used effectively as a benchmark in assisting major actors in examining their own beliefs and assumptions about the future, in deciding what roles they can and should play, in coping with anticipated changes, and in designing a better and more affordable system of long-term care for tomorrow.

It seems inevitable that long-term care will change significantly. This is indicated by the results from Project 2010. The implications of these changes are broad and far reaching. The challenges are how to maximize the most desirable aspects of these future trends and developments and how to encourage the various stakeholders to make the right decisions.

Long-term care should be shaped by conscious choices about future directions, rather than being fated by seemingly random and uncontrollable events. As society ponders long-term care, it should not squander the future as it has the past.

References

Brody, S., Poulshock, S., and Masciocchi, C. (1978). The family caring unit: A major consideration in the long-term support system. *Gerontologist* 18:556–61.
Cornish, E. (1977). *The Study of the Future*. Bethesda, Md.: World Future Society.
Helmer, O. (1983). *Looking Forward: A Guide to Futures Research*. Beverly Hills, Calif.: Sage.

Horowitz, A. (1985). Family caregiving to the frail elderly. In C. Eisdorfer, ed., *Annual Review of Gerontology and Geriatrics* (vol. 1). New York: Springer Publishing.

Kodner, D. (1993). The future of long term care: Results and implications of a Delphi study. Ph.D. diss., Union Institute, 1993. *Dissertation Abstracts International* 54:5401A.

Linstone, J., and Turoff, M., eds. (1975). *The Delphi Method: Techniques and Applications*. Reading, Mass.: Addison-Wesley.

Manton, K., Corder, L., and Stallard, E. (1993). Estimates of change in chronic disability and institutional incidence and prevalence rates in the U.S. elderly population from the 1982, 1984 and 1989 National Long-Term Care Survey. *Journal of Gerontology* 47 (4): S153-66.

Millet, S., and Honton, E. (1991). *A Manager's Guide to Technology Forecasting and Strategy Analysis Methods*. Columbus, Oh.: Batelle.

Rowe, G., Wright, G., and Bolger, F. (1991). Delphi: A reevaluation of research and theory. *Technological Forecasting and Social Change* 39:235–51.

Soldo, B., Agree, E., and Wolf, D. (1989). The balance between formal and informal care. In M. Ory and K. Bond, eds., *Aging and Health Care: Social Science and Policy Perspectives*. New York: Routledge.

Stone, R., Cafferata, G., and Sangl, J. (1987). Caregivers of the elderly: A national profile. *Gerontologist* 27:616–26.

U.S. General Accounting Office (1982). The elderly should benefit from expanded home health care but increasing these services will not insure cost reductions (IPE-83-1). Washington, D.C.: U.S. Government Printing Office.

Index

Library of Congress Cataloging-in-Publication Data

The future of long-term care : social and policy issues / edited by Robert H. Binstock,
Leighton E. Cluff, and Otto von Mering.
 p.   cm.
Includes index.
ISBN 0-8018-5320-6 (alk. paper)
 1. Long-term care of the sick—United States.   2. Aged—Long-term care—United
States.   I. Binstock, Robert H.   II. Cluff, Leighton E.   III. Von Mering, Otto.
  RA997 .F87   1996
  362. 1'6'0973—dc20   96-2146